PSYCHIATRY/
NEUROLOGY

PRETEST® SELF-ASSESSMENT AND REVIEW

PSYCHIATRY/ NEUROLOGY

PRETEST® SELF-ASSESSMENT AND REVIEW

Third Edition

Joseph H. Friedman, M.D.

Chief, Division of Neurology
Memorial Hospital of Rhode Island
Pawtucket, Rhode Island

Professor of Clinical Neurosciences
Brown University School of Medicine
Providence, Rhode Island

James D. Duffy, M.D.

Director, Division of Neuropsychiatry
Assistant Professor, Department of Psychiatry
University of Connecticut School of Medicine
Farmington, Connecticut

McGraw-Hill
Health Professions Division
PreTest® Series

New York   St. Louis   San Francisco   Auckland   Bogotá   Caracas   Lisbon   London   Madrid
Mexico City   Milan   Montreal   New Delhi   San Juan   Singapore   Sydney   Tokyo   Toronto

McGraw-Hill

A Division of The McGraw·Hill Companies

Psychiatry/Neurology: PreTest® Self-Assessment and Review, Third Edition
Copyright © 1997, 1992, 1982 by the McGraw-Hill Companies, Inc. All rights reserved. Printed in the United States of America. Except as permitted under the United States Copyright Act of 1976, no part of this publication may be reproduced or distributed in any form or by any means, or stored in a data base or retrieval system without the prior written permission of the publisher.

2 3 4 5 6 7 8 9 DOCDOC 9 8

ISBN 0-07-052535-8

The editors were John Dolan and Bruce MacGregor.
The production supervisor was Helene G. Landers.
This book was set in Times Roman by V&M Graphics.
The printer was R.R. Donnelley & Sons, Company.

Library of Congress Cataloging-in-Publication Data

Psychiatry/neurology : PreTest self-assessment and review.—3rd ed.
/ [edited by] Joseph H. Friedman, James D. Duffy.
    p.   cm.
  ISBN 0-07-052535-8
  1. Psychiatry—Examinations, questions, etc. 2. Neurology—
Examinations, questions, etc. 3. Neuropsychiatry—Examinations,
questions, etc. I. Friedman, Joseph H. II. Duffy, James D.
  [DNLM: 1. Psychiatry—examination questions. 2. Neurology—
  examinations, questions. WM 18.2 P9735 1997]
RC457.P774 1997
616.8′0076—dc21
DNLM/DLC
for Library of Congress   97-72
                                                                   CIP

CONTENTS

Part One   NEUROLOGY

Part Two   PSYCHIATRY

PREFACE

This text contains 750 questions and answers to test neurologists and psychiatrists preparing for Part I of their specialty Board examinations. Part I of the American Board of Psychiatry and Neurology tests the basic sciences pertinent to clinical practice. Part I does not purport to test clinical skills as such, which are tested on Part II. Candidates must pass Part I to become eligible to take Part II.

When taking Part I of the Board examination, the neurology candidates will answer approximately 270 questions in neurology and 90 in psychiatry, for a total of 360 questions. Psychiatry candidates will answer 250 questions in psychiatry and 90 in neurology, for a total of 340 questions. The actual proportion of questions devoted to each basic science in this text approximates the proportion that will appear on the Board examination.

The questions in this text are arranged according to subject matter. In this way candidates can readily score themselves in each field to determine the adequacy of their preparation. On the actual Board examination the questions will be arranged randomly rather than by subject matter. Within any given field in this text, as well as on the Board examination, the sequence of questions is meaningless. Do not look for any order or meaning in the sequence of the questions.

We wish to thank Drs. Harry W. Fischer, Leena Ketonen, Mary Ambler, Mehdi Abedi, and Julie Armada for providing illustrations. We are particularly indebted to Dr. Haruo Okazaki for generously providing illustrations for the chapter on neuropathology.

Joseph H. Friedman, M.D
James D. Duffy, M.D.

INTRODUCTION

Psychiatry/Neurology: PreTest® Self-Assessment and Review, 3/e, has been designed to provide physicians with a comprehensive, relevant, and convenient instrument for self-evaluation and review within the broad areas of psychiatry and neurology. Although it should be particularly helpful to residents preparing for the American Board of Psychiatry and Neurology certification examination, it should also be useful for physicians in practice who are simply interested in maintaining a high level of competence in psychiatry or neurology. Study of this self-assessment and review book should help to (1) identify areas of relative weakness; (2) confirm areas of expertise; (3) assess knowledge of the sciences fundamental to psychiatry and neurology; (4) assess clinical judgment and problem-solving skills; and (5) introduce recent developments in psychiatry and neurology.

This book consists of 750 multiple-choice questions that parallel the format and degree of difficulty of the questions on the above-mentioned Board examinations. The questions in each chapter are followed by answers, paragraph-length explanations, and specific page references to either textbooks or journal articles. The bibliography at the end of this book is divided into neurology and psychiatry sections.

We have assumed that the time available to the reader is limited; as a result, this book can be used profitably a chapter at a time. By allowing no more than two and a half minutes to answer each question, you can simulate the time constraints of the actual Board examinations. When you finish answering all the questions in a chapter, spend as much time as necessary verifying answers and carefully reading the accompanying explanations. If after reading the explanations for a given chapter, you feel a need for a more extensive and definitive discussion, consult the references listed.

Based on our testing experience, examinees on most medical examinations who answer half the questions correctly would score around the 50th or 60th percentile. A score of 65 percent would place the examinee above the 80th percentile, while a score of 30 percent would rank him or her below the 15th percentile. In other words, if you answer fewer than 30 percent of the questions correctly, you are relatively weak in that area. A score of 50 percent would be approximately average, and 70 percent or higher would be honors.

We have used three basic question types in accordance with the format of the American Board of Psychiatry and Neurology certification and recertification examinations. Considerable editorial time has been spent trying to ensure that each question is clearly stated and discriminates between those physicians who are well prepared in a subject and those who are less knowledgeable.

This book is a teaching device that provides readers with the opportunity to objectively evaluate and update their clinical expertise, their ability to interpret data, and their ability to diagnose and solve clinical problems. We hope that you will find this book interesting, relevant, and challenging. The authors, as well as the PreTest staff, would be very happy to receive your comments and suggestions.

NEUROLOGY

NEUROANATOMY

Directions: Each item below contains five suggested responses. Select the **one best** response to each item.

1. The red nucleus receives afferent projections from two major sources. These are

(A) the oculomotor nucleus and the deep cerebellar nuclei
(B) the thalamus and the deep cerebellar nuclei
(C) the thalamus and the rubrospinal tract
(D) the deep cerebellar nuclei and the cerebral cortex
(E) the cerebellar cortex and the cerebral cortex

2. The optic tract ends primarily in the lateral geniculate body. Fibers also terminate in which one of the following structures?

(A) Pretectal area
(B) Medial geniculate body
(C) Inferior colliculus
(D) Red nucleus
(E) Onuf's nucleus

3. True statements about the olfactory nerve include all the following EXCEPT

(A) it has crossed and uncrossed projections
(B) it projects first to the medial dorsal thalamus and then to the amygdala
(C) it is the only sensory nerve to reach the cortex directly
(D) it directly projects to the prepyriform area
(E) it is closely linked to emotional and memory functions

4. The great cerebral vein (Galen) empties into the

(A) rectus sinus
(B) transverse sinus on each side
(C) jugular vein on each side
(D) internal cerebral vein (Rosenthal) on each side
(E) superior cerebellar vein

5. The term *thalamic fasciculus* is most closely synonymous with

(A) field H of Forel
(B) field H_1 of Forel
(C) field H_2 of Forel
(D) all three fields of Forel
(E) none of the above

6. A mass in the jugular foramen would cause all the following EXCEPT

(A) hoarseness
(B) Horner's syndrome
(C) dysphagia
(D) weakness of the sternomastoid muscle
(E) deviation of the soft palate to the opposite side

7. The neocortex consists of how many relatively discrete levels?

(A) 3
(B) 4
(C) 5
(D) 6
(E) 7

8. Hemiballismus is typically associated with infarctions of the

(A) ipsilateral subthalamic nucleus
(B) contralateral subthalamic nucleus
(C) ipsilateral pars reticulata of the substantia nigra
(D) contralateral pars reticulata of the substantia nigra
(E) red nucleus

9. The ansa lenticularis is correctly described by which of the following statements?

(A) It is a nucleus between the internal and external segments of the globus pallidus
(B) It connects the subthalamic nucleus to the putamen
(C) It starts in the medial globus pallidus and eventually joins the thalamic fasciculus, terminating in the thalamus
(D) It connects the putamen to the globus pallidus
(E) It is a fiber bundle originating in the medial thalamus and terminating in the pars reticulata of the substantia nigra

10. Which one of the following statements concerning the cavernous sinus is true?

(A) It is an irregular network of veins adjacent to the internal carotid artery and cranial nerves III, IV, V, and VI
(B) It drains the rectus sinus
(C) It is an arteriovenous structure
(D) It drains directly into the internal jugular vein
(E) It is distinct on each side and does not communicate with its partner

11. Which one of the following statements concerning the cerebellum is correct?

    (A) The mossy fibers it receives terminate on Purkinje cells
    (B) Its input is primarily from the red nucleus and the inferior olive
    (C) Its input is primarily climbing fibers and its output is via mossy fibers
    (D) It receives mossy fibers, climbing fibers, and aminergic fibers
    (E) Its output is primarily climbing fibers and its input is via mossy fibers

12. The median raphe nuclei of the pons contain high percentages of

    (A) gamma-aminobutyric acid (GABA)
    (B) dopamine
    (C) endogenous benzodiazepine-like substance
    (D) epinephrine
    (E) serotonin

13. Which one of the following statements concerning the pyramidal tract is true?

    (A) It derives entirely from Betz cells
    (B) About 40 percent of the cell bodies that send axons into it are located in the parietal lobe
    (C) It crosses entirely in the lower medulla
    (D) It is distinct from the corticobulbar tract
    (E) It contains about 25,000 to 50,000 axons

14. A herpes zoster vesicular eruption that involves the external auditory canal alone might be associated with an abnormality of cranial nerve(s)

    (A) VII
    (B) VIII
    (C) IX and X
    (D) XI
    (E) XII

15. All the following statements concerning cranial nerve VII are true EXCEPT

    (A) lesions proximal to the geniculate ganglion cause weakness of muscles of facial expression, hyperacusis, impaired taste, and impaired tearing
    (B) lesions distal to the geniculate ganglion cause hyperacusis and may cause taste loss but no problem with tearing
    (C) a partial lesion of the VIIth nerve at the stylohyoid foramen may cause only facial weakness
    (D) aberrantly regenerating parasympathetic fibers following a VIIth nerve injury proximal to the geniculate ganglion are the cause of crocodile tears
    (E) patients with Bell's palsy often experience numbness because there are facial cutaneous sensory areas supplied by the facial nerve

16. All the following statements concerning the inferior olive (oliva) are true EXCEPT

    (A) uncrossed olivocerebellar fibers form the largest part of the inferior cerebellar peduncle

    (B) it projects widely through the cerebellar cortex

    (C) it projects to the deep cerebellar nuclei

    (D) afferents to it arise from the cerebral cortex

    (E) afferents to it arise from the red nucleus

17. The intermediolateral nucleus of the spinal cord

    (A) receives input from dorsal root ganglia

    (B) modulates proprioceptive input

    (C) sends out preganglionic sympathetic fibers

    (D) receives unmyelinated pain fibers

    (E) is the origin for gamma motor neurons

Directions: Each item below contains four suggested responses of which **one or more** is correct. Select:

A	if	**1, 2, and 3**	are correct
B	if	**1 and 3**	are correct
C	if	**2 and 4**	are correct
D	if	**4**	is correct
E	if	**1, 2, 3, and 4**	are correct

18. The IVth cranial nerve may correctly be described as

(1) being the only cranial nerve to attach to the dorsal aspect of the brainstem

(2) having the smallest diameter of all the cranial motor nerves

(3) undergoing complete internal decussation

(4) containing no myelinated fibers

19. The locus ceruleus is the major brain source of which of the following neurotransmitters?

(1) Serotonin

(2) Substance P

(3) Epinephrine

(4) Norepinephrine

20. Regarding the figure shown below, correct statements include which of the following?

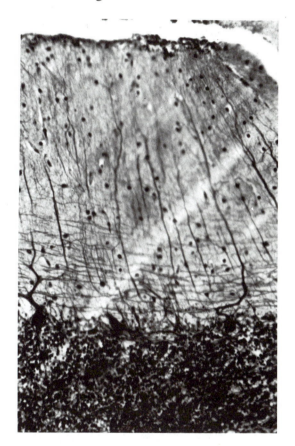

(1) Large neurons appear in the plexiform layer

(2) Purkinje cells are seen at the upper margin of the granular layer

(3) The external granular layer is evident at the bottom of the photograph

(4) This section could be from the posterior lobe of the cerebellum

SUMMARY OF DIRECTIONS

A	B	C	D	E
1,2,3	1,3	2,4	4	All are
only	only	only	only	correct

21. The spinal cord is supplied by which of the following arteries?

(1) Recurrent artery of Heubner
(2) Artery of Adamkiewicz
(3) Posterior inferior cerebellar artery
(4) Vertebral arteries

22. True statements concerning the anatomy of the anterior choroidal artery include

(1) it arises from the internal carotid artery proximal to the posterior communicating artery
(2) it supplies the hippocampal formation
(3) it supplies the head of the caudate nucleus
(4) it has a long subarachnoid course

23. A lesion of the nerve shown by the arrow in the figure below would produce which of the following clinical signs?

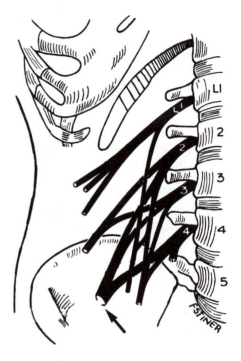

Adapted from Adams, Victor, and Ropper, 6/e, Fig. 46-6, with permission.

(1) Absence of the quadriceps muscle stretch reflex
(2) Atrophy of the posterior muscles of the calf
(3) Reduction in the circumference of the thigh
(4) Loss of sensation over the posterior aspect of the thigh

24. Major, well-established components of the thalamic fasciculus include the

(1) medial lemniscus
(2) dentatorubrothalamic tract
(3) pallidal efferent fibers
(4) corticothalamic fibers

25. Electron microscopy characteristically shows which of the following structural features at synapses?

   (1) Small, round vesicles
   (2) Endoplasmic reticulum
   (3) Electron-dense material along the pre- and postsynaptic membranes
   (4) No mitochondria

26. Horner's syndrome may be caused by

   (1) infarctions in the distribution of the posterior inferior cerebellar artery
   (2) compressive spinal cord lesions at C7–T1
   (3) intrinsic spinal cord lesions in the upper thoracic segments
   (4) an ipsilateral hypothalamic lesion

27. The deep cerebellar nuclei may be characterized by which of the following statements?

   (1) They receive inhibitory input from the cerebellar cortex
   (2) They receive excitatory input from pontine nuclei
   (3) They provide a major feedback system to the cerebellar cortex
   (4) They provide most of the cerebellar outflow via the superior cerebellar cortex

28. Pallidothalamic fibers terminate in significant numbers on which of the following nuclei?

   (1) Ventralis posterolateralis
   (2) Ventralis lateralis
   (3) Medialis dorsalis
   (4) Ventralis anterior

Directions: Each group of questions below consists of lettered options followed by a set of numbered items. For each numbered item select the **one** lettered option with which it is **most** closely associated. Each lettered option may be used **once, more than once, or not at all.**

Items 29–33

The following clinical syndromes can be caused by stroke. Match each syndrome with the appropriate artery.

  (A) Anterior inferior cerebellar artery
  (B) Paramedian branch of upper basilar artery
  (C) Superior cerebellar artery
  (D) Vertebral artery leading to medial medulla
  (E) Posterior inferior cerebellar artery

29. Oscillopsia, facial weakness, paralysis of conjugate gaze, deafness, ataxia, facial numbness, and crossed body numbness

30. Skew deviation, ipsilateral Horner's syndrome, ipsilateral conjugate gaze paresis, and crossed body numbness

31. Ipsilateral ataxia, internuclear ophthalmoplegia, palatal myoclonus, and contralateral face, arm, and leg weakness

32. Ipsilateral tongue atrophy with crossed arm and leg weakness and numbness

33. Ipsilateral Horner's syndrome, hoarseness, unilateral ataxia, vertigo, and contralateral numbness below the face

Items 34–37

For each of the statements listed below, select the region of the hypothalamus most closely involved.

    (A) Ventromedial nucleus in tuberal region
    (B) Supraoptic nuclei
    (C) Posterior hypothalamus
    (D) Preoptic region
    (E) Arcuate nucleus

34. This area is concerned with water balance

35. Body heat is increased by this region when core temperature declines

36. Destruction of this area bilaterally results in hyperphagia

37. This region is important in controlling release of gonadotropic hormones from the pituitary

Items 38–42

For each lesion listed below, match the visual field defect (if any) to which it is most closely related.

    (A) Partial contralateral superior homonymous quadrantanopia
    (B) Superior altitudinal hemianopia of both eyes
    (C) Partial contralateral inferior homonymous quadrantanopia
    (D) Complete contralateral homonymous hemianopia without macular sparing
    (E) No visual field defect

38. Complete destruction of the calcarine cortex of one occipital lobe

39. Destruction of the anterior part of the temporal lobe

40. Bilateral destruction of the inferior bank of the calcarine fissure

41. Unilateral destruction of the inferior part of the parietal lobe

42. Destruction of the splenium of the corpus callosum

NEUROANATOMY

A N S W E R S

1. The answer is D. (Carpenter, 4/e, p 210.) The red nucleus is a prominent midbrain structure. It contains, in addition to neurons, myelinated fibers to the superior cerebellar peduncle and the oculomotor nerve. Its major input arises from the deep contralateral cerebellar nuclei after crossing in the caudal midbrain. The cerebral cortex projection arises from the precentral and premotor cortex.

2. The answer is A. (Carpenter, 4/e, p 285.) The optic tract projects to the superior colliculus and the pretectal area, where the consensual pupillary reflex arc is located, and to the superior colliculus. The superior colliculus is important in visual tracking and voluntary eye movements. In many animals an additional connection to the suprachiasmatic nucleus in the thalamus has been detailed. This connection is undoubtedly important in circadian rhythmicity.

3. The answer is B. (Adams RD, 5/e, pp 199–200.) The olfactory nerve has a unique structure and projection. It is the only sensory input that goes directly to cortex without a relay. It has a crossed portion that travels in the anterior commissure and an uncrossed portion that innervates the amygdala and the prepyriform cortex, which is considered the primary olfactory cortex and is located in the hippocampal gyrus.

4. The answer is A. (Carpenter, 4/e, pp 259–460.) The great cerebral vein (Galen) is a short midline vein that receives paired feeders from each side, including the basal internal veins (Rosenthal), the internal cerebral veins, the occipital veins, and the posterior callosal vein. It empties into the rectus sinus, another midline structure.

5. The answer is B. (Carpenter, 4/e, p 342.) Field H_1 of Forel is the lamina of myelinated fibers between the zona incerta and the thalamus. This lamina of fibers is also termed the *thalamic fasciculus*. It receives fibers from fields H and H_2, but is most nearly synonymous with field H_1.

This field conveys sensory fibers from the lemnisci and motor fibers of cerebellar and pallidal origin. Therefore, it is not a unitary tract with a single function. The thalamic fasciculus forms a shell of myelinated fibers around the ventral surface of the thalamus and becomes continuous with the shell of myelinated fibers around the lateral aspect of the thalamus, known as the *external medullary lamina.* The myelinated capsule extends continuously across the dorsum of the thalamus, where it is designated the *striatum zonale.* The medial border of the thalamus, which forms the boundary of the third ventricle, contains few myelinated fibers. Thus the thalamus is surrounded by myelinated fibers that form a capsule ventrally, laterally, and dorsally, but not medially.

6. **The answer is B.** (Adams RD, 5/e, p 1172.) Cranial nerves IX, X, and XI exit the skull via the jugular foramen. Lesions of the IXth and Xth nerves cause unilateral vocal cord weakness, dysfunction of swallowing, and soft palate weakness. The XIth nerve innervates the sternomastoid and the upper trapezius. Horner's syndrome is caused by interruption of the sympathetic fibers between the hypothalamus and the upper thoracic cord and then between the cord and the face along the carotid artery.

7. **The answer is D.** (Carpenter, 4/e, pp 390–393.) The neocortex consists of six layers. The molecular layer is most superficial, followed by the external granular, the external pyramidal, the internal granular, the internal pyramidal, and the multiform layers. The olfactory cortex (paleopallium), the hippocampal formation, and the dentate gyrus (archipallium) contain only three layers. The cerebellar cortex also has only three layers, but is composed of different cells than those of the paleopallium or archipallium.

8. **The answer is B.** (Adams RD, 5/e, p 71. Carpenter, 3/e, p 317.) *Ballismus* refers to flinging, throwing, or kicking movements caused by involuntary contractions of proximal muscles. This is often considered a proximal form of chorea. In the primate, surgical lesions of the subthalamic nucleus (nucleus of Luys) produce contralateral hemiballismus. Because the ballismus is abolished if further lesions are made in the ipsilateral globus pallidus, the fascicularis lenticularis or the ventral lateral thalamic nuclei, it is thought that the subthalamic nucleus exerts an inhibitory influence on the globus pallidus and the ventral thalamus. In humans, hemiballismus usually arises from lesions of the subthalamic nucleus but may rarely arise from other structures of the basal ganglia or the thalamus.

9. **The answer is C.** (Carpenter, 4/e, p 341.) The term *ansa* designates a looplike structure. In this case it is a fiber bundle that originates in the lateral portion of the medial segment of the globus pallidus. It sweeps around the posterior limb of the internal capsule, enters field H of Forel, and then enters the thalamic fasciculus, which terminates in the rostral ventral thalamic nuclei.

10. **The answer is A.** (Carpenter, 4/e, pp 439, 457.) The cavernous sinus is an irregular network of veins that encases the internal carotid artery and cranial nerves III, IV, V, and VI. The two sinuses communicate with each other via the basilar venous plexus and then drain into the petrosal sinuses. Blood then enters the transverse sinus and the internal jugular vein.

11. The answer is D. (Adams RD, 5/e, p 78.) There are three types of input to the cerebellum: the mossy fibers, which originate in the spinocerebellar tracts and the pontine, reticular, and vestibular nuclei; the climbing fibers, which originate in the inferior olive; and the aminergic fibers, comprising dopaminergic, noradrenergic, and serotoninergic axons that originate in the midbrain, the locus ceruleus, and the raphe nuclei. The mossy fibers end in the granule cell layer. Climbing fibers terminate on contralateral Purkinje cells, and aminergic fibers end in Purkinje and granule cells.

12. The answer is E. (Carpenter, 4/e, p 186.) The median raphe nuclei extend from the medulla to the pons and contain large amounts of serotonin (5-hydroxytryptamine, 5-HT) although several other neurotransmitters, including dopamine, substance P, and enkephalin also are present, sometimes in the same neuron. The median raphe nuclei project to the frontal lobe, the substantia nigra, the lateral geniculate body, the olfactory bulb, the amygdala, the neostriatum, and the pyriform lobe.

13. The answer is B. (Adams RD, 5/e, p 42.) The corticospinal tract consists of about 1 million axons, far more than rise from the 25,000 to 35,000 Betz cells in the motor cortex. About 40 percent of the cells that send axons into the corticospinal tract arise in the parietal lobe, and the rest are about evenly divided between the motor cortex and the premotor cortex. The corticobulbar tract intermingles with the pyramidal tract in the brainstem. Most corticospinal fibers cross in the lower medulla, some cross higher up, and a number, with considerable individual variation, are uncrossed.

14. The answer is A. (Adams RD, 5/e, p 1176.) The Ramsay Hunt syndrome, thought due to herpes zoster involvement of the geniculate ganglion, is a lower motor neuron VIIth nerve palsy associated with a shingles eruption in the ear. The VIIth nerve provides sensory innervation to a very limited portion of the ear, hence the association with the Bell-like palsy.

15. The answer is E. (Carpenter, 4/e, pp 172–173.) The VIIth nerve contains some innervation from the spinal trigeminal tract (Vth nerve), which supplies the external auditory meatus and a patch in the retroauricular region. When herpes zoster causes a VIIth nerve paresis, vesicles are evident either behind the ear or on the external ear, not on the face. This is called the *Ramsay Hunt syndrome*. The VIIth nerve exits the stylohyoid foramen and includes fibers from the superior salivatory nucleus and the nucleus fasciculus solitarius. Nerves from the geniculate ganglion supply taste to the anterior two-thirds of the tongue and terminate in the gustatory nucleus. Preganglionic neurons in the salivatory nucleus supply the chorda tympani, the lacrimal glands, and the submandibular and sublingual salivary glands.

16. The answer is A. (Carpenter, 4/e, p 125.) The inferior olive is the most prominent structure in the medulla and has the appearance of a folded bag. It is a major source of input to the cerebellum and constitutes the single largest portion of the contralateral inferior cerebellar peduncle. It projects widely through the cerebellar cortex and to the deep cerebellar nuclei and receives input from the cerebral cortex, red nucleus, periaqueductal gray, and the central tegmental tract.

17. The answer is C. (Carpenter, 4/e, p 70.) The intermediolateral nucleus is found in the thoracic and lumbar portions of the spinal cord, where it sends out preganglionic sympathetic fibers. These leave the cord via the ventral roots and synapse in the sympathetic ganglia, which then send fibers to the non-nervous-system end organ. Parasympathetic regions of the spinal cord lie in the cervical and sacral regions.

18. The answer is A (1, 2, 3). (Carpenter, 4/e, p 194–195.) The IVth cranial nerve is the only nerve to exit from the dorsal surface of the brainstem. It has the smallest diameter of any cranial nerve. The IVth cranial nerve undergoes a complete internal decussation before exiting at the junction of the superior medullary velum with the inferior colliculus. It conveys myelinated motor axons to the superior oblique muscle. After exiting from the dorsal aspect of the brainstem, the IVth nerve runs through the lateral wall of the cavernous sinus before entering the orbit through the superior orbital fissure. Interruption of the IVth cranial nerve at any site along its course causes paralysis of only one ocular rotatory muscle. The superior oblique muscle is the only muscle that the nerve supplies. The patient has diplopia on looking downward and inward with the affected eye. Patients sometimes compensate by keeping their head tilted, causing a pseudotorticollis.

19. The answer is D (4). (Carpenter, 4/e, pp 132, 184.) The locus ceruleus is a small, pigmented nucleus in the medulla that has the largest concentration of norepinephrine in the brain. It projects throughout the neuraxis, including the spinal cord, cerebral cortex, and cerebellar cortex. It is affected in Parkinson's disease, but the effects of its dysfunction are not known.

20. The answer is C (2, 4). (Carpenter, 4/e, pp 225–232.) This photomicrograph is of normal cerebellar cortex. The histology of the cerebellar cortex, unlike that of the cerebral hemisphere cortex, is uniform throughout, so that this particular section could represent any part of the cerebellar cortex. The cortex consists of three layers, which are, from the outside in, the molecular, Purkinje cell, and granular cell layers. The most striking features of the cerebellar cortex are the densely packed cells in the granular cell layer and the large Purkinje cells at the upper margin of this layer with their long processes extending perpendicularly to the surface of the cortex. The plexiform and external granular layers exist in the cerebral cortex, which has six layers, not three.

21. The answer is C (2, 4). (Carpenter, 4/e, pp 436–437.) The spinal cord is supplied in the rostral region by branches of the vertebral arteries and radicular arteries. The paired anterior spinal arteries, one from each of the vertebral arteries, join to form a single, midline anterior spinal artery, which is also supplied by the segmental arteries. The anterior spinal artery branches into anterior radicular arteries. The posterior aspect of the cord is supplied by paired posterior radicular arteries that derive from segmental arteries. The artery of Adamkiewicz is the largest anterior radicular artery and generally travels with a lower thoracic or upper lumbar spinal root. The PICA supplies the medulla and cerebellum. The recurrent artery of Heubner supplies portions of the basal ganglia.

22. The answer is C (2, 4). (Carpenter, 4/e, p 446.) The anterior choroidal artery is a small-caliber vessel that arises from the internal carotid artery distal to the posterior communicating artery. It has a long subarachnoid course and enters the choroidal fissure and then the inferior horn of the lateral ventricle. The anterior choroidal artery supplies the hippocampal formation and the border region of the medial lateral segments of the globus pallidum (anterior choroidal artery ligation was used for a time in treating Parkinson's disease, helpful possibly because of the pallidal lesion).

23. The answer is B (1, 3). (Adams RD, 5/e, p 1162.) In the figure accompanying the question, the arrow indicates the femoral nerve, a major branch of the lumbosacral plexus. The femoral nerve arises from lumbar roots 2, 3, and 4. It supplies motor fibers to the quadriceps femoris muscle, composed of the rectus femoris, vastus lateralis, vastus medialis, and vastus intermedius muscles. These muscles occupy the anterior compartment of the thigh and extend the leg at the knee. A lesion of the femoral nerve would cause weakness of knee extension and atrophy of the quadriceps muscles, with a reduction in the circumference of the thigh and absence of the stretch reflex of the quadriceps femoris muscle. An affected patient would lose sensation over the anteromedial aspect of the thigh. The lateral femoral cutaneous nerve mediates sensation on the anterolateral aspect of the thigh. One of the commonest causes of femoral neuropathy is diabetes mellitus.

24. The answer is A (1, 2, 3). (Carpenter, 4/e, p 342.) The thalamic fasciculus consists of the lamina of myelinated fibers that runs along the ventral or inferior aspect of the thalamus, between it and the zona incerta. It conveys those axons that synapse in the thalamus from the lemnisci, dentatorubral system, and globus pallidus. It lacks corticothalamic axons, which approach the thalamus from other directions via the thalamic peduncles, rather than the thalamic fasciculus. Thus, the thalamic fasciculus serves to connect the thalamus with infracortical structures rather than with the cerebral cortex. A synonym for the thalamic fasciculus is field H_1 of Forel.   V A + VL Nucleus.

25. The answer is B (1, 3). (Kandel, 2/e, pp 168–172.) Electron microscopy shows that synapses contain small, round structures called *synaptic vesicles* that are presumed to contain neurotransmitters. Synapses have electron-dense materials called *synaptic bars* along the membrane of the pre- and postsynaptic cell. The synapses contain many mitochondria, but as a rule they show few microtubules. Microtubules are numerous along the axon and in the perikaryon and dendrites. Endoplasmic reticulum is abundant in the perikaryon but lacking in the axon and synapse.

26. The answer is E (all). (Adams RD, 5/e, p 242. Carpenter, 4/e, pp 209–210.) Horner's syndrome consists of the triad of ptosis, miosis, and facial anhidrosis, although not all three are present with partial lesions. It results from interruption of sympathetic innervation to the face and eye. The fibers originate in the hypothalamus and descend ipsilaterally through the brainstem tegmentum to the intermediolateral columns of the eighth cervical segment and upper three thoracic segments. They then exit the cord and travel with the common and then internal carotid arteries. Interruption of the pathway at any point, such as in the medulla with a Wallenberg stroke (PICA syndrome) or cord lesions at the level of the intermediolateral columns, can cause the syndrome.

27. The answer is E (all). (Carpenter, 4/e, pp 234–236.) The four deep cerebellar nuclei—the dentate, emboliform, globose, and fastigial—receive afferent innervation from the cerebellar cortex as well as from the rest of the brain, primarily from pontine nuclei. Cerebellar input flows through the inferior and middle cerebellar peduncles, whereas cerebellar output travels primarily from the dentate, emboliform, and globose nuclei via the superior cerebellar peduncle. There is an intricate connection in both directions between the cerebellar cortex and the deep nuclei. Since the cerebellar cortex provides only inhibitory projections and the deep nuclei have been found to be active, it has been assumed that the pontine projections to the deep nuclei are excitatory in nature.

28. The answer is C (2, 4). (Carpenter, 4/e, p 267.) The pallidothalamic fibers project to the ventral intermediate and anterior parts of the thalamus, where they end in nucleus ventralis lateralis and nucleus ventralis anterior. These connections help to bring the thalamus into the extrapyramidal motor circuits. The most posterior nucleus of the ventral tier is a sensory relay nucleus. The pallidothalamic fibers loop under the internal capsule as the ansa lenticularis or run directly across the capsule as the fasciculus lenticularis. The fibers of the two fasciculi curve upward into the thalamus by joining the thalamic fasciculus, from which they enter the ventral tier of thalamic nuclei. These ventral tier nuclei then distribute to the motor cortex of the frontal lobe to form a link between the pyramidal and extrapyramidal circuits.

29–33. The answers are 29-A, 30-C, 31-B, 32-D, 33-E. (Adams RD, 5/e, pp 691–695.) The medial medullary syndrome may be caused by vertebral occlusion or more distal branch occlusion. This causes XIIth nerve weakness, leading to atrophy, weakness of the contralateral arm and leg due to pyramidal tract interruption, and tactile and proprioceptive impairment due to medial lemniscus interruption.

The Wallenberg (lateral medullary) syndrome of posterior inferior cerebellar artery (PICA) occlusion can be caused by more proximal blockage as well, down to the vertebral artery. The syndrome includes an ipsilateral Horner's syndrome (all elements of the triad), vertigo, diplopia, oscillopsia or nystagmus due to vestibular dysfunction, unilateral ataxia, facial numbness due to the Vth nucleus interruption, hoarseness or dysphagia from IXth and Xth nuclear involvement, and contralateral sensory loss below the face from spinothalamic tract impairment.

The anterior inferior cerebellar artery (AICA) syndrome causes vestibular dysfunction (nystagmus, vertigo, nausea, oscillopsia,), VIIth nerve or nuclear interruption producing lower motor neuron facial weakness, ataxia from middle cerebellar peduncle involvement, impaired facial sensation from descending Vth tract, and contralateral spinothalamic dysfunction (pain and temperature).

The superior cerebellar artery syndrome causes a lateral superior pontine syndrome affecting the middle and superior cerebellar peduncles, superior surface of the cerebellar dentate nucleus, vestibular nuclei, and sympathetic pathway, which causes ipsilateral conjugate gaze paresis, skew deviation, Horner's syndrome, vertigo, and dysfunction of the contralateral spinothalamic tract (pain and temperature) and medial lemniscus (touch, vibration, and position sense).

The medial superior pontine syndrome (involving paramedian branches of the upper basilar artery) causes an internuclear ophthalmoplegia due to medial longitudinal fasciculus injury, ataxia from middle and superior cerebellar peduncle ischemia, and rhythmic myoclonus of the palate, pharynx, or vocal cords from central tegmental bundle injury. Contralateral face, arm, and leg weakness results from corticospinal and corticobulbar tract interruption.

34–37.   The answers are 34-B, 35-C, 36-A, 37-D. (Carpenter, 4/e, pp 317–321.) The hypothalamus is important in exerting control over a large number of behavior-related functions, such as autonomic functions, sexual and reproductive functions, sleep cycles, appetite, water and electrolyte balance, and rage. The anterior hypothalamus is important in cooling the body and responds to temperature increases; the posterior aspect does the opposite. Bilateral destruction of the anterior regions results in hyperthermia; bilateral destruction of the posterior regions results in poikilothermia. The supraoptic nucleus secretes vasopressin, which is important in water balance. Decreased vasopressin release results in diabetes insipidus. The ventromedial nucleus is important in satiety and anger. Its destruction results in increased eating due to the loss of satiety. The preoptic area is one region, including the amygdaloid complex, that is important in controlling ovulation.

38–42.   The answers are 38-D, 39-A, 40-B, 41-C, 42-E. (Adams RD, 4/e, pp 220–222.) Complete destruction of the calcarine cortex of one occipital lobe causes a complete contralateral homonymous hemianopia without macular sparing. This cortex receives the pathway originating in the temporal half of the ipsilateral eye and nasal half of the contralateral eye.

Destruction of the anterior part of the temporal lobe destroys the portion of the geniculocalcarine tract that loops around the temporal ventricle (Meyer's loop). These fibers convey the pathway originating in the inferior temporal quadrant of the ipsilateral retina and the inferior nasal quadrant of the contralateral retina, causing a contralateral superior field defect. The quadrantic field defect is usually incomplete but fairly homonymous.

Bilateral destruction of the inferior bank of the calcarine fissure causes a superior altitudinal visual field defect in both eyes. The inferior bank of each calcarine fissure receives the pathway that originates in the inferior temporal quadrant of the ipsilateral retina and the inferior nasal quadrant of the contralateral retina. Joining the two superior quadrantic field defects gives a superior altitudinal hemianopia.

Destruction of the inferior part of the parietal lobe causes a partial contralateral inferior homonymous quadrantanopia. The lesion destroys the superior fibers of the geniculocalcarine radiation. These fibers mediate the inferior homonymous fields contralaterally.

Interruption of the corpus callosum fails to cause a visual field defect per se. The lesion might, however, also encroach on the calcarine cortex located posterior to the splenium of the corpus callosum and cause a field defect in this way. A lesion extending laterally from the corpus callosum, such as a butterfly glioblastoma, would be very unlikely to cause a field defect because the geniculocalcarine tract, which conveys optic impulses, passes lateral to the wall of the lateral ventricle, separating it a considerable distance from the splenium.

NEUROPATHOLOGY

Directions: Each item below contains five suggested responses. Select the **one best** response to each item.

43. All the following disorders are associated with neurofibrillary tangles EXCEPT

(A) postencephalitic parkinsonism
(B) progressive supranuclear palsy
(C) dementia pugilistica
(D) Down's syndrome
(E) Shy-Drager syndrome

44. Periodic paralysis, paroxysmal ataxia, and familial hemiplegic migraines share a common pathophysiology. Which one of the following mechanisms has been implicated in each of these inherited disorders?

(A) Glutamate toxicity
(B) Abnormality of the gamma-aminobutyric acid (GABA) receptor
(C) Excitotoxicity
(D) Oxidative phosphorylation deficit in mitochondria
(E) Ion channel disorder

45. The most common intracranial mass lesion in the American adult with AIDS is due to

(A) CNS lymphoma
(B) Kaposi's sarcoma
(C) staphylococcal abscess
(D) polymicrobial abscess
(E) toxoplasmosis

46. Brain abscesses in association with congenital heart disease usually are

(A) solitary
(B) polymicrobial
(C) frontal in location
(D) occipital in location
(E) cerebellar in location

47. All the following disorders are due to excess CAG nonsense repeats EXCEPT

(A) Huntington's disease
(B) juvenile (Westphal variant) Huntington's disease
(C) Machado-Joseph (Azorean) disease
(D) fragile X syndrome
(E) myotonic dystrophy

48. An alcoholic patient shows severe dystaxia of gait with little involvement of the arms and no dysarthria or nystagmus. These findings result from which of the following lesions?

(A) Degeneration of the spinocerebellar tracts
(B) Degeneration of the flocculonodular lobe
(C) Atrophy of the anterior vermis
(D) Diffuse Purkinje cell loss in the entire cerebellum
(E) Diffuse granule cell loss in the entire cerebellum

49. Mitochondrial disorders may cause all the following laboratory abnormalities EXCEPT

(A) ragged red fibers in skeletal muscle biopsy
(B) sensorineural loss in hearing tests
(C) slowed conduction in nerve conduction studies
(D) axonal changes on EMG and nerve conduction studies
(E) psychosis

50. Tropical spastic paraparesis has been associated with which one of the following etiologies?

(A) Canine distemper virus
(B) Human T-cell leukemia virus type I (HTLV-I)
(C) Ingestion of chick peas (*Lathyrus sativus*)
(D) Ingestion of machine oil
(E) An inherited enzyme deficiency

51. The pathogenesis of arthrogryposis multiplex congenita is best described as being

(A) overwhelmingly acknowledged as an expression of myelodysplasia
(B) overwhelmingly acknowledged as myopathic
(C) related to a defect in connective tissue
(D) a congenital peripheral neuropathy
(E) a symptom complex of varied causes

52. A muscle biopsy of a patient affected by the Kearns-Sayre syndrome of ophthalmoplegia with retinitis pigmentosa is likely to show

(A) giant mitochondria with excessive quantities of lipids
(B) dense central portions of muscle fibers that stain positively with the periodic acid–Schiff reaction
(C) bacillus-like rods in the muscle fibers
(D) ragged red type I fibers in the Gomori stain
(E) central nuclei

53. An AIDS patient with an encephalitis but no mass lesions has unilaterally impaired vision. The fundus shows a white exudate with surrounding hemorrhage and edema. The most likely cause is

(A) cytomegalovirus (CMV)
(B) metastatic Kaposi's sarcoma
(C) lymphoma
(D) human immunodeficiency virus (HIV)
(E) cryptococcus

54. All the following statements about the neurologic complications of subacute infective endocarditis are true EXCEPT

(A) mycotic aneurysms tend to occur distally rather than proximally as with berry aneurysms
(B) acute encephalopathy is common
(C) aseptic meningitis is common
(D) brain abscesses are common
(E) seizures are common

55. The following low-power photomicrograph shows dilated vessels with thrombosis. Which one of the following correctly identifies the abnormality?

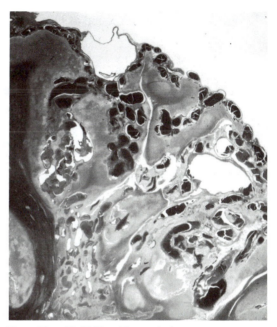

From Okazaki, 1989, with permission.

(A) Old infarct with partial revascularization
(B) Glioblastoma multiforme
(C) Hemangioblastoma
(D) Metastatic hypernephroma
(E) Arteriovenous malformation

56. Prions cause which one of the following diseases?

(A) Gerstmann-Straussler syndrome
(B) Rasmussen's encephalitis
(C) Familial paroxysmal ataxia
(D) Machado-Joseph disease
(E) Limbic encephalitis

57. A patient known to drink large quantities of beer was admitted to the hosptial within weeks of starting a diuretic. His sodium level on admission was 105 meq/L. After a good initial response to rapid correction of his electrolytes, he began to develop progressive quadriparesis. The photo-micrograph reveals the lesion. Which of the following is the correct diagnosis?

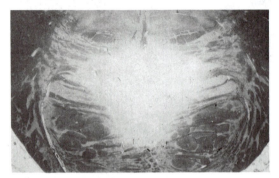

From Okazaki, 1989, with permission.

(A) Marchiafava-Bignami syndrome
(B) Wernicke-Korsakoff syndrome
(C) Central pontine myelinolysis
(D) Multiple sclerosis
(E) Syringomyelia

58. Lead poisoning in *adults* is LEAST likely to cause which of the following problems?

(A) Encephalopathy
(B) Proximal weakness
(C) Footdrop
(D) Wristdrop
(E) Motor neuropathy

59. The brain of a teenager shown below is best described as illustrating

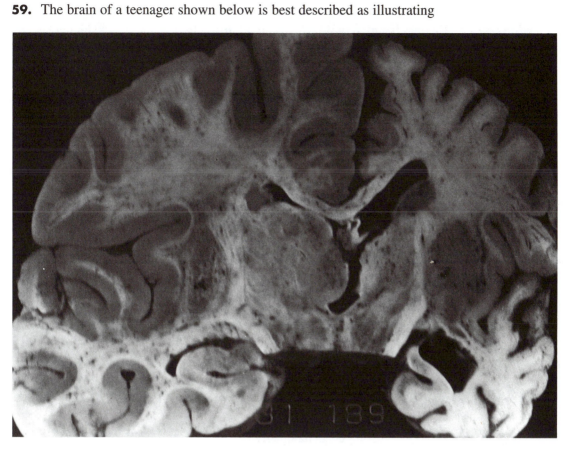

(A) respirator brain
(B) hemiatrophy
(C) Alexander's disease
(D) metastatic cancer
(E) progressive multifocal leukoencephalopathy (PML)

60. A 30-year-old woman presents with weight loss, poor concentration, and depression developing over a month and a mildly unsteady but difficult to characterize gait disorder. The lesions below illustrate her diagnosis. The correct diagnosis is

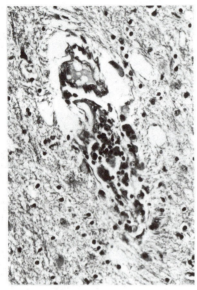 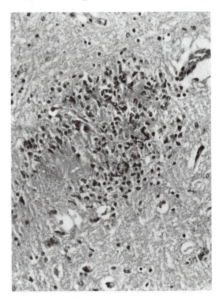

From Okazaki, 1989, with permission.

(A) multiple sclerosis
(B) Epstein-Barr encephalitis
(C) progressive multifocal leukoencephalopathy (PML)
(D) Lyme encephalitis
(E) acquired immunodeficiency syndrome (AIDS)

61. An AIDS patient develops a progressive hemiparesis affecting her leg more than her arm. There is a mild dementia as well. The CT scan of the brain with contrast reveals no abnormality. The photograph below shows the lesion. The correct diagnosis is

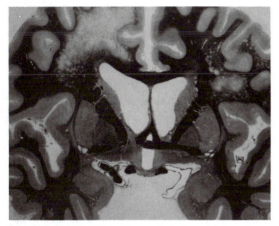

From Okazaki, 1989, with permission.

(A) toxoplasmosis
(B) tuberculosis
(C) multiple metastases from Kaposi's sarcoma
(D) progressive multifocal leukoencephalopathy (PML)
(E) Creutzfeldt-Jakob disease

62. This tumor occurs in several histologic types but is of glial origin. The figure shows the epithelial type. It has a predilection for the ventricles but does not always have an intraventricular portion. Which of the following is the correct identification?

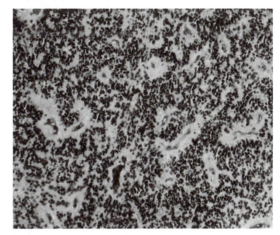

From Okazaki, 1989, with permission.

(A) Astrocytoma
(B) Ependymoma
(C) Chordoma
(D) Lymphoma
(E) Metastatic germ cell tumor

63. The photomicrograph below depicts which of the following nutritional disorders?

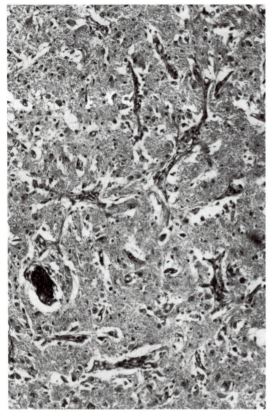

From Okazaki, 1989, with permission.

(A) Subacute combined degeneration
(B) Pyridoxine deficiency
(C) Wernicke's encephalopathy
(D) Lathyrism
(E) Lead encephalopathy

64. This mass was found in an elderly man who had suffered focal motor seizures for at least 5 years. Which abnormality is the correct description of the figure?

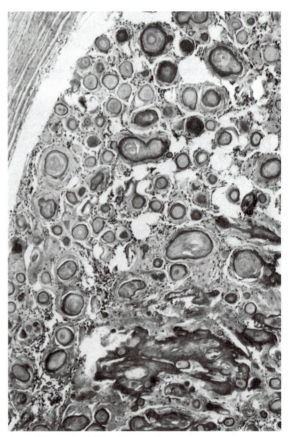

From Okazaki, 1989, with permission.

(A) Meningioma
(B) Arteriovenous malformation
(C) Vascularized lining of a chronic subdural hematoma
(D) Cavernous hemangioma
(E) Capillary venous malformation

65. The two figures are sections from different parts of the same neoplasm. Which is the correct diagnosis?

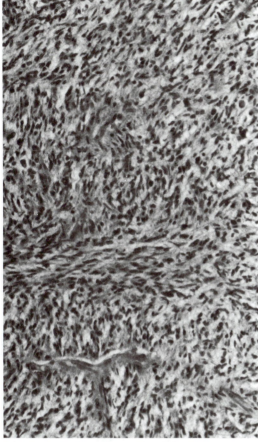 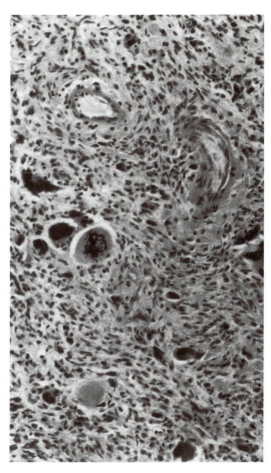

From Okazaki, 1989, with permission.

(A) Astrocytoma grade II
(B) Glioblastoma
(C) Metastatic Kaposi's sarcoma
(D) Medulloblastoma
(E) Craniopharyngioma

Directions: Each item below contains four suggested responses of which **one or more** is correct. Select:

A	if	**1, 2, and 3**	are correct
B	if	**1 and 3**	are correct
C	if	**2 and 4**	are correct
D	if	**4**	is correct
E	if	**1, 2, 3, and 4**	are correct

66. The electron photomicrograph of peripheral nerve below exhibits

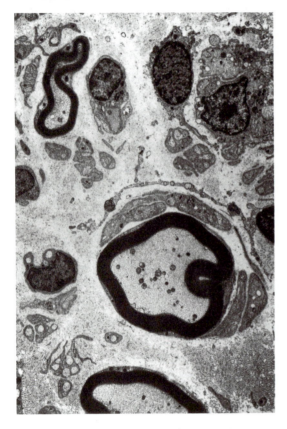

(1) an absence of myelinated fibers
(2) numerous inflammatory cells
(3) active wallerian degeneration
(4) onion-bulb formation

67. A patient with cardiac arrest resulting in brain death is maintained on a respirator for 72 h. At autopsy, the brain would typically show which of the following?

(1) Collapse of the ventricles with extreme swelling
(2) Extreme firmness of the white matter to palpation
(3) Universal necrosis of neurons
(4) Thrombosis of most or all large cerebral arteries

68. The Dandy-Walker syndrome is associated with which of the following anomalies?

(1) Agenesis of the cerebellar vermis
(2) Occipital meningocele
(3) Agenesis of the splenium of the corpus callosum
(4) Spina bifida

69. Focal slowing of nerve conduction velocity at sites of chronic nerve entrapment, with normal conduction velocities distally, is related histologically to which of the following pathologic changes?

(1) Lymphocytic infiltration
(2) Nerve trunk edema
(3) Atrophy of the endoneurium
(4) Segmental demyelination

70. True statements concerning cerebral amyloid angiopathy include

(1) it spares the basal ganglia
(2) it is unrelated to systemic amyloidosis
(3) it is a recognized cause of lobar hemorrhages
(4) it is uncommon in older patients

71. Which of the following will occur as a result of aging in the human brain?

(1) Increase in lipofuscin and neuro-melanin within neurons
(2) Massive acetylcholine loss in the hippocampus
(3) Decrease in D_2 dopamine receptors in the striatum
(4) Loss of neurons in all brain regions

72. Findings common in von Hippel-Lindau disease include

(1) retinoblastoma
(2) cerebellar hemangioblastoma
(3) subungual fibromas
(4) retinal hemangioblastoma

73. In the pathology of the AIDS-dementia complex, common findings include

(1) multiple foci of microglia, macro-phages, and multinucleated giant cells
(2) white matter pallor
(3) reactive gliosis
(4) amyloid deposition around blood vessels

74. Neuropathies with predominantly Schwann cell degeneration rather than primary axonal degeneration include

(1) acute idiopathic polyneuritis (Landry Guillain-Barré syndrome)
(2) most cases of Charcot-Marie-Tooth peroneal muscular atrophy
(3) diphtheria
(4) uremic neuropathy

Directions: Each group of questions below consists of lettered options followed by a set of numbered items. For each numbered item, select the **one** lettered option with which it is **most** closely associated. Each lettered option may be used **once, more than once, or not at all.**

Items 75–77

For each diagnosis listed below, select the figure to which it is most closely related. If none of the figures apply, answer (E) None of the above.

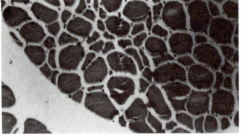

A

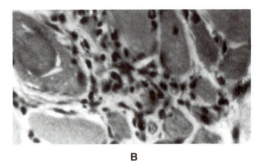

B

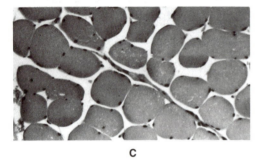

C

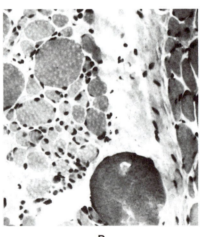

D

75. Normal muscle

76. Neurogenic atrophy in an adult

77. Muscular dystrophy

Items 78–82

For each pattern of demyelination or dysmyelination described below, select the disease to which it is most closely related.

    (A) Pelizaeus-Merzbacher disease (aplasia axialis congenita)
    (B) Sudanophilic leukodystrophy
    (C) Metachromatic leukodystrophy
    (D) Krabbe's globoid cell leukodystrophy
    (E) Adrenoleukodystrophy

78. The absence of myelin affects the parieto-occipital region most prominently but does extend into the frontal regions, often somewhat asymmetrically. The lesion shows three zones, visible on cut section and by CT scan

79. Typically, the brain shows more or less symmetrical tigroid patches of myelinated fibers against an unmyelinated background of white matter. No enzymatic deficiencies are known

80. The centrum ovale shows diffuse demyelination tending to affect the periventricular region maximally and sparing the arcuate fibers. No enzymatic abnormalities are recognized

81. The brain and peripheral nerves contain an excess of sulfatides that stain brown with basic dyes

82. The brain shows a diffuse demyelination, and the peripheral nerves show a segmental demyelination. Microscopic sections of cerebral white matter show accumulations of large spherical cells, many of which contain more than one nucleus

NEUROPATHOLOGY

A N S W E R S

43. The answer is E. (Rowland, 9/e, pp 438, 536, 718, 730.) Neurofibrillary tangles (NFTs) are most commonly associated with Alzheimer's disease but are characteristic of other disorders as well. The NFTs of progressive supranuclear palsy are composed of paired straight filaments, which are different from the paired helical filaments found in the other disorders. The NFTs are associated with neuronal dropout and sometimes astrocytic gliosis in each of the disorders. The etiology of the NFTs in these varied disorders is unknown. The Shy-Drager syndrome is one of the "multisystem atrophies," which include striatonigral degeneration and olivopontocerebellar atrophy. Their pathology is characterized primarily by neuronal loss and gliosis in brainstem, basal ganglia, and cerebellar structures. In Shy-Drager syndrome there is involvement of autonomic structures as well.

44. The answer is E. (Browne, Nature-Genetics 8:136–140, 1994.) All of these inherited disorders, clinically and genetically distinct from each other, are examples of "ion channelopathies" that lead to dysfunction. Why the syndromes are episodic is, as yet, unexplained, but the abnormal genes have been located. Most of the patients with hyperkalemic and hypokalemic periodic paralysis, as well as paroxysmal ataxia, improve with acetazolamide.

45. The answer is E. (Simpson, Ann Intern Med 121:769–785, 1994.) In general, the most common cause of intracranial masses in American adult patients with AIDS is cerebral toxoplasmosis. In other areas, tuberculosis is more common. Diagnosis of toxoplasmosis is based on biopsy; serologic studies are usually not helpful since a high percentage of adults are serologically positive for the infection. Although all the other listed pathogens cause intrabrain masses, they are less common than toxoplasmosis.

46. The answer is A. (Adams RD, 5/e, p 613.) Brain abscesses associated with congenital heart disease usually are solitary. The number and distribution of brain abscesses provide some clue as to the cause. Therefore, knowledge of distributional patterns becomes important. Abscesses from mastoiditis or sinusitis tend to be adjacent to the site of infection. Thus, a frontal lobe abscess would be unlikely to have originated in the mastoid. Such an abscess would most likely be blood-borne and the clinician should suspect the lungs or heart as the organ of origin. Many chronic lung conditions serve as a source of brain abscesses. Lung abscesses themselves and bronchiectasis, for example, may provide the primary source of an infected embolus that could travel to the brain. In most cases a single organism is responsible for the infection.

47. The answer is D. (Swanson, J Neurol Neurosurg Psychiatry 59:460–470, 1995.) The CAG triplet repeat is the cause of the first three listed disorders plus spinocerebellar ataxia type I, dentatorubral pallidoluysial atrophy, and probably others as well. Yet not all inherited neurologic disorders are due to this abnormality. In these inherited disorders the number of CAG repeats determines the presence or absence of disease. There is an inverse correlation, which is general and not applicable to individual cases, between the number of repeats and disease onset. In general the larger the number of repeats, the earlier the disease onset; however, the number of repeats does not necessarily predict the exact phenotype of the disease and each disease has its own specific minimum number of repeats that determines disease presence. Fragile X syndrome has been associated with excess trinucleotide repeats, but not CAG.

48. The answer is C. (Adams RD, 5/e, pp 868–870. Okazaki, 2/e, p 193.) A particular syndrome characterized by unsteadiness of gait, little or no dystaxia on formal testing of the legs, and sparing of the arms, eyes, and speech is related to degeneration of the anterior and superior parts of the vermis and adjacent parts of the anterior lobe. All neurons of this region are affected, the Purkinje neurons perhaps more so than others. This syndrome is the closest approximation to an anterior lobe syndrome in humans. The clinical appearance is similar to that of the cerebellar aspect of the Wernicke-Korsakoff syndrome. Adams and Victor maintain that alcoholic cerebellar degeneration is probably the same process as the ataxia of Wernicke-Korsakoff syndrome.

49. The answer is E. (Johns, N Engl J Med 333:638–644, 1995.) Mitochondria are present in most human cells, so their dysfunction may be expected to cause a wide spectrum of disorders. Most phenotypic abnormalities are in muscles and the nervous system and include the syndromes of progressive external ophthalmoplegia (Kearns-Sayre being the best known); the MELAS syndrome (myoclonic epilepsy, lactic acidosis, and strokes); myoclonic epilepsy with ragged red fibers; the syndrome of neuropathy, ataxia, and retinitis pigmentosa (which includes proximal weakness, sensory neuropathy, developmental delay, seizures, dementia, and the syndromic descriptions); maternally inherited Leigh disease; and Leber's hereditary optic neuropathy. Non-nervous system abnormalities also occur, including diabetes, cardiac conduction abnormalities, cataracts, liver and kidney dysfunction, and others. While most mitochondrial disorders are hereditary, zidovudine, an AIDS antiviral drug, causes a myopathy by depleting mitochondrial DNA from muscles cells, leading to mitochondrial loss. This observation suggests the possibility of other toxic causes of mitochondrial disorders. Retardation and dementia may occur with mitchondrial disorders but not a psychosis.

50. The answer is B. (Rowland, 9/e, pp 738–739.) Tropical spastic paraparesis is a subacute disease restricted to tropical regions around the world. It has been associated with antibodies to the retrovirus HTLV-I (note that HTLV-III is the AIDS virus, also labeled as HIV-1) in about 80 percent of cases throughout the world. However, exposure to HTLV-I does not imply the presence of neurologic disease and the virus has not been shown to be causal as of this time. Clinically the illness is usually of subacute onset with corticospinal tract, posterior column, and bladder dysfunction and thus resembles a spinal cord form of multiple sclerosis. Lathyrism has a similar clinical picture but is due to chronic ingestion of the chick pea.

51. The answer is E. (Adams RD, 5/e, p 1243.) Arthrogryposis multiplex congenita refers to the condition of an infant born with more than one joint in a fixed position. Thus, it is a descriptive clinical term instead of a true diagnosis. Arthrogryposis is a symptom complex of varied causes rather than a disease entity with a specific, universally acknowledged pathogenesis. Any mechanism that interferes with mobility during intrauterine development may produce the clinical picture of multiple fixed joints. Oligohydramnios, which hampers intrauterine motility, or prolonged paralysis of the fetus by curare-like drugs may cause the syndrome in experimental animals. The pathogenetic mechanisms may involve hypoplasia or destruction of ventral horn neurons, destruction of nerves, and disease of muscle or connective tissue. Children born with their legs fixed in flexion and adduction are likely to have the myopathic variety of the arthrogrypotic syndrome.

52. The answer is D. (Adams RD, 5/e, pp 1246–1247.) The muscle biopsy of a patient affected by the Kearns-Sayre syndrome of ophthalmoplegia, retinitis pigmentosa, and heart block shows ragged red type I fibers in the Gomori stain of muscle. These ragged red fibers are typical of mitochondrial myopathies. The syndrome may include retardation, hearing loss, and cerebellar and vestibular dysfunction. The other biopsy findings mentioned in the question occur in one of the various congenital myopathies, several of which may also affect the ocular or cranial nerve muscles. In central core disease, the central parts of the fibers stain positively with the periodic acid-Schiff reaction for carbohydrates. In nemaline myopathy, bacillus-like rods occur in the muscle fibers. The muscle biopsy shows central nuclei in centronuclear myopathy. These various biopsy findings are virtually diagnostic of the disease in question.

53. The answer is A. (Simpson, Ann Intern Med 121:769–785, 1994.) CMV is present in most AIDS patients and is transmitted in routes similar to those of HIV. It has a predilection for the retina, often involving one first rather than the two simultaneously. While toxoplasmosis also involves the retina, the coexistent encephalitis makes CMV a more likely pathogen. CMV can be cultured from blood or urine in over 80 percent of cases. Twenty-five percent of patients dying with CMV retinitis also have CMV in the brain.

54. The answer is D. (Jones, Brain 112:1295–1315, 1989. Pruitt, Medicine 57:329–343, 1978.) Brain abscesses are uncommon with endocarditis, especially in the subacute forms, and tend to be microscopic. Mycotic aneurysms may occur anywhere but tend to occur in distal parts of the vascular tree so that many aneurysmal ruptures result in intraparenchymal hemorrhages. Seizures are relatively common, presumably because of microemboli to the cortex. Acute encephalopathy and aseptic meningitis, with a granulocytic or lymphocytic pleocytosis, are common. Both are probably due to multiple microemboli. CSF may or may not grow the bacterial pathogen even when a granulocytic pleocytosis is present.

55. The answer is E. (Okazaki, 2/e, pp 76–82.) An arteriovenous malformation (AVM) is a tangled collection of thick-walled, abnormal blood vessels that are structurally between veins and arteries. These malformations occur predominantly in the cerebrum (90 percent) and half occur in the middle section of the brain. As in the photomicrograph, they tend to have a wedgelike appearance with the wider base in the cortex. Neurologic damage and seizures occur on the basis of ischemia, compression, and hemorrhage; the last is proportional to the size of the AVM. Treatment of the AVM is somewhat controversial.

56. The answer is A. (Rowland, 9/e, pp 169–173.) Prions are proteins that are transmissible agents associated with a number of sporadic and familial diseases. The most commonly recognized are kuru and Creutzfeldt-Jakob disease, which cause dementing spongiform degenerations. Kuru is transmitted by ingestion of the protein. In Creutzfeldt-Jakob disease, transmission may occur by direct insertion of the protein into the host's body (e.g., corneal implantation, injection of purified growth hormone from cadaver brains), but most cases have no known exposure. Prions act by inserting themselves into the host DNA and thus become part of the host's genome, producing certain rare familial disorders, which include Gerstmann-Straussler syndrome and fatal insomnia. Some of these illnesses, such as Creutzfeldt-Jakob disease and kuru, had been classified as "slow virus" disorders prior to a better understanding of the pathogenesis.

57. The answer is C. (Okazaki, 2/e, p 194.) Central pontine myelinolysis (CPM) is a severe disorder affecting the pons primarily, but also the striatum, thalamus, internal capsule, and cerebellum. It is a demyelinating disorder with relative preservation of axons and neurons that has been strongly associated with rapid correction of severe hyponatremia of multiple causes. That CPM does not occur routinely with rapid correction of sodium level argues against this as the sole causal factor.

58. The answer is A. (Adams RD, 5/e, p 1134.) Lead poisoning (plumbism) causes different syndromes in adults and children. Children develop encephalopathy and cognitive dysfunction, whereas adults develop a predominantly motor neuropathy with a predilection for the radial nerves and for arms to be more affected than legs. Footdrop and weakness of the shoulder and hip girdle may also occur. Diagnosis is confirmed by elevated blood lead levels or by increased urinary lead excretion after administration of $CaNa_2$ EDTA, a chelating agent.

59. The answer is B. (Poirier, 3/e, pp 207–208.) A teenager's brain should have small ventricles and very tight sulci. The brain presented shows an obvious asymmetry but no other abnormality. The age of the patient clearly indicates that the "full" side is the normal side and the other side is atrophic. This generally occurs as the result of a perinatal brain insult that is often difficult to identify but is often ascribed to vascular occlusion or obstetric trauma. Respirator brain and Alexander's disease are diffuse processes affecting both sides. Progressive multifocal leukoencephalopathy does not cause a significant change in brain size.

60. The answer is E. (Okazaki, 2/e, p 141.) The figures reveal multinucleated giant cells (left) and a microglial nodule (right). These are pericapillary in distribution and are typical of the lesions seen in AIDS encephalopathy (AIDS-dementia complex). The history is not uncommon for the onset of the AIDS-dementia complex, which is a result of the HIV virus itself rather than of a secondary infection. Clinically one cannot easily distinguish this from CMV encephalitis. There is widespread demyelination and there may be vacuolar degeneration as well, particularly in the white matter of the spinal cord.

61. The answer is D. (Okazaki, 2/e, p 140. Poirier, 3/e, p 120.) Progressive multifocal leukoencephalopathy (PML) is one of the many secondary infections that occur in AIDS patients. First described in patients with lymphomas and later in other severely immunocompromised hosts, it now may be most commonly seen in AIDS patients. It is the result of infection with a papovavirus, the JC virus (not the agent of Creutzfeldt-Jakob disease, which is itself a slow virus, or prion). This disorder causes large, confluent areas of demyelination that are usually asymmetric and have a predilection for the subcortical hemispheric white matter. On histology there are discrete areas of inflammation with giant astrocytes, abnormal oligodendroglia with viral particles, and macrophages.

62. The answer is B. (Okazaki, 2/e, pp 224–225. Poirier, 3/e, pp 27–29.) Ependymomas usually occur in children and have a predilection for the fourth ventricle. They are of glial origin, and of gliomas in the spinal cord, ependymomas form the majority and tend to occur in the caudal portion. The tumors tend to be highly cellular and may form tubules and perivascular pseudorosettes. In this photomicrograph the tumor has formed true rosettes.

63. The answer is C. (Okazaki, 2/e, pp 191–192.) This figure is a high-power view of the mamillary body, the site most often involved in Wernicke's encephalopathy, a deficiency of thiamine occurring in the context of an inherited transketolase deficiency. The major lesions occur in the periventricular gray around the third and fourth ventricles and aqueduct of Sylvius. The capillaries are prominent both in number and in size, and petechial hemorrhages are very common. Neurons themselves are relatively well preserved although some degenerative changes do occur. Myelinated axons are more affected.

64. The answer is A. (Okazaki, 2/e, pp 224–225. Poirier, 3/e, pp 27–29.) The figure shows a meningioma with characteristic epithelial-like cells clustered in tightly wrapped whorls around a hyalinized, calcified center called a *psammoma body*. Meningiomas occur in two major histologic types: the endotheliomatous type, composed of cells with an epithelial appearance, and the fibroblastic type, which looks similar to fibrous tissue. Both may have psammoma bodies, although they are more common in the endotheliomatous type. In cases where the psammoma bodies are profuse, the tumor is often called a *psammomatous meningioma.*

65. The answer is B. (Okazaki, 2/e, pp 204–219.) It is common to find different pathologies in different parts of a glioblastoma multiforme. Different regions often have different degrees of mitoses and cellular abnormalities. With immature cell types, special staining with glial fibrillary acidic protein may be required to demonstrate the glial origin of the cells.

66. The answer is D (4). (Poirier, 3/e, pp 240–241.) The electron photomicrograph is a cross-section of an onion-bulb formation of a peripheral nerve. These occur with repeated bouts of segmental demyelination and remyelination. When extensive, as occurs in many hereditary neuropathies such as Charcot-Marie-Tooth and Dejerine-Sottas, these cause hypertrophic changes that may be clinically evident. The endoneurium has a loose appearance and contains increased amounts of collagen. There is an increase in the concentric whorling of the Schwann cells around the axon sheath.

67. The answer is B (1, 3). (Okazaki, 2/e, pp 61–62.) The so-called respirator brain typically shows extreme swelling of the gray and white matter accompanied by collapse of the cerebral ventricles. Although in some instances the tissue feels fairly firm, typically it is very soft. Usually, the brain shows transforaminal and transtentorial herniation. Microscopically, the brain shows universal death of all neurons. The endothelial cells swell tremendously, occluding the smaller vessels. While the veins and venous sinuses typically contain thrombi, the larger arteries usually remain patent. The necrosis of tissue and absence of blood flow may or may not involve the spinal cord. Thus, in patients with a dead brain, some spinal reflexes may remain, although these patients will, of course, lack evidence of reflexes mediated through the brainstem.

68. The answer is A (1, 2, 3). (Poirier, 3/e, p 203.) The Dandy-Walker syndrome describes a congenital malformation in which the outflow from the fourth ventricle is blocked, causing massive dilatation. Frequently associated anomalies are occipital meningocele and agenesis of the cerebellar vermis. A less common association is agenesis of the splenium of the corpus callosum. Lumbar spina bifida is commonly associated with an Arnold-Chiari malformation.

69. The answer is D (4). (Adams RD, 5/e, p 1074.) Focal slowing of conduction velocity at entrapment sites, with preserved distal conduction, is related to segmental or local demyelination of the nerve. The preservation of the distal axons and their myelin sheaths accounts for the preserved conduction velocity. The nerve trunk edema and lymphocytic infiltration that may be seen in various peripheral neuropathies are not the usual lesions at entrapment sites. The endoneurium undergoes proliferation and thickening rather than atrophy. Surgical treatment by decompression or transposition of the nerve trunk may allow restoration of function, regeneration of the myelin sheaths, and an increase in conduction velocity across the lesion site.

70. The answer is A (1, 2, 3). (Okazaki, 2/e, p 170.) Primary cerebral amyloid angiopathy is a common finding in older patients. It is almost always seen in conjunction with senile plaques. Medium-sized cortical vessels frequently develop aneurysms leading to intraparenchymal hemorrhages (lobar hemorrhages). The deep gray structures of the basal ganglia are unaffected by the disorder. Cerebral amyloid is completely unrelated to either primary or secondary systemic amyloid.

71. The answer is B (1, 3). (Siegel, 5/e, pp 629–633, 636.) Lipofuscin and neuromelanin accumulate with normal aging. These are intracellular deposits that also accumulate outside the CNS. These pigments are thought to be nontoxic, even in large deposits. Age-related changes of neurochemicals are relatively minor compared with disease-related changes, such as dopamine loss in Parkinson's disease or acetylcholine loss in Alzheimer's disease. There is a decline in dopamine and D_2 receptors in the striatum with age, but it is unclear what other neurochemical alterations occur in the brain due to large variations beween subjects and between different regions in the same subject. Most brain atrophy is actually due to neuronal shrinkage rather than neuronal dropout. The inferior olive, for example, does not suffer age-related neuronal dropout. It is uncertain if acetylcholine declines with normal aging.

72. The answer is C (2, 4). (Poirier, 3/e, p 206.) Von Hippel-Lindau disease, an inherited disorder, is also called retinocerebellar angiomatosis because of the hemangioblastomas found most often in the retina and cerebellum. Hemangioblastomas may also be found in the spinal cord and other locations. In addition, tumors of the kidney and pancreas may occur. Subungual fibromas are found in tuberous sclerosis. Retinoblastomas are not associated with other nervous system tumors.

73. The answer is A (1,2,3). (Simpson, Ann Intern Med 121:769–785, 1994.) The AIDS-dementia complex is the most frequent neurologic complication of AIDS. The clinico-pathologic correlation is problematical in that the pathology shows less severe changes than the clinical situation would predict. Key components of the pathology are multiple foci of microglia, macrophages, and multinucleated giant cells. However, reactive gliosis and diffuse white matter pallor are common. HIV-infected cells may also be seen. In addition, a significant percentage of patients with AIDS dementia also have cytomegalovirus, (CMV) infection of the brain.

74. The answer is A (1, 2, 3). (Adams RD, 5/e, p 1074.) Acute idiopathic polyneuritis, most cases of peroneal muscular atrophy, diphtheria, infantile metachromatic leukodystrophy, and Krabbe's disease produce segmental demyelination. The loss of myelin accounts for the extremely low nerve conduction velocities that characterize these conditions. The advent of nerve biopsy, usually performed on the sural nerve (a purely sensory nerve), has served to clarify the pathogenesis of a variety of neuropathies predominantly affecting either myelin sheaths or axons. Some neuropathies predominantly affect distal parts of axons with the demyelination secondary to wallerian degeneration of the axon. In these conditions, such as uremia and nutritional deficiency states, the nerve conductions may or may not be slow and are therefore not helpful indices.

75–77. The answers are 75-C, 76-A, 77-D. (Rowland, 9/e, pp 766–767.) Figure C shows normal muscle. All muscle fibers have a uniform coloration and show faint stippling, indicating minimal ice crystal artifact. The fibers have a fairly uniform size. The outline of each fiber has a gently polyhedral or polygonal shape in the trichrome-stained frozen section. The nuclei are all subsarcolemmic in location. Very little endomysial connective tissue is present, but the perimysium is evident and contains blood vessels. Inflammatory cells are absent. A segment of normal peripheral nerve appears at the left of the section.

Figure A shows neurogenic atrophy in an adult. The muscle fibers stain fairly uniformly. The large fibers have the usual polyhedral outline, and their nuclei maintain a subsarcolemmic location. Inflammatory cells are absent. The abnormal feature consists of groups of collapsed profiles of atrophic muscle fibers. These appear in clusters and may show some rounding of their nuclei, which do not appear flattened against the sarcolemma as in the normal fibers. This pattern indicates a neurogenic atrophy in mature muscle. It contrasts with figure B, which shows the typical pattern of neurogenic atrophy in a child. In this case, the child exhibits Werdnig-Hoffmann disease, and the customary feature of neurogenic atrophy in infants is the rounding of the atrophic fibers rather than the polyhedral flattening as seen in figure A.

Figure D shows muscular dystrophy. The diagnostic features consist of some variation in fiber size with enlargement of some fibers and rounding of the contour. The increased space between the individual muscle fibers indicates an accompanying fibrosis. Later, much more necrosis and inflammation may occur with fatty replacement. The serum creatine phosphokinase (CPK) will be highest during the early stages of dystrophy. Histochemical stains in dystrophy will show a poor differentiation of fiber types. Although the microscopist can suspect Duchenne's muscular dystrophy from the section, the same features may occur in other dystrophies. Thus, the final diagnosis of the type of dystrophy depends on a blending of the total clinical information and genetic history with the physical findings and the muscle biopsy.

78–82. The answers are 78-E, 79-A, 80-B, 81-C, 82-D. (Poirier, 3/e, pp 133–138. Rowland, 9/e, pp 558–561, 599–600.) The demyelinating diseases are a heterogeneous group of disorders, often genetic in origin, in which the pattern of myelin deficiency differs from one disease to another—often differing so much as to constitute a decisive diagnostic feature. However, the pathologic distribution of the demyelination is only one feature in the nosology of the disease.

In adrenoleukodystrophy, a sex-linked recessive disorder and the commonest form of leukodystrophy in males, the loss of myelin predominantly affects the parieto-occipital regions of the brain but does extend frontally. The demyelination shows three zones. The central zone exhibits little or no myelin and appears quiescent histologically, showing only glial scarring. The second zone contains some surviving myelin and preserved axons and displays a prominent perivascular inflammatory reaction. The most peripheral of the three zones shows scattered demyelination with axonal preservation and the presence of numerous para-amino-salicylic acid (PAS)-positive and sudanophilic macrophages. In adrenoleukodystrophy, the localization of the most intense inflammation in the second zone differs from multiple sclerosis, which exhibits the most intense inflammation at the periphery of the lesion. Clinically, the male child with adrenoleukodystrophy usually appears normal at birth and in early infancy and begins to show neurologic retrogression between 3 and 12 years of age. The bronze skin, reflecting the adrenal insufficiency, provides a clinical clue to the type of neurologic disorder present.

In Pelizaeus-Merzbacher disease, a sex-linked recessive disorder, the brain classically shows patches of myelinated fibers scattered through otherwise amyelinated white matter; but some brains that are genetically and clinically associated with this disorder lack myelin entirely. Thus, the classic pathologic finding of tigroid patches of myelin constitutes only one link in the chain of diagnostic evidence for identifying the disease. The absence of myelin probably represents a failure of myelin formation rather than demyelination as such. Pelizaeus-Merzbacher disease is manifested in the neonatal period by oscillating eye movements. Cases of so-called adult-onset Pelizaeus-Merzbacher disease, which at autopsy show tigroid patches of preserved myelinated fibers, probably have little relation to the classic entity; nor does Cockayne's syndrome, which shows similar preserved myelin patches.

In sudanophilic leukodystrophy, the demyelination affects the centrum ovale diffusely but tends to concentrate in the periventricular zone and to spare the arcuate fibers. The arcuate fibers consist of the short association fibers of a hemisphere that connect one area of cortex with the neighboring areas. These short association fibers curve around the depth of the gyri, from which they receive the name *arcuate*. The arcuate fibers are preserved in some other types of leukodystrophy, such as globoid cell leukodystrophy. In sudanophilic leukodystrophy, the myelin degeneration products stain orthochromatically with dyes and, as implied in the name *sudanophilic*, the degeneration products have an affinity for sudan black. The sudanophilia by itself fails to constitute a pathognomonic feature. The sudanophilic material has a high content of esterified cholesterol. Similar sudanophilic degradation products of myelin occur in a variety of disorders ranging from phenylketonuria to head injuries.

In metachromatic leukodystrophy, a metabolic product accumulates in the central and peripheral nervous systems. This substance appears brownish in cresyl violet or thionin stains, which ordinarily produce a blue color. The prefix *meta-* indicates this alteration in tinctorial reaction. The basic defect usually is a deficiency in the lysosomal enzyme arylsulfatase A. In other cases, multiple sulfatases are deficient. The metabolic substance that accumulates in the tissues consists of sulfatides, which are sulfuric acid esters of cerebrosides. The discovery of the fact that the metachromatic substance consisted of a lipid led to the renaming of metachromatic leukodystrophy as sulfatide lipidosis, placing it with the disorders of lipid metabolism rather than with the demyelinating diseases. The disease typically manifests in infants or children and has a sex-linked recessive inheritance pattern.

In Krabbe's globoid cell leukodystrophy, demyelination affects the central and peripheral nervous systems. Affected patients have a defect in galactocerebroside β-galactosidase. The outstanding pathologic feature is the presence of globoid cell macrophages that appear as clumps in the white matter and often have multiple nuclei. The macrophages and Schwann cells contain abnormal tubules on electron-microscopic sections. Globoid leukodystrophy follows a recessive inheritance pattern. It usually manifests by neurologic retrogression in the young infant, and the patient is usually dead by 4 years of age.

NEUROPHYSIOLOGY

Directions: Each item below contains five suggested responses. Select the **one best** response to each item.

83. Stimulation of the supplementary motor area produces movements that are

(A) more discrete and isolated than those produced in area 4
(B) more consistently contralateral than those produced in area 4
(C) complex and bilateral, involving trunk and legs
(D) restricted to the face and hand
(E) restricted to release of sphincters

84. Cerebellar dysfunction is most severe when the lesion involves the

(A) spinocerebellar tracts
(B) frontopontine tract
(C) temporopontine tract
(D) pontocerebellar tract
(E) superior cerebellar peduncle

85. The troponin-tropomyosin system has which of the following actions?

(A) It excites the myosin to contract
(B) It inhibits the contractile protein actin
(C) It unites with excess magnesium ions
(D) It splits adenosine triphosphate (ATP)
(E) None of the above

86. The innervation for taste sensation involves cranial nerve(s)

(A) VII
(B) VII and IX
(C) IX and X
(D) VII, IX, and X
(E) VII, IX, and XII

87. In the neuropathies that primarily affect axons, as contrasted to those that primarily cause Schwann cell degeneration, the nerve conduction velocity is usually

(A) 10 to 15 meters per second (m/s)
(B) 35 to 40 m/s
(C) 50 to 80 m/s
(D) more than 80 m/s
(E) too variable to have diagnostic significance

88. Central neuronal hyperventilation is most likely to be seen in comatose patients with which one of the following brainstem regions affected?

(A) Bilateral thalamus
(B) Dorsomedial medulla
(C) Lower pons
(D) Upper midbrain
(E) Lower midbrain and upper pontine tegmentum

89. If an EMG was performed on a patient with asterixis whose arms were raised in front with the hands extended, one would expect to see which one of the following?

(A) A brief contraction in the extensors of the hand
(B) Simultaneous contractions in the extensors and flexors of the hand
(C) A brief silence in the extensors of the hand
(D) Irregular contractions and silences in the extensors and flexors of the hand
(E) None of the above

90. A 25-year-old woman sees her doctor because of headaches and weight loss. Her examination is remarkable for papilledema, impaired upward gaze, light-near dissociation, and retraction nystagmus. Which of the following is the LEAST likely diagnosis?

(A) Germinoma
(B) Teratoma
(C) Medulloblastoma
(D) Glioma
(E) Epidermoid cyst

91. The sternocleidomastoid muscle acts to turn the head

(A) contralaterally, tilt it contralaterally, and flex it
(B) contralaterally, tilt it ipsilaterally, and protrude it
(C) contralaterally, tilt it contralaterally, and retract it
(D) ipsilaterally, tilt it ipsilaterally, and extend it
(E) ipsilaterally, tilt it ipsilaterally, and protrude it

92. The EEG below is most compatible with which one of the following diagnoses?

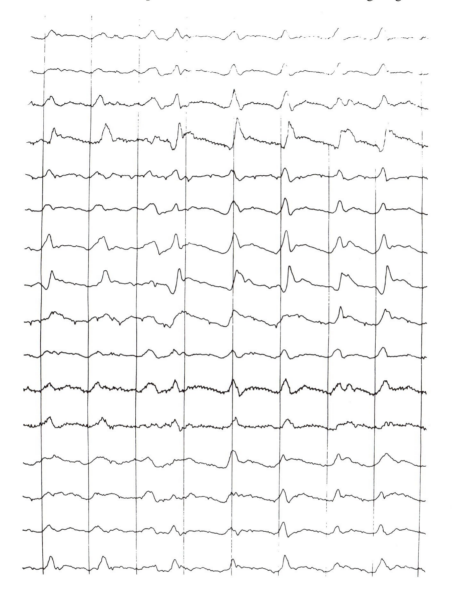

(A) EEG artifact
(B) Multifocal myoclonus
(C) Hypoxic ischemia
(D) Rasmussen's encephalitis
(E) Creutzfeldt-Jakob disease

93. An 18-month-old child, previously normal in all respects, develops a seizure disorder with the following EEG. The treatment of choice is

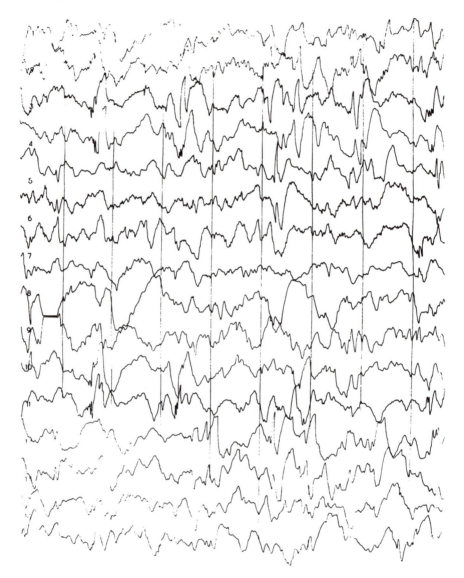

(A) valproic acid
(B) carbamazepine
(C) adrenocorticotropic hormone (ACTH)
(D) phenobarbital
(E) lamotrigine

94. The tonic neck reflex consists of

(A) extending the ipsilateral arm and leg and flexing the contralateral arm and leg

(B) extending the contralateral arm and leg and flexing the ipsilateral arm and leg

(C) extending the ipsilateral arm and contralateral leg

(D) extending the contralateral arm and ipsilateral leg

(E) displaying none of the above reflexes

95. After caloric-induced nystagmus, volitional visual fixation has which of the following effects on nystagmus?

(A) It augments the nystagmus

(B) It inhibits the nystagmus

(C) It increases the slow component

(D) It increases the fast component

(E) None of the above

96. The accommodation, or "near reflex," of the eyes consists of

(A) pupillodilation, convergence, and lens thickening

(B) pupillodilation, intorsion, and lens thickening

(C) pupilloconstriction, divergence, and lens thickening

(D) pupilloconstriction, convergence, and lens thickening

(E) pupilloconstriction, extorsion, and ptosis

97. The ulnar nerve conduction study below is suggestive of

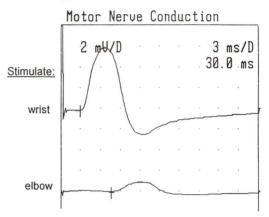

(A) ulnar entrapment in the elbow

(B) ulnar injury in the wrist

(C) brachial plexus injury

(D) Guillain-Barré syndrome

(E) diphtheric neuropathy

Directions: Each item below contains four suggested responses of which **one or more** is correct. Select:

A	if	**1, 2, and 3**	are correct
B	if	**1 and 3**	are correct
C	if	**2 and 4**	are correct
D	if	**4**	is correct
E	if	**1, 2, 3, and 4**	are correct

98. Contraction myoedema (slow waves of contraction that ripple over the muscle during a postural change) is very likely to be associated with

(1) complaints of stiffness and tightness in the muscles
(2) percussion myoedema
(3) slow relaxation after voluntary contraction of muscles
(4) delayed relaxation of muscles involved in stretch reflexes

99. Relaxation of muscle depends on

(1) union of troponin-tropomyosin with calcium
(2) enzymatic hydrolysis of the actin-myosin complex
(3) union of magnesium with the myosin
(4) calcium uptake by the sarcoplasmic reticulum

100. Characteristics of conduction aphasia include which of the following?

(1) Fluent paraphasia with retention of prosody
(2) Retention of comprehension and awareness of word errors
(3) Striking inability to repeat words or nonsense syllables
(4) Interruption of the arcuate fasciculus and overlying cortex

101. Cardiac rhythm disturbances thought to arise as a result of a cerebral infarct include which of the following?

(1) Atrial fibrillation
(2) Premature ventricular contractions
(3) Bradycardia
(4) Heart block

102. An elderly patient, on no medications and with no known psychiatric problems, complains of the recent onset of persistent auditory hallucinations that sound "like an organ." What associated signs should be looked for on neurologic examination?

(1) Unilateral deafness
(2) Hemiparesis
(3) Limb ataxia
(4) Impaired smell

103. A temporary increase in muscle strength on repetitive contractions may be seen with some frequency in

(1) myotonic dystrophy
(2) McArdle's phosphorylase deficiency
(3) myasthenia gravis
(4) small cell carcinoma of the lung

104. Stimulation of autonomic neurons in the sacral cord segments 2 through 4 should produce which of the following?

(1) Contraction of the detrusor muscle
(2) Catecholamine production
(3) Acetylcholine production
(4) Relaxation of detrusor muscle

105. True statements regarding gamma motoneurons include that they

(1) innervate intrafusal muscle fibers
(2) are subject to inhibition of the descending pathway
(3) are smaller than alpha motoneurons
(4) innervate extrafusal muscle fibers

106. During sleep most movement disorders either improve considerably or resolve completely. Which of the following movement abnormalities will usually persist during sleep?

(1) The chorea of Huntington's disease
(2) The tics of Gilles de la Tourette syndrome
(3) The tremor of Parkinson's disease
(4) Palatal myoclonus

107. Pain is mediated through which of the following?

(1) Unmyelinated C fibers
(2) Dorsal horn of the spinal cord
(3) Myelinated A (A delta) fibers
(4) Serotonin-containing neurons

108. Conditions that may produce or enhance fasciculations include

(1) severe dehydration
(2) organophosphate poisoning
(3) exercise in untrained persons
(4) hypocalcemia

109. In benign positional vertigo, the Hallpike maneuver will induce which of the following?

(1) Torsional (rotatory) nystagmus
(2) Nystagmus that lasts usually less than 15 s
(3) Vertigo that habituates rapidly
(4) Reversal of nystagmus and vertigo on sitting up

110. Use of the VER (visual evoked response) to evaluate a patient with suspected factitious blindness is subject to certain precautions. Abnormal test results do not always indicate organic pathology because patients may have

(1) been humming during testing
(2) kept their eyes closed during testing
(3) taken barbiturates
(4) converged their eyes or altered their fixation

111. Which of the following would be INCOMPATIBLE with a clinical diagnosis of brain death in a patient who suffered a witnessed cardiopulmonary arrest?

(1) Oval or irregularly shaped pupils that are unresponsive to light
(2) Cough induced by suctioning
(3) "Lazarus sign" during apnea testing
(4) Core temperature of 31.5°C (88.7°F)

SUMMARY OF DIRECTIONS

A	B	C	D	E
1,2,3	1,3	2,4	4	All are
only	only	only	only	correct

112. In the early evaluation of a patient with suspected Guillain-Barré syndrome, which of the following electrophysiologic tests would be likely to reveal an abnormality?

    (1) Repetitive nerve stimulation
    (2) H reflex
    (3) Central conduction velocity
    (4) F wave

113. Common findings in brainstem auditory evoked responses (BAER) in patients with an acoustic neuroma include

    (1) no recordable BAER
    (2) delayed interval between waves I and V
    (3) delayed interval between waves I and III
    (4) normal findings

114. A homonymous altitudinal hemianopia (a defect of the upper or lower field that involves both sides) may be due to lesions of

    (1) the lateral geniculate body
    (2) the retina
    (3) the visual association area
    (4) the posterior cerebral artery

Directions: Each group of questions below consists of lettered options followed by a set of numbered items. For each numbered item, select the **one** lettered option with which it is **most** closely associated. Each lettered option may be used **once, more than once, or not at all.**

Items 115–118

Match each clinical condition with the appropriate EEG finding.

    (A) Periodic lateralized epileptiform discharges (PLEDs)
    (B) Burst suppression
    (C) Triphasic waves
    (D) Pseudoperiodic generalized sharp waves
    (E) Temporal beta rhythm

115. Creutzfeldt-Jakob disease

116. Large hemispheric stroke

117. Axonic encephalopathy

118. Herpes encephalitis

Items 119–122

For each description below, choose the tremor that most accurately describes the movement.

    (A) Rubral tremor
    (B) Psychogenic tremor
    (C) Parkinsonian tremor
    (D) Cerebellar tremor
    (E) Essential tremor

119. Tremor of the hands at about 4 Hz at rest, with sustentation and with action

120. Tremor of the hands at rest and with sustentation but not with action

121. Shaking of the head "no" at times, "yes" at other times; the hands are silent at rest, but there is tremor at 8 Hz with sustentation and also tremor with action

122. Tremor of the right hand and foot at rest with a frequency of about 5 Hz while the left side is normal, then tremor of the left hand and foot at about 5 Hz while the right side is quiet; no tremor with sustentation or action

NEUROPHYSIOLOGY

ANSWERS

83. The answer is C. (Kandel, 2/e, pp 494–496.) The supplementary motor area produces complex, frequently bilateral movements of the axial muscles and legs, although a full somatotopic representation does exist. The most discrete contralateral movements come from area 4. Isolated sphincter movements cannot be obtained from the supplementary area. The role of the supplementary area in brain function remains to be determined. It may be responsible for some return of voluntary function after pyramidal tract destruction because it has bilateral projections. Blood flow studies show an increased activity of the supplementary motor area during complex volitional movements, and aphasia has been reported after infarction of the region.

84. The answer is E. (Adams RD, 5/e, p 78.) Lesions of the afferent systems to the cerebellum cause relatively little clinical dysfunction. For example, a high cervical cordotomy that is performed to relieve pain and involves sectioning of the entire ventral spinocerebellar tract on one side results in little, or merely transient, dysfunction. Some damage may occur to the cerebellar cortex or white matter, with little clinical defect. The most severe signs of cerebellar dysfunction are due to lesions of the efferent system (such as destruction of the superior cerebellar peduncle), or with large, severely destructive lesions of the cerebellar cortex and deep white matter. As with lesions elsewhere, the clinical expression of the lesion will vary with the age of the person when the lesion occurs, the size of the lesion, and the rate of tissue destruction.

85. The answer is B. (Adams RD, 5/e, pp 1060–1062.) The troponin-tropomyosin system inhibits the contractile protein actin and prevents its union with myosin. The latter event leads to muscular contraction. After depolarization (induced by the action potential) spreads to the interior of the muscle fiber, calcium is released from the sarcoplasmic reticulum, where it is stored. Calcium binds to the troponin-tropomyosin protein that inhibits the combination of actin and myosin. The interaction of actin and myosin leads to the rapid release of energy by splitting of ATP, a reaction that provides the energy for contraction. Muscle relaxation, which is an active process, occurs when calcium reunites with the sarcoplasmic reticulum.

86. The answer is D. (Kandel, 2/e, pp 520–521.) Taste is modulated by taste buds located on the anterior and posterior tongue, the palate, pharynx, epiglottis, and upper esophagus. The anterior third of the tongue and the palate taste buds are innervated by the VIIth cranial nerve. The epiglottal and esophageal taste buds are innervated by the vagus nerve. Taste in the posterior tongue is innervated by the glossopharyngeal nerve.

87. The answer is B. (Adams RD, 5/e, pp 1073–1074.) In the primary neuropathies with "dying-back" (retrograde) or wallerian (orthograde) degeneration, the conduction velocity is usually in the range of 35 to 40 m/s and thus only slightly reduced from normal. Those nerve fibers that remain conduct at approximately their normal rate. In the neuropathies that cause primarily Schwann cell degeneration, the conduction velocity is profoundly reduced, often to the range of 10 to 15 m/s. This fact is in keeping with the supposition that one role of the myelin sheath is to increase conduction velocity. Both toxic-metabolic neuropathies and heredofamilial neuropathies may be associated with primarily axonal or myelin sheath degeneration.

88. The answer is E. (Adams RD, 5/e, p 310.) Central hyperventilation is an upper brainstem respiratory pattern that may be seen in awake, sleeping, and comatose patients with lesions of the lower midbrain and upper pontine tegmentum. It is a sign of early herniation in the Plum and Posner model. Central hyperventilation induces a respiratory alkalosis. Low pontine lesions (a preterminal condition in the cerebral herniation model) cause apneustic breathing, and dorsomedial medullary lesions cause an irregular breathing pattern. These breathing patterns are interpretable only in patients with normal lungs.

89. The answer is C. (Adams RD, 5/e, p 88.) Asterixis is frequently called *negative myoclonus.* It is evaluated by having the patient extend a limb, usually the arms with the hands extended. When pronounced it may be seen proximally as well as distally in the arms and the legs. During prolonged muscle contraction there is a brief period of electrical silence during which the muscle relaxes. When the hands are extended, this sudden silence causes the hands to flap. It is often not understood that to evaluate asterixis the patient must be conscious, as the muscle contractions must be voluntary.

90. The answer is C. (Adams RD, 5/e, p 578.) Parinaud's syndrome of impaired upgaze, light-near dissociation, and retraction nystagmus is due to compression of the tegmentum of the midbrain. This may be caused by the tumor itself or, more commonly, third ventricular obstruction with resultant hydrocephalus. Typically this syndrome is caused by pineal tumors, which may be malignant or benign. Medulloblastoma is a cerebellar tumor, whereas the others are all plausible disorders of the pineal region.

91. The answer is B. (Haerer, 5/e, p 244.) The sternocleidomastoid muscle acts to turn the head contralaterally, tilt it ipsilaterally, and protrude it. One can readily confirm the role of the muscle by palpating it during these actions. The usual clinical test for the action of the muscle is to test contralateral head rotation, but the muscle's strength in the other maneuvers is also easily tested and its action easily observed. Knowledge of its other actions sometimes helps in the analysis of hysterical paralysis. In involuntary movement disorders with spasmodic torticollis, the overaction of the sternocleidomastoid muscle frequently causes head tilt as well as rotation. However, the other neck muscles also frequently are involved in head turning and head tilting. Hence, surgical section of the sternocleidomastoid alone fails in the treatment of spasmodic torticollis. The head may continue to tilt and turn in the absence of this muscle.

92. The answer is E. (Daly, 2/e, pp 413–415.) The EEG in early Creutzfeldt-Jakob disease is disorganized and slow. This corresponds to the phase of the illness with mild to moderate dementia and multisystem brain dysfunction. As the illness progresses and the patient becomes more demented, with bilateral pyramidal and extrapyramidal signs and myoclonus, the EEG reveals bilaterally synchronous, periodic, high-voltage, diphasic and triphasic sharp waves, 200 to 500 msec in duration. With time the complexes may become more complex. The period between the sharp waves is about 1 s but is not exact. The complexes are not time-locked to the myoclonus.

93. The answer is C. (Adams RD, 5/e, p 282.) *Hypsarrhythmia* is the term invented for this type of EEG, which consists of continuous multifocal spikes and high-voltage slow waves. While not specific to a single seizure disorder, it is seen in children, often previously normal, who develop flexion or extension movements of the trunk and limbs, producing a "jack-knife" movement, also called a "salaam attack" or infantile spasm. These spells respond well to ACTH or benzodiazepines.

94. The answer is A. (Adams RD, 5/e, p 509.) An infant whose head is turned to one side extends the ipsilateral arm and leg and flexes the contralateral arm and leg. While normal infants in the age range of 2 to 4 months will spend considerable amounts of time in the tonic neck reflex (TNR) posture and will, to some degree, exhibit the TNR when the examiner turns the infant's head, the normal infant readily struggles out of it and the response fatigues. This reflex may be briefly obtained in 60 percent of normal infants 1 to 2 months old and then becomes less common. In older children it is generally a sign of abnormality. Abnormality is evidenced by a machinelike response that persists. Such an infant has some disturbance in cerebral control of movement and generally will have some form of cerebral palsy. The TNR also may appear in infants with degenerative diseases of the cerebrum.

95. The answer is B. (Adams RD, 5/e, pp 237–240.) Deliberate visual fixation inhibits caloric or vestibular nystagmus. The cortical influence thus overrides the vestibular mechanisms. A dancer uses this phenomenon to inhibit vestibular symptoms induced by a series of spins or pivots. The dancer deliberately fixes the eyes on some stationary point, then retains fixation as long as possible while the body turns. Then the dancer snaps the head around to resume fixation as long as possible, while the body turns independently of the head. Thus, during most of the turn, the eyes and head remain fixed while the body turns. Both the inhibitory effect of visual fixation and the brief time occupied by turning the head reduce the vestibular stimulation. Therefore, one can best elicit vestibular nystagmus using Frenzel glasses to inhibit fixation. Brainstem and cerebellar nystagmus are elicited better through fixation.

96. The answer is D. (Newell, 7/e, pp 409–411.) To accommodate for near vision requires the eyes to converge, the lens to thicken, and the pupils to constrict. Convergence aims the visual axis of each eye at the near target. Thickening of the lens increases its ability to focus the more divergent rays from the near object on the retina, and pupilloconstriction narrows the aperture that admits light rays to the retina, producing a pinhole camera effect. The nervous system coordinates these three actions into a single reflex. However, as a person reaches the fifth decade, loss of lens elasticity prevents the normal thickening that should occur to accommodate for near vision. The affected person then complains of blurred vision for near objects, a condition called *presbyopia*.

97. The answer is A. (Adams RD, 5/e, p 1073.) The nerve conduction study reveals a reduced amplitude and mild delay of the compound motor action potential from the elbow but a normal response at the wrist. This implies a problem between the elbow and the wrist, most likely a cubital tunnel or other elbow-related syndrome. The conduction velocity in such situations is usually reduced.

98. The answer is E (all). (Adams RD, 5/e, p 1235.) Contraction myoedema and percussion myoedema, stiffness of muscles, and slow relaxation of muscles all occur together in hypothyroidism, in association with complaints of weakness. These findings, in association with the classic symptoms of dry skin and husky voice, establish a diagnosis of hypothyroid myopathy. The physical findings in hypothyroidism separate hypothyroid myopathy from conditions involved in the differential diagnosis of muscular diseases such as dystrophy, polymyositis, and the myotonias.

99. The answer is D (4). (Adams RD, 5/e, pp 1060–1064.) Muscle relaxation is an active metabolic process that requires the union of calcium with the sarcoplasmic reticulum. Deficiency of calcium or of the energy mechanisms that bind it to the sarcoplasmic reticulum interferes with muscular relaxation. Contraction of muscle as seen in certain disorders with exercise intolerance may reflect a disturbance in the metabolism of the ionic binding required for muscle relaxation. This process, like contraction itself, is ATP-dependent.

100. The answer is E (all). (Adams RD, 5/e, p 420.) The characteristics of conduction aphasia include fluent paraphasia with retention of prosody, retention of comprehension, awareness of word errors, striking inability to repeat words or nonsense syllables, and a lesion that usually interrupts the arcuate fasciculus. Wernicke proposed a major center for the reception of language in the posterior superior temporal region and a center for expression in the posterior inferior frontal region. Separation of these two regions by interruption of the intervening cortex of the supramarginal gyrus and inferior parietal lobule and of the interconnecting white matter, predominantly the arcuate fasciculus, produces conduction aphasia. The arcuate fasciculus is a large bundle of fibers, which, as the name implies, arc around the sylvian fissure from the temporal lobe to the frontal lobe. A major distinction between conduction aphasia and Wernicke's aphasia is that the ability to comprehend speech and to recognize word errors is lost in Wernicke's aphasia and retained in conduction aphasia.

101. **The answer is C (2, 4).** (Meyers, Stroke 13:838–842, 1982.) Cardiac arrhythmias are relatively common in the setting of an acute cerebral infarct and are thought to be mediated by increased sympathetic output. Observed rhythms have been premature ventricular contractions and all three types of heart block. Cardiac necrosis with elevated CPK has also been noted. Atrial fibrillation is often a cause of stroke rather than an outcome. Bradyarrhythmias are not believed to be induced by strokes.

102. The answer is B (1, 3). (Adams RD, 5/e, pp 253–254.) Auditory hallucinations may occur with pontine lesions. These are partly, not fully, formed sounds like a siren, or buzzing, or an orchestra tuning that are usually associated with hearing loss and signs of pontine damage. Auditory hallucinations may also occur in the elderly with hearing loss as a release phenomenon. Unlike the auditory hallucinations of psychomotor epilepsy, these are relatively persistent, not episodic.

103. **The answer is D (4).** (Adams RD, 5/e, p 1187.) A paradoxical increase in the strength of muscular contraction may occur in patients with small cell carcinoma of the lung. Affected patients complain of weakness that increases with use; but they may show a temporary increase in strength, measurable both clinically and by electromyography. This feature helps to distinguish the myasthenic state of affected patients from true myasthenia gravis, in which continuous use of a muscle reduces its strength.

104. **The answer is B (1, 3).** (Adams RD, 5/e, pp 473–476.) The parasympathetic system is cholinergic and arises from cranial nerve nuclei and the sacral cord. Its role in bladder function and sexual function is crucial. The parasympathetics from S2, S3, and S4 innervate the detrusor, and parasympathetic activity causes the detrusor to contract. Parasympathetic activity also relaxes the bladder neck, which allows the contracting bladder muscles to force the urine into the urethra.

105. **The answer is A (1, 2, 3).** (Kandel, 2/e, pp 566–567.) Intrafusal muscle fibers are those muscle fibers within the muscle spindle. Extrafusal fibers are those outside, in the bulk of the muscle. Alpha motoneurons are large in size and control extrafusal contraction. Beta motoneurons innervate both types of muscle fibers and are important in controlling spindles. Gamma motoneurons are small and innervate the intrafusal muscles only. They control spindle length and thus the response of the sensory nerves to muscle stretch.

106. **The answer is D (4).** (Adams RD, 5/e, p 89.) It is uncommon for movements to persist during sleep. If one sees the bed of a patient with Huntington's disease in the morning, it will be markedly disturbed, but this is the result of movements before and after sleep. During sleep virtually all tremors, tics, and choreic movements resolve regardless of the etiology. Palatal myoclonus and epilepsia partialis continua do not change during sleep, which separates them from the other disorders. In the dystonic disorders, the associated tremor resolves during sleep but the sustained abnormal muscle contractions may persist or resolve, so that observation during sleep in a dystonic patient is a relatively useless exercise.

107. **The answer is A (1, 2, 3).** (Kandel, 2/e, pp 388–390.) Myelinated A and unmyelinated C fibers carry nociceptive stimuli to lamina I in the dorsal horn of the spinal cord. The A fibers project directly to lamina I, while the C fibers project to lamina II and are connected via interneurons to lamina I. Lamina V also receives direct input from A and C fibers. Both A and C fibers are thought to secrete an excitatory amino acid, probably glutamate, and a neuropeptide, probably substance P.

108. The answer is E (all). (Adams RD, 5/e, p 1194.) Conditions that produce fasciculations range from exercise to organophosphate poisoning. Exercise in untrained persons and severe dehydration are intrinsic causes of the membrane instability that results in the motor unit discharges that constitute the fasciculations. Organophosphates are extrinsic anticholinesterase agents that increase the amount of acetylcholine. Low calcium blood levels likewise increase membrane instability. These nonneurologic causes of fasciculations need to be distinguished from the primarily neurologic disorders associated with fasciculations. Benign fasciculations, which are fasciculations appearing in otherwise healthy persons, also must be differentiated from fasciculations due to neuronal disease. In patients with benign fasciculations, there is no known evidence of toxic-metabolic disorder, atrophy or weakness, or EMG indications of denervation.

109. The answer is E (all). (Adams RD, 5/e, p 264.) The Hallpike maneuver consists of placing a patient supine from a seated position with the head tilted backwards by 30 degrees and then rotated to one side by 30 degrees. With vestibular dysfunction the patient develops vertigo after a few seconds along with a rotatory nystagmus that is proportional to the severity of the vertiginous symptoms. The rotation is due to simultaneous contractions of vertical and horizontal eye muscles and typically involves the twelve o'clock point of the eye beating toward the floor. This phenomenon fatigues after a few trials, but while changing positions, the nystagmus and symptoms reverse directions as the patient reverses positions.

110. The answer is D (4). (Daly, 2/e, pp 607–608.) During routine VER testing the technician performing the study watches the subject to insure compliance. In testing, a patient who was overtly noncompliant would be easily identified. Taking barbiturates and making noise (humming) should not alter the VER, but poor fixation and convergence (crossing the eyes) can severely alter a VER in a normal subject. Since one eye is patched, the crossed eyes are not discovered by the technician. The cause of the delay is uncertain.

111. The answer is C (2,4). (Quality Standard Subcommittee of the American Academy of Neurology, Neurology 45:1012–1014, 1995. Wijdicks, Neurology 45:1003–1011, 1995.) The criteria for brain death are clinical, although laboratory tests such as EEG, conventional angiography or isotope angiography (showing no flow to the brain), single photon emission computed tomography (SPECT), or transcranial Doppler ultrasonography may be added. Certain determinations should be made before declaring brain death. These include a core temperature above $32°$ C ($89.6°$F) and the absence of potentially significant sedatives, neuromuscular blocking agents, and potentially confounding medical conditions. Unresponsive pupils are accepted as an absent brainstem reflex regardless of their shape. Certain movements are considered of spinal reflex origin. These include the "Lazarus sign," which may occur during apnea testing, as well as other unusual movements. Coughing and gagging, however, are considered to be brainstem reflexes and, if present, are inconsistent with death.

112. The answer is C (2, 4). (Adams RD, 5/e, pp 1126–1130.) Acute idiopathic polyneuritis, the Guillain-Barré syndrome (GBS), is an ascending sensorimotor neuropathy that affects people of all ages. It follows viral illnesses in a majority of cases and causes a progressive problem starting in the feet with numbness, tingling, and, to a more profound degree, weakness. Deep tendon reflexes are lost early on. The pathologic process is quite patchy but has a predilection for ventral and dorsal roots and is demyelinating in nature. Nerve conduction studies show slowing of conduction velocity due to the demyelination, but the patchy nature of the process makes distal conduction velocities unreliable. F and H responses test the motor and sensory nerves along their entire course and are therefore the tests most likely to reveal an abnormality early on. EMG is useless early in the course and central conduction velocity would probably be normal.

113. The answer is A (1, 2, 3). (Daly, 2/e, pp 647–651.) BAER findings are rarely normal with acoustic neuromas. About one-third of patients have no recordable potentials, making interpretations impossible. Absent responses may also occur in patients who are deaf from any cause. Most patients, however, do have a wave I, which is generated by the spiral ganglion, whereas wave II is generated by the VIIIth nerve exiting the internal acoustic meatus, the usual site of the tumor. The intervals between I and III or I and V are usually delayed. Wave III is often not easily distinguished. It is important to realize that the acoustic stimulus produces impulses that travel in parallel pathways, so that brainstem lesions may not slow the response.

114. The answer is D (4). (Newell, 7/e, p 30.) Altitudinal defects in one eye are due to retinal disease. The retinal vessels travel vertically so that proximal ischemia will infarct the upper or lower halves of the retina, or both. To have a homonymous deficit the lesion must be in the brain. To have visual losses homonymously in both fields means the brain lesion must be bihemispheric so that isolated lesions of the occipital cortex caused by posterior cerebral artery ischemia are the only explanation.

115–118. The answers are 115-D, 116-A, 117-B, 118-A. (Daly, 2/e, pp 353, 413–415, 429–430.) Almost all patients with Creutzfeldt-Jakob disease eventually display pseudoperiodic generalized sharp waves that are diphasic or triphasic in appearance. These changes may only occur late in the disease but are helpful diagnostically when present. PLEDs are a distinctive EEG finding that correlates with many large, rapidly developing cortical abnormalities. While stroke is the most common, PLEDs may be seen with brain abscesses, rapidly growing tumors, and herpes encephalitis. The finding of PLEDs is very helpful in confirming the last diagnosis, although other encephalitides can, on occasion, also cause PLEDs. PLEDs may or may not be associated with focal seizures. *Burst suppression* describes a pattern of sudden spikes, slow waves, and sharp waves followed by a relatively flat waveform pattern. This is most commonly seen with anoxic encephalopathy but may be seen with other encephalopathies and drug overdoses. It generally carries a poor prognosis for anoxic patients. Triphasic waves are present with toxic encephalopathies. While most often associated with hepatic encephalopathy, they may be present in uremia or other toxic states; on the other hand, they may not be present in hepatic coma.

119–122. The answers are 119-A, 120-C, 121-E, 122-B. (Elble, pp 60–61, 143–144, 155–157.) Rubral tremor is caused by lesions in and around the red nucleus. It consists of a low, 2- to 5-Hz tremor of proximal and distal muscles (hence, it is a large-amplitude tremor) present at rest, with sustentation, and with action. It can be thought of as a combined parkinsonian and cerebellar tremor. It is not responsive to medications but is, luckily, uncommon.

Parkinsonian tremor is present at rest. It may or may not be present on sustentation but resolves with movement. It is usually asymmetric to some degree, often present only on one side. It typically involves the fingers and hands and may involve the feet and jaw but rarely the head. Often the tremor resolves completely when the patient is calm and relaxed. It always worsens with anxiety.

Essential tremor usually involves the hands, head, and voice, in that order of frequency. It is usually quite symmetric, causing tremor on sustentation and with movement, but is absent at rest. The tremor often varies in quality. In the hands it may be flapping at one time and more supination-pronation at others. The head may shake "no" or "yes" at different times.

Psychogenic tremor is often highly variable, with a history that distinguishes it from other tremors. Psychogenic tremors often begin precipitously without apparent cause and may fluctuate in ways that organic tremors do not. It is important to note that most patients with psychogenic tremor do not have hysterical personalities and do not exhibit belle indifférence.

NEUROCHEMISTRY

Directions: Each item below contains five suggested responses. Select the **one best** response to each item.

123. To achieve release of acetylcholine from a nerve ending, which of the following is necessary?

(A) Sodium influx
(B) Potassium efflux
(C) Sodium influx and potassium efflux
(D) Calcium influx
(E) Sodium efflux and potassium influx

124. The biochemical abnormality that is shared by the inborn errors of the urea cycle and that has neurologic manifestations is which of the following?

(A) A great increase in urea excretion
(B) Large amounts of prehepatic bilirubin in the blood
(C) High blood ammonia levels
(D) High serum uric acid levels
(E) Deficiency of brain carbamoyl-phosphate synthetase

125. All the following are neuroactive peptides EXCEPT

(A) somatostatin
(B) substance P
(C) neurotensin
(D) serotonin
(E) dysnorphin

126. Myelin is made up of several chemical components. Which one of the following constitutes the smallest percentage of its weight?

(A) Phosphatidylinositol
(B) Water
(C) Protein
(D) Lecithin
(E) Cerebroside

127. Maple syrup urine disease can be partially treated by which one of the following dietary alterations?

  (A) Restriction of phenylalanine, alanine, and glycine
  (B) Restriction of ketogenic compounds
  (C) Addition of branched-chain amino acids
  (D) Restriction of valine, leucine, and isoleucine
  (E) Addition of "Lorenzo's oil"

128. The rate of transport of metabolic substances from the perikaryon to the periphery in peripheral nerves is estimated to be in the range of

  (A) 1 mm to 1 m/day
  (B) 1 to 10 m/day
  (C) 1 m/min
  (D) 10 to 100 m/min
  (E) 45 to 60 m/s

129. An 8-year-old child experiences several episodes of extreme irritability, unsteadiness of gait, and a skin rash in response to sunlight. His parents are second cousins. The single most important diagnostic test would be

  (A) an EEG with photic stimulation
  (B) a CT scan
  (C) a urinary amino acid screen
  (D) a serum lipid profile
  (E) a liver biopsy

130. The most important mechanism for inactivating or terminating the action of catecholamine neurotransmitter released at the synaptic cleft is thought to be

  (A) irreversible binding of the catecholamine with the postsynaptic membrane
  (B) energy-dependent reuptake of the transmitter by the presynaptic neuron
  (C) inherent instability of the neurotransmitter
  (D) addition of sulphate radical by sulphatases
  (E) isomerization from the D to the L form

131. After release into the synaptic cleft, acetylcholine is removed mainly by

  (A) passive diffusion into the interstitial fluid and CSF
  (B) engulfment into the postsynaptic membrane by pinocytosis
  (C) return to the presynaptic ending by passive diffusion
  (D) enzymatic hydrolysis with presynaptic uptake of choline
  (E) long-term binding to the presynaptic surface

132. Striatal dopamine is located in highest concentration in the

  (A) perikarya of striatal neurons
  (B) glia
  (C) dendrites
  (D) synapses
  (E) perivascular space

133. The "second messenger" theory of the mechanism of action of neurotransmitters (and other signaling substances such as hormones) suggests that the primary messenger substance

(A) releases a second substance into the synaptic cleft
(B) releases a second substance that inactivates the degradative enzymes for the neurotransmitter
(C) activates the enzyme-controlled metabolism of cyclic nucleotides
(D) blocks the energy-dependent expulsion of sodium
(E) acts on the DNA to alter the encoded genetic constitution of the cell

134. Abetalipoproteinemia (Bassen-Kornzweig syndrome) results in

(A) deficiency of vitamin E
(B) increased high-density lipoproteins
(C) decreased levels of vitamins B_6 and B_{12}
(D) increased serum levels of lecithin
(E) abnormally increased levels of vitamins A and K

135. The problem in identifying glutamic acid as a neurotransmitter is that

(A) none of the enzymes that could act on it can be isolated from the nervous system
(B) it fails to pass the blood-brain barrier
(C) it may also have a significant role in intermediary metabolism
(D) it cannot be demonstrated in the CNS
(E) it cannot be shown by iontophoresis to have any effect on neuronal polarization

136. The rate-limiting enzyme for catecholamine synthesis is

(A) dopa decarboxylase
(B) phenylalanine hydroxylase
(C) tyrosine hydroxylase
(D) aromatic amino acid decarboxylase
(E) dopamine β-hydroxylase

Directions: Each item below contains four suggested responses of which **one or more** is correct. Select:

A	if	**1, 2, and 3**	are correct
B	if	**1 and 3**	are correct
C	if	**2 and 4**	are correct
D	if	**4**	is correct
E	if	**1, 2, 3, and 4**	are correct

137. Correct statements about the metabolism of acetylcholine include which of the following?

(1) An active uptake system returns acetylcholine to the interior of the presynaptic neuron
(2) The cholinergic neurons manufacture both the acetyl group and the choline group
(3) The rate-limiting factor is the availability of acetyl groups
(4) Acetylcholinesterase hydrolyzes acetylcholine to acetic acid and choline

138. True statements concerning acetylcholine receptors include

(1) nicotinic receptors are found on Renshaw cells in the spinal cord
(2) both muscarinic and nicotinic receptors are found in the brain
(3) muscarinic receptors are not found on skeletal muscle endplates
(4) stimulation of muscarinic receptors peripherally causes contraction of smooth muscle

139. Glutamate functions in the brain as

(1) a putative excitatory neurotransmitter
(2) a precursor of γ-aminobutyric acid
(3) an ammonia scavenger in detoxification
(4) an energy source in coupled phosphorylation

140. Major differences between serotonin and catecholamine metabolism include no apparent

(1) feedback inhibition of serotonin synthesis
(2) active uptake mechanism for serotonin
(3) activation of a secondary messenger by serotonin as contrasted to catecholamines
(4) depletion of serotonin by reserpine

141. Neurologic diseases that may be associated with red or brown urine include

(1) McArdle's disease
(2) porphyria
(3) alcoholic myopathy
(4) polymyositis

142. The neurosecretory granules isolated from catecholaminergic neurons of the peripheral and central nervous system are characterized by

(1) having a high concentration of dopamine or norepinephrine
(2) having the complete system of enzymes for synthesis of catecholamines
(3) containing high concentrations of ATP and ATPase
(4) lacking a distinct membrane under electron microscopy

143. Correct statements concerning serotonin, norepinephrine, and histamine include which of the following?

(1) The metabolic pathway to each begins with an essential amino acid

(2) The precursor undergoes decarboxylation

(3) Monoamine oxidase is involved in their inactivation or degradation

(4) Each of the substances has a potent vasoactive effect

144. Second messengers in the nervous system include

(1) cyclic adenosine monophosphate (cAMP)

(2) nitric acid

(3) cyclic guanosine monophosphate (cGMP)

(4) substance P

145. Characteristics of monoamine oxidase (MAO) include which of the following?

(1) It converts catecholamines to their corresponding aldehydes by oxidative deamination

(2) It exists only in a single unique form specific for catecholamines

(3) It is located in high concentration in mitochondria

(4) It is the rate-limiting enzyme in the catecholamine metabolic pathway

146. In its metabolic pathway, γ-aminobutyric acid (GABA) may be described as

(1) being derived from glucose and glutamic acid

(2) undergoing transamination and subsequently entering the Krebs cycle

(3) undergoing a rapid increase in concentration in postmortem tissues

(4) producing many derivatives that could act as neuromodulators or neurotransmitters

147. In regard to its distribution, γ-aminobutyric acid may correctly be described as

(1) being confined to the CNS

(2) being present in much higher concentrations in the ventral than dorsal horns

(3) having a very low concentration in white matter

(4) having a very low concentration in the basal ganglia and substantia nigra

148. Central cholinergic pathways are thought to include which of the following?

(1) Collaterals from the ventral horn motor neurons to the Renshaw cells

(2) Afferents to the hippocampus from the septum and diagonal band

(3) Cranial nerves IX, XI, and XII

(4) Projections from the majority of the raphe nuclei

SUMMARY OF DIRECTIONS

A	B	C	D	E
1,2,3	1,3	2,4	4	All are
only	only	only	only	correct

149. There are differences between central nervous system (CNS) and peripheral nervous system (PNS) myelin involving

    (1) lipid composition
    (2) protein composition
    (3) barrier to blood-borne chemicals
    (4) percentage of collagen

150. Evidence that glycine may be a neurotransmitter is reflected in which of the following statements?

    (1) It hyperpolarizes the postsynaptic membrane in spinal motor neurons
    (2) Its inhibitory action is blocked by strychnine but not by other blockers of amino acid receptors
    (3) Stimulation of dorsal spinal cord roots produces glycine release in the cord
    (4) Anoxia of the lumbar spinal cord produces a marked decline both in spinal interneurons and in glycine concentrations

151. An inborn deficiency of the enzyme biotinidase leads to developmental retardation, hearing loss, cerebellar signs, and skin and hair changes. True statements about this condition include which of the following?

    (1) Oral replacement of biotin may reverse some of the neurologic abnormalities
    (2) Some urinary organic acids are increased
    (3) Determination of biotinidase levels in fibroblasts may be necessary to confirm the diagnosis
    (4) The serum ammonia level is elevated

152. In one animal model of multiple sclerosis, experimental allergic encephalitis, true statements include which of the following?

    (1) It is caused by attenuated virus
    (2) Myelin basic protein can trigger the demyelinating lesions
    (3) The illness can be transferred from one animal to another via cell free plasma
    (4) The illness can be transferred from one animal to another via T cells

Directions: Each group of questions below consists of lettered options followed by a set of numbered items. For each numbered item, select the **one** lettered option with which it is **most** closely associated. Each lettered option may be used **once, more than once, or not at all.**

Items 153–156

For each locale in the CNS, match the correct chemical.

    (A) Gamma-aminobutyric acid (GABA)
    (B) Dopamine
    (C) Acetylcholine
    (D) Serotonin
    (E) Epinephrine

153. Medium spiny neurons in the striatum

154. Large spiny neurons in the striatum

155. Dorsal raphe nuclei

156. Putamen

Items 157–160

For each of the neurotransmitters listed below, choose the precursor with which it is most closely associated.

    (A) Tyrosine
    (B) Tryptophan
    (C) Glutamic acid
    (D) Glucose or citrate
    (E) Alanine

157. Acetyl group of acetylcholine

158. Serotonin

159. Dopamine

160. γ-Aminobutyric acid (GABA)

Items 161–164

Match each description with the appropriate term.

    (A) Intron
    (B) Exon
    (C) Initiation codon
    (D) Stop codon
    (E) Knockout

161. A section of DNA in a gene that ultimately is expressed as part of functional mRNA

162. A section of DNA in a gene that does not appear in the translated functional mRNA

163. A section of mRNA that starts translation from nucleic acid into protein

164. A section of mRNA that stops translation from nucleic acid into protein

Items 165–168

Match the disorder with the biochemical defect.

    (A) Abnormal amino acid transport
    (B) Disorder of phenylalanine hydroxylase
    (C) Lack of hypoxanthine-guanine phosphoribosyltransferase
    (D) Deficient activity of cystathionine reductase
    (E) Deficiency of hexosaminidase B

165. Early vomiting followed by delayed development, then seizures in a blond, blue-eyed child

166. Childhood strokes and ectopic lens

167. Renal tubular acidosis, rickets, retardation, and myopathy

168. Retardation, choreoathetosis, and self-mutilation

NEUROCHEMISTRY

123. **The answer is D.** (Kandel, 2/e, pp 120–125.) Using an experimental preparation that blocked sodium channels, Katz and Miledi demonstrated that electrical depolarization still resulted in acetylcholine release proportional to the magnitude of the depolarization. Blocking both sodium and potassium channels produced a similar result. Thus, although sodium influx and potassium efflux are necessary for a normal action potential, they are not required to release neurotransmitters. Calcium is required, however, and the quantity of neurotransmitter released depends on the amount of calcium influx that occurs during depolarization.

124. **The answer is C.** (Rowland, 9/e, pp 575–576.) A biochemical abnormality that is shared by the inborn errors of the urea cycle is an increase in the blood ammonia level. The formation of urea via the urea cycle is both the only known metabolic pathway for urea synthesis in humans and the major pathway for ammonia detoxification. Patients with an inborn error of the urea cycle have a deficiency of one of the five enzymes that lead to the biosynthesis of urea. When urea fails to be produced because of a block along the pathway of urea production, ammonia will accumulate in the body tissues and fluids. Ammonia accumulation leads to vomiting, lethargy, convulsions, hypotonia, coma, and mental retardation. Exacerbations may be related to the ingestion of large amounts of dietary protein. Although hepatomegaly may occur, there is no evidence of jaundice. The best single screening test for a urea cycle disorder is a determination of blood ammonia level. The specific defect is subsequently identified by the abnormal pattern of amino acid excretion in the urine and direct demonstration of the particular enzyme defect by biochemical assay of the patient's cells.

125. The answer is D. (Cooper, 7/e, p 418.) Serotonin is an indolealkyl amine, related chemically to LSD, and not a peptide, which is composed of amino acids. Neuroactive peptide-secreting neurons are different from neurons that secrete monoamines (glycine and GABA) in that they do not resorb the secreted substance and are first synthesized as prohormones. The neuropeptides are often found in the same neurons known to secrete other neurotransmitters, such as dopamine and acetylcholine. For example, dopamine colocalizes with CCK and neurotensin, acetylcholine with VIP and substance P, and so on. Most peptides have not yet been proved to be transmitters but are clearly involved in modulating synaptic transmission.

126. The answer is A. (Siegel, 5/e, p 127.) Myelin is about 40 percent water in the brain. The dry weight is mainly lipid (70 to 80 percent) and protein (15 to 30 percent); of the lipid part, the largest components are cholesterol and cerebroside. Lecithin constitutes more than 10 percent of the dry weight of myelin. Phosphatidylinositol makes up less than 1 percent of the dry weight of human myelin.

127. The answer is D. (Adams, 5/e, p 804.) Maple syrup urine disease is an autosomal recessive disorder caused by an abnormality of branched amino acid catabolism. The branched-chain amino acids are valine, leucine, and isoleucine. Restriction of the diet results in "reasonably normal mental development." Without dietary restriction, the child develops respiratory irregularities, opisthotonos, and hypertonicity within a week, followed by seizures, coma, and death in 2 to 4 weeks.

128. The answer is A. (Kandel, 2/e, pp 57–61.) The rate of axoplasmic transport of substances is variously estimated as 1 mm/day to 1 m/day. Interestingly, the rate of regeneration of axons is in the range of 1 to 5 mm/day, which approximates the rate of slow axoplasmic flow. Whether axoplasmic flow increases or decreases during regeneration remains in dispute. The rate of transport of metabolic substances down the axon (1 mm/day to 1 m/day) contrasts with the rate of propagation of the nerve impulse, which is in the range of 45 to 60 m/s. This vastly greater rate of impulse propagation underscores its electrical nature in contrast with axoplasmic flow, which involves the movement of ions, molecules, or even macromolecules.

129. The answer is C. (Rowland, 9/e, pp 544–545.) The combination of intermittent episodes of unsteady gait (ataxia), emotionality, and a photosensitive skin rash in a patient coming from a consanguineous mating suggests Hartnup disease. This disease is a recessively inherited error of metabolism characterized by a deficiency in the gastrointestinal and renal transport of tryptophan and certain other monoaminomonocarboxylic amino acids. The critical diagnostic test for Hartnup disease is the demonstration of the pattern of excessive excretion of monoaminomonocarboxylic acids in the urine. The direct selection of this single, simple urine screening test eliminates the need for further laboratory testing.

130. The answer is B. (Cooper, 7/e, pp 254–255.) Probably the most important mode of inactivation of catecholamine neurotransmitter at the synaptic cleft is an energy-dependent reuptake of the substance into the presynaptic neuron. Whatever the mechanism, apparently it is efficient because little of a catecholamine such as norepinephrine overflows into the circulation, in spite of strong stimulation of sympathetic nerves. While degradation by monoamine oxidase (MAO) or catechol-*O*-methyltransferase (COMT) accounts for much of the inactivation of released catecholamine neurotransmitter, the inhibition of these enzymes fails to potentiate the effect of nerve stimulation. In favor of the importance of active reuptake is the fact that a sympathetic neuron can concentrate catecholamines from surrounding media by a ratio as great as 10,000 to 1.

131. The answer is D. (Cooper, 7/e, pp 206–208.) The removal and inactivation of acetylcholine after its release appears to be mainly dependent on enzymatic hydrolysis. The choline part of the molecule is then actively transported back into the presynaptic cell by an energy-dependent mechanism. The availability of choline appears to be the limiting factor in acetylcholine synthesis, and this mechanism of active return of choline may be a mechanism for conservation of a rate-limiting metabolite. In some instances, the entire neurotransmitter molecule is taken up by the presynaptic ending and presumably can be recycled many times without undergoing degradation or resynthesis.

132. The answer is D. (Siegel, 5/e, pp 902–903.) Fractionation of the striatum with subsequent chemical analysis shows the highest concentrations of dopamine in the synaptosomal fraction. This observation indicates that the striatum, rather than producing its own dopamine, receives it from elsewhere via axonal transport and via reuptake mechanisms. Its accumulation in the synaptosomes suggests that it plays a neurotransmitter role. The nigrostriatal pathway apparently provides the majority of dopaminergic synapses for the striatum. Interruption of this pathway or degeneration of the substantia nigra is associated with a severe decrease in the dopamine content of the striatum.

133. The answer is C. (Siegel, 5/e, p 430.) Just how the primary chemical messenger, whether neurotransmitter or hormone, activates the target cell to do its job of secreting, contracting, or firing an impulse is one of the fundamental questions of cell biology. Current data suggest that the neurotransmitter coupled with its receptor activates nucleotide cyclases (cAMP, cGMP), Ca^{2+}, nitric oxide, and other chemicals, setting into play a series of enzymatically dependent events that provide the energy for the subsequent actions of the target cell. A whole series of "Koch's postulates" has been developed to justify the recognition of a second messenger mechanism, just as they have been developed to justify recognition of a particular substance as a primary neurotransmitter.

134. The answer is A. (Rowland, 9/e, pp 594–596.) Abetalipoproteinemia is a rare disorder of children that was one of the first hereditary ataxias described. The child is unable to synthesize the apoprotein of beta-lipoprotein, which results in a decrease in plasma levels of chylomicrons, low-density lipoproteins, very low-density lipoproteins, cholesterol, triglycerides, lecithin, cephalin, and sphingomyelin. Fat-soluble vitamins A, E, and K are markedly reduced because of fat malabsorption. The clinical syndrome consists of progressive ataxia, areflexia, weakness, retinitis pigmentosa, impaired proprioception, and ophthalmoparesis. Acanthocytes account for over 50 percent of the red blood cells seen on a peripheral blood smear. The neuropathology is widespread and includes segmental demyelination in peripheral nerves, demyelination in spinal cord posterior columns, and loss of neurons in the cerebellar cortex and anterior horns of the spinal cord. The neuropathologic explanation for the ophthalmoparesis is still unknown.

135. The answer is C. (Cooper, 7/e, pp 171–176.) Glutamic acid can be demonstrated to have excitatory effects on crustacean muscle and mammalian neurons. It and the enzymes that metabolize it can be isolated from nervous tissue. The main problem in identifying glutamic acid as a neurotransmitter is that it has a role in intermediary metabolism, which gives it a much more ubiquitous distribution in comparison to other putative neurotransmitters like dopamine, which can be localized to specific neurons and specific tracts.

136. The answer is C. (Cooper, 7/e, pp 226–227.) The term *catecholamine* refers to compounds composed of a benzene ring with two adjacent hydroxyl moieties (the catechol nucleus) plus an amine group. The term refers to dopamine, epinephrine, and norepinephrine. The synthesis of catecholamines starts with tyrosine or with phenylalanine, which is converted to tyrosine and then metabolized to L-dopa, dopamine, norepinephrine, and epinephrine in that order. The rate-limiting enzyme is tyrosine hydroxylase, which converts L-dopa to dopamine. It is this fact that allows L-dopa to be successful in treating Parkinson's disease; that is, the rate-limiting synthesis step has been bypassed.

137. The answer is D (4). (Cooper, 7/e, pp 197–199, 206–208.) In the metabolism of acetylcholine, the rate-limiting factor is the availability of choline, which apparently is manufactured mostly in the liver and transported to the neurons. Acetylcholinesterase hydrolyzes acetylcholine to acetic acid and choline. An active transport mechanism returns choline, but not the entire acetylcholine molecule, to the neuron. One stumbling block in acetylcholine research has been the lack of a drug that specifically blocks the uptake of choline.

138. The answer is A (1, 2, 3). (Siegel, 5/e, pp 253–258.) Nicotinic and muscarinic receptors are found throughout the body. The skeletal muscle motor endplate is nicotinic and does not involve muscarinic receptors. The optic tectum is primary nicotinic. Renshaw cells in the spinal cord are stimulated by activation of nicotinic receptors. Both nicotinic and muscarinic receptors are found in the brain, as well as in muscle. Muscarinic receptors have different functions in different smooth muscles. Muscarinic activation of GI smooth muscle causes depolarization of the membrane and contraction, whereas it causes hyperpolarization and relaxation of sphincters.

139. The answer is E (all). (Cooper, 7/e, pp 171–176.) Glutamate has numerous roles in the CNS. It is a putative excitatory neurotransmitter, a precursor of GABA, and an ammonia scavenger and is involved in energy metabolism. It also is a structural amino acid for protein synthesis. Glutamine and other putative amino acid neurotransmitters can be derived from glucose, and glutamate is involved in many other metabolic reactions including production of proline, glutathione, and *N*-acetylaspartate.

140. The answer is B (1, 3). (Cooper, 7/e, p 359.) Although serotonin and catecholamine metabolism share many features, serotonin synthesis differs in its apparent freedom from feedback inhibition. There is strong evidence for activation of a secondary messenger by catecholamines, as has been demonstrated in the effect of stimulation of the nucleus locus ceruleus on the Purkinje cells. Reserpine depletes both catecholamines and serotonin, which has confounded the correlation between neurohumoral levels and behavior.

141. The answer is E (all). (Rowland, 9/e, pp 788–790.) A number of neurologic diseases may produce reddish brown discoloration of the urine. The color results from hemoglobin or myoglobin pigments. The pigmented urine in most instances of neuromuscular disease results from necrotic or injured muscle, which liberates myoglobin, or from the biosynthesis of heme. The liberated pigment damages the kidney and leads to renal failure. Renal failure poses a threat to survival in many neuromuscular diseases that might not, in themselves, be fatal, including McArdle's disease, porphyria, alcoholic myopathy, and polymyositis.

142. The answer is B (1, 3). (Cooper, 7/e, pp 34, 247.) Subcellular particles called *neurosecretory granules* isolated from catecholaminergic neurons have high concentrations of dopamine or norepinephrine and of ATP and ATPase. The ATP may bind the norepinephrine within the granules by means of a salt linkage. The granules lack the complete enzyme systems for the synthesis of the catecholamines. Electron microscopy shows that the granules have a dense core and a well-developed outer membrane. The very structure of these neurosecretory granules raises questions as to whether they could fuse with the presynaptic membrane and release their neurotransmitter contents rapidly enough to account for synaptic transmission. Older data suggest this is unlikely, whereas newer data support the possibility.

143. The answer is E (all). (Cooper, 7/e, pp 352–359.) The metabolic pathway to serotonin begins with tryptophan, to norepinephrine with phenylalanine or tyrosine, and to histamine with histidine. Tryptophan, phenylalanine, and histidine all are essential amino acids. Each of the amino acids undergoes decarboxylation. Monoamine oxidase may be involved in the activation or degradation of serotonin, norepinephrine, and histamine. All three substances produce vasoactive agents. Tryptophan produces tryptamine and tyramine, and phenylalanine produces norepinephrine and epinephrine, all of which are vasopressors (as is serotonin), whereas histamine is a vasodilator.

144. The answer is A (1, 2, 3). (Siegel, 5/e, pp 430–442.) The concept of the second messenger system explains how many chemicals outside the cell alter intercellular function. The first established intracellular second messenger was cyclic AMP (adenosine 3[1], 5[1]-cyclic monophosphate). Cyclic GMP (guanosine 3[1],5[1]-cyclic monophosphate) is another second messenger system widely present in the CNS. Calcium ions, metabolites of phosphatidylinositol and arachidonic acid, and nitric oxide are other second messengers. The first messenger binds to a receptor in the external cell membrane, which then triggers a response in a protein bound to the inner surface of the cell membrane, which in turn activates the second messenger. With the exception of synaptic transmission and ion channels, almost all exterior-interior interactions occur via G (guanine nucleotide-binding) proteins.

145. The answer is B (1, 3). (Cooper, 7/e, pp 251–254.) Monoamine oxidase (MAO) converts catecholamines to their corresponding aldehydes by oxidative deamination. It exists in more than one form and lacks specificity for catecholamines, acting on a number of other substances including serotonin, tryptamine, and tyramine. It is generally regarded as existing in highest concentration in the mitochondria. It is not a rate-limiting enzyme in the catecholamine pathways. In spite of the presumed role of MAO in inactivating various biogenic amines that could serve as neurotransmitters, the action of these transmitters appears to be unaffected by the inactivation of MAO.

146. The answer is E (all). (Cooper, 7/e, pp 126–130.) GABA has an amino acid precursor, glutamic acid, but also can be derived from glucose. It undergoes transamination and then may enter the Krebs cycle. A striking fact about GABA is that it can produce a large number of compounds that may have neuromodulator or neurotransmitter actions. It can produce compounds that have anesthetic action or that may depress or excite some neurons. Thus, the metabolic derivatives of GABA are under intensive study at this time. One problem in assessing GABA levels or the effects of chemical manipulations on the GABA content of the CNS is that GABA undergoes a very rapid rise in concentration in postmortem tissues, which may result from activation of glutamic acid decarboxylase at death.

147. The answer is A (1, 2, 3). (Cooper, 7/e, pp 127–128.) GABA and its synthesizing enzyme, glutamic acid decarboxylase, are confined to the CNS, including the retina, which is embryologically derived from the CNS. GABA is found in much higher concentrations in the gray matter than in the white matter, in keeping with its presumed role as a neurotransmitter. It is found in high concentrations in the ventral horns, where inhibitory effects do occur, rather than in the dorsal horns, where excitatory neurotransmitters predominate. A GABA pathway is believed to run from the striatum to the pallidum and substantia nigra; the synthesizing enzyme for GABA (glutamic acid decarboxylase) and its degradative enzyme (GABA-transaminase) are in high concentration in these regions.

148. The answer is A (1, 2, 3). (Cooper, 7/e, pp 210–213.) Although technical difficulties prevent the establishment of acetylcholine as a neurotransmitter in central pathways as firmly as in the peripheral nervous system, some central pathways are thought to be cholinergic.

The most likely pathways include Renshaw collaterals from the ventral horn motor neurons, hippocampal afferents from the diagonal band and septum, the habenulointerpenduncular tract, the ascending reticular activating system, and cranial nerves containing voluntary motor fibers (III through VII, IX, XI, and XII). Several other central cholinergic pathways are suggested. On the other hand, many central pathways lack evidence of being cholinergic; many, such as the raphe nuclei, which appears to be serotoninergic, have other putative neurotransmitters.

149.   The answer is C (2, 4). (Siegel, 5/e, pp 763–764.) Both CNS and PNS consist of large amounts of myelin, which serves a similar purpose in each setting. The protein composition is considerably different. A far higher percentage of the PNS protein is collagen. Several proteins, such as P0, the major structural protein in the PNS, are not present in the CNS, whereas myelin-associated glycoprotein (MAG) is much more common in CNS myelin than in the PNS. Both CNS and PNS have blood-nervous system barriers, which while not exactly identical, are similar.

150.   The answer is E (all). (Cooper, 7/e, pp 162–171.) Glycine has been determined to fulfill the requirements for a neurotransmitter in the spinal cord and is a candidate neurotransmitter at other sites as well, including the retina, cerebellar Golgi cells, brainstem afferents to dopaminergic cells in the substantia nigra, and others. It hyperpolarizes the membrane of spinal motor neurons, which causes a fall in membrane resistance and a rise in chloride ion permeability. Its action is blocked by strychnine but not bicuculline, a GABA blocker. The localization of glycine follows the localization of strychnine binding, which again suggests a neurotransmitter role. Glycine is localized primarily to the ventral and dorsal gray in the spinal cord in interneurons. When the thoracic aorta is clamped, the resultant ischemia/anoxia preferentially destroys most spinal interneurons and brings with it a similar drop in glycine concentration. In a perfused cord preparation, stimulation of the dorsal roots brings about glycine release.

151.   The answer is A (1,2,3). (Siegel, 5/e, pp 836–837.) Biotin is a cofactor in amino acid metabolism, for gluconeogenesis in the pyruvate carboxylase reaction and for acetyl-CoA carboxylase in fatty acid synthesis. Deficiency of biotin therefore leads to a buildup of organic acids. Biotinidase cleaves biotinyl residues from the enzyme to which biotin binds, allowing it to be recycled. A deficiency of biotinidase leads to a depletion of biotin, which can be overcome by oral supplements. Restoration of biotin levels will halt the progression of disease and will lead to partial reversal of neurologic abnormalities. The disorder can usually be diagnosed by measuring urinary levels of organic acids, but sometimes biotinidase levels in fibroblasts or blood cells must be measured. Serum levels of biotinidase are usually low as well.

152. The answer is C (2, 4). (Siegel, 5/e, pp 778–779.) There are acute, chronic, and chronic relapsing forms of experimental allergic encephalitis (EAE). The acute form occurs with the injection of myelin basic protein (MBP) and Freund's adjuvant. This leads to widespread demyelination in the brain. This disorder is transferred via CD4+ T cells from animal to animal and not by a serum-borne substance. The chronic form is brought on by the addition of other myelin chemicals to MBP. The relapsing form occurs with the addition of non-MBP components of myelin or after the transfer of certain T-cell clones from an animal with the acute form.

153–156. The answers are 153-A, 154-C, 155-D, 156-B. (Siegel, 5/e, 287–290, 902–906.) Most striatal neurons are medium spiny neurons that contain GABA. These GABA-secreting neurons project to the substantia nigra and to the external segment of the globus pallidum. These pallidal neurons project to the subthalamic nucleus, forming the so-called indirect path in the basal ganglia, which connects the striatum to the internal segment of the globus pallidum. GABA is a widely present neurotransmitter in the central nervous system and is inhibitory.

Large spiny neurons in the striatum function primarily as interneurons, receiving impulses from cortex, substantia nigra, and medium spiny neurons. They project mainly within the striatum. Only about 5 percent of striatal neurons are of this type, however. They are acetylcholine-secreting neurons and stain positively for choline acetyl transferase, indicating synthesis of acetylcholine within the neuron.

Serotonin-containing neurons project widely throughout the brain, but the cell bodies are localized to discrete clusters in the midline of the upper brainstem. The caudal neurons project to brainstem and spinal areas and the rostral neurons project to the forebrain and limbic system.

The putamen received 90 percent of the nigrostriatal projection. Although the pars compacta neurons are the dopamine-containing neurons, most synthesis and all the secretion takes place in the synapse, located primarily in the putamen. In the studies of dopamine distribution in Parkinson's disease, the dopamine loss is greatest in the putamen.

157–160. The answers are 157-D, 158-B, 159-A, 160-C. (Cooper, 7/e, pp 171, 195, 297, 355.) The precursor of the acetyl group of acetylcholine is glucose or citrate; of serotonin, tryptophan; of dopamine, tyrosine; and of GABA, glutamic acid. These precursor substances, occurring in the diet, undergo several metabolic transformations to gain activity as neurotransmitters. With some further slight metabolic transformation, the neurotransmitter loses its capacity to excite or inhibit the postsynaptic neuron. The elaborate metabolic pathway involved insures that only the exact substance, rather than a substance that happens to enter the blood, will affect the function of the neurons.

The precursors of acetylcholine differ from the other precursors in this group. The precursors of serotonin, dopamine, and GABA are all amino acids. The acetyl group of acetylcholine is readily available from the catabolism of glucose. The choline that comes from the diet is the rate-limiting moiety of acetylcholine synthesis. Choline is taken up for recycling by the presynaptic ending, after the splitting of acetylcholine by cholinesterase at the synapse.

The recycling of one moiety of a transmitter, choline, appears to be unusual. The biogenic amines are transformed by undergoing methylations or hydroxylations. In the case of amino acid–related transmitters, inactivation may ultimately involve deamination. Serotonin is inactivated by both oxidation and deamination. The end product of this process is 5-hydroxy-indoleacetic acid. The carboxyl group of the acetic acid replaces the amino grouping on the terminal carbon of the aliphatic portion of the molecule.

161–164. The answers are 161-B, 162-A, 163-C, 164-D. (Siegel, 5/e, p 495.) Introns, or intervening sequences, are interruptions in the DNA gene sequence that code for RNA sequences that are removed before functional mRNA is formed. The part of the DNA gene sequence coding for RNA that ultimately ends up being incorporated into functional mRNA is called an exon. Once DNA is transcribed into RNA, RNA is cut and spliced per instructions contained on that very same RNA and thus converted into "mature," or functional, mRNA. The way in which this rearrangement of the RNA occurs varies in different types of cell tissues. Genes also contain sequences that are not translated and help regulate gene expression. The initiation site thus selects the section of mRNA where the ribosome translates the RNA message and sets the phase (the sets of three) for translation. In addition there is a "cap" and a "tail," which are added to the mRNA after transcription and are not coded for in the original DNA. A knockout is an organism that lacks a particular gene, thus allowing investigators to evaluate the effect of a gene's absence.

165–168. The answers are 165-B, 166-D, 167-A, 168-C. (Rowland, 9/e, pp 538–544, 546–547.) Phenylketonuria is caused by a deficiency of phenylalanine hydroxylase, which is normally found in organs outside of the brain. As a result of this, the normal hydroxylation of phenylalanine to tyrosine does not take place. If not recognized, a normal diet will lead to accumulations of large amounts of phenylalanine. In the brain there is a delay of maturation, defective myelination, and decreased pigmentation of the substantia nigra. Affected children have deficient pigmentation. They are irritable and vomit early on before showing delayed milestones. By 18 months seizures are common.

Homocystinuria is the most common disorder of metabolism of sulfur-containing amino acids. In most cases, cystathionine synthetase is lacking. The enzyme synthesizes the catabolism of cystathionine from homocysteine and serine. As a result, increased levels of homocysteine and methionine accumulate. Patients have strokes in the first year or two of life and invariably have ectopic lenses.

There are a few different disorders of amino acid transport. The oculocerebrorenal syndrome of Lowe is sex-linked recessive. Patients have elevated lysine levels in urine. The kidney defect is an aminoaciduria with renal tubular acidosis and rickets. Neurologically there is severe retardation and growth delay.

Lesch-Nyhan syndrome is a disorder of purine metabolism due to a lack of hypoxanthine-guanine phosphoribosyltransferase. This leads to increased purine metabolism with a buildup of uric acid that may simulate gout. The neurologic syndrome that differentiates it from most other disorders is the uniform presence of self-mutilation. Severe dementia, spasticity, and choreoathetosis start in the first year.

NEUROPHARMACOLOGY

Directions: Each item below contains five suggested responses. Select the **one best** response to each item.

169. A postganglionic Horner's syndrome can be distinguished from a preganglionic or central one using which one of the following drugs?

(A) Cocaine
(B) Atropine
(C) Hydroxyamphetamine
(D) Pilocarpine
(E) Timolol

170. The most effective preventative of seizure in eclampsia is

(A) nitroprusside
(B) phenytoin
(C) magnesium sulfate
(D) calcium chloride
(E) diazepam

171. Abrupt discontinuation of chronic cocaine use leads to which one of the following sequences of behavioral changes?

(A) Tremors, diaphoresis, and seizures followed by profound sleepiness
(B) Depression, anxiety, and drug craving followed by hypersomnolence possibly lasting for days
(C) A brief period of well being followed by drug craving, hallucinations, and psychosis
(D) An agitated global confusional state
(E) An akinetic rigid syndrome lasting days followed by chorea ("crack dancing")

172. A patient lacking available history is brought in off the street with delirium; pupillodilatation; dry, flushed skin and mucous membranes; peculiar myoclonus-like twitchings; tachycardia; and fever. The clinical condition appears to be deteriorating during a period of 45 min of observation. The drug of choice for treatment would be which of the following?

(A) Edrophonium
(B) Thiamine
(C) Phenobarbital
(D) Physostigmine
(E) Metocurine iodide (Metubine)

173. Local anesthetic agents like procaine are thought to act by

(A) inhibiting cyclic AMP
(B) inhibiting the oxidative enzymes of the mitochondria in the perikaryon and synaptic endings
(C) blocking pyridoxal-dependent enzymes of the catecholamine metabolic pathway
(D) blocking the voltage-dependent transient rise in membrane permeability to sodium
(E) completing depolarization

174. A 60-year-old man takes a monoamine oxidase inhibitor for depression and lithium for mania. After several months, his depression recurs and sertraline, a serotonin reuptake inhibitor, is added to the regimen. Two days later he is brought to the emergency room and is found to have a temperature of 38.33°C (101°F). He is obtunded, confused, rigid, and myoclonic. Treatment of the most likely explanation for this problem would be

(A) hydration
(B) bromocriptine
(C) dantrolene
(D) pancuronium bromide
(E) diazepam

175. Which of the following statements regarding botulinum toxin (botulin) A is true?

(A) It is the treatment of choice for blepharospasm and hemifacial spasm
(B) It is not helpful in torticollis
(C) It weakens muscles by blocking the motor end plate
(D) It acts by uncoupling myofibrils
(E) It interrupts acetylcholine synthesis

176. The most widely accepted theory to explain tachyphylaxis by sympathomimetic drugs is which of the following?

(A) Irreversible binding of the neurotransmitter at the receptor site
(B) Stimulation of degradative enzymes
(C) Increased flushing of intercellular fluid through the synapse
(D) Displacement of neurotransmitter from the presynaptic terminals
(E) Release of dopamine β-hydroxylase

177. You wish to provide proper anticoagulation to maximally reduce the cardioembolic stroke rate in a patient with nonrheumatic atrial fibrillation while keeping bleeding complications to a minimum. The current recommendation is administration of

(A) warfarin and maintenance of an International Normalized Ratio (INR) of 2.0 to 3.9
(B) warfarin and maintenance of an INR of 1.5 to 2.5
(C) aspirin 1300 mg per day
(D) ticlopidine 500 mg per day
(E) aspirin 325 mg per day and warfarin with an INR of 1.5

178. When ethanol is ingested after disulfiram, the subject experiences

(A) nausea and vomiting from acute vestibular toxicity
(B) vomiting, headache, and abdominal pain from acute ileus
(C) dyspnea, headache, and vomiting from acetaldehyde toxicity
(D) itching, confusion, and dyspnea from ammonium toxicity
(E) dysphoria and nausea from blocked opiate receptors

179. When added to other anticonvulsant drugs, gabapentin causes

(A) elevation of carbamazepine plasma levels
(B) elevation of phenytoin plasma levels
(C) increased metabolism of valproic acid and decreased plasma levels
(D) elevation of phenobarbital levels
(E) no changes in plasma levels in any of the anticonvulsants listed above

180. Malignant hyperthermia is correctly characterized by which of the following statements?

(A) It can be induced by antipsychotic drugs
(B) It can be precipitated by halothane
(C) It is best treated with a paralyzing agent like succinylcholine
(D) It responds to intravenous diazepam
(E) It is rarely familial

181. A patient with active pulmonary tuberculosis complains of tingling and numbness in the feet and hands about 1 month into therapy with isoniazid, rifampin, and ethambutol. The best treatment for this is to

(A) administer pyridoxine
(B) administer pantothenic acid
(C) replace ethambutol with an alternative
(D) replace rifampin with an alternative
(E) replace isoniazid with an alternative

182. A young woman receives an injection of 4.8 million units of penicillin G procaine for treatment of gonorrhea. She returns to the office minutes later complaining of tinnitus, headaches, and hallucinations. She then has a generalized seizure. The most likely explanation is

(A) a reaction to the procaine
(B) penicillin allergy
(C) toxicity from use of or withdrawal from unrelated drugs of abuse
(D) a psychogenic reaction to the treatment
(E) an AIDS-related brain disorder

183. A manic-depressive patient recently started on lithium treatment develops diarrhea, ataxia, fasciculations, tremor, overactive muscle stretch reflexes, and seizures. The blood lithium level is 1.5 meq/L. The best interpretation of these findings is that the

(A) correct diagnosis of delirium tremens was overlooked
(B) symptoms and lithium blood level are compatible with lithium intoxication
(C) patient has acute hyperthyroidism
(D) lithium has precipitated a catecholaminergic crisis
(E) patient must have received a stimulant medication and should have a toxicology screening

184. MPTP is a toxin that causes parkinsonism in humans. All the following statements about MPTP are true EXCEPT that it

(A) must be converted in glial cells to MPP+ to become toxic
(B) is prevented from becoming toxic if MAO-B is blocked
(C) destroys striatal as well as nigral neurons
(D) primarily affects dopaminergic neurons
(E) produces an opiate "high"

185. A striking difference in the response of the nigrostriatal system to mechanical or pharmacologic interruption of impulse flow, as contrasted to the other catecholaminergic systems, is that the interruption results in

(A) increased storage of dopamine in the axonal terminals and increased production
(B) great increase in acetylcholine in the striatum
(C) immediate switch to serotonin neurotransmission
(D) no change in the production or storage of dopamine because of steady-state kinetics of the system
(E) extreme depletion of dopamine in the striatum

186. Infantile spasms are most likely to respond to which one of the following medications?

(A) Valproic acid
(B) Carbamazepine
(C) Clonazepam
(D) ACTH
(E) Bromide

187. An overdose of which one of the following drugs can cause fixed and unequal pupils?

(A) Phenobarbital
(B) Glutethimide
(C) Amphetamine
(D) Lithium
(E) Imipramine

188. Deprenyl (selegiline; Eldepryl) may be characterized by which of the following statements?

(A) It has been demonstrated to slow the progression of disability in Parkinson's disease
(B) It is a potentially dangerous drug because it blocks the enzyme MOA
(C) It has a major symptomatic effect in otherwise untreated patients with Parkinson's disease
(D) It improves memory function in Parkinson's disease
(E) It is useful in Parkinson's disease because of its antidepressant effects

189. Which one of the following statements concerning the pharmacokinetics of phenytoin is true?

(A) Brain concentration equals the protein-bound concentration in the blood
(B) Only small amounts bind to plasma protein
(C) In the therapeutic range, the plasma half-life increases with the concentration
(D) At low plasma concentrations, the drug has a longer half-life than at high concentrations
(E) There is little variability in the plasma half-life

190. Meperidine (Demerol) may have a fatal interaction with

(A) lithium
(B) benztropine
(C) tricyclic antidepressants
(D) MAO antidepressants
(E) phenytoin

191. Chronic use of which one of the following drugs may lead to auditory hallucinations in an otherwise clear sensorium?

(A) Levodopa
(B) Phenobarbital
(C) Cocaine
(D) Ethanol
(E) Alprazolam

192. Which one of the following drugs causes a syndrome of visual hallucinations in an otherwise clear sensorium?

(A) Amphetamine
(B) Methanol
(C) Ethanol
(D) Cocaine
(E) Levodopa

193. A man with leukemia is admitted with mild confusion, a lower motor neuron facial palsy on one side, and biceps weakness on the contralateral side. His brain CT scan is normal but spinal fluid reveals a lymphocytic pleocytosis with a mildly low glucose and mildly elevated protein. No leukemic cells are seen initially, but fungal and bacterial cultures are negative. Which drug is most likely to be beneficial?

(A) Methotrexate
(B) Dexamethasone
(C) Amphotericin
(D) Isoniazid
(E) Cisplatin

Directions: Each item below contains four suggested responses of which **one or more** is correct. Select:

A	if	**1, 2, and 3**	are correct
B	if	**1 and 3**	are correct
C	if	**2 and 4**	are correct
D	if	**4**	is correct
E	if	**1, 2, 3, and 4**	are correct

194. Dexamethasone has been proved to be effective in reducing the edema associated with which of the following conditions?

(1) Cerebral infarction
(2) Glioma
(3) Cerebral trauma
(4) Abscess

195. Pseudotumor cerebri has been linked to which of the following medications?

(1) Ferrous sulfate
(2) Tetracycline
(3) Pyridoxine
(4) Vitamin A

196. Manipulations that increase the action of tyrosine hydroxylase in catecholaminergic neurons include which of the following?

(1) Administration of MAO inhibitors
(2) Administration of tyramine
(3) Administration of 6-hydroxydopamine or α-methyl-ρ-tyrosine (AMPT)
(4) Increased activity of the catecholaminergic neurons

197. Petit mal (three cycles per second spike and wave) seizures can be treated with which of the following medications?

(1) Valproic acid
(2) Phenobarbital
(3) Ethosuximide
(4) Phenytoin

198. Which of the following statements would apply to the pharmacology of tardive dyskinesia?

(1) It is thought to result from hypersensitivity of cholinergic receptors
(2) It may resolve when the offending agent is stopped
(3) The dyskinesia will worsen within days of increasing the offending drug
(4) It may be masked by antidopaminergic drugs

199. Tacrine, an anticholinesterase drug, has certain common side effects that limit its use. These are mainly

(1) sleep anomalies
(2) nausea and vomiting
(3) more frequent myasthenic crises than with physostigmine
(4) elevations of transaminase

200. Tricyclic antidepressants may cause which of the following cardiac rhythm disturbances?

(1) Prolonged conduction between the sinus and AV nodes
(2) Flattened T waves
(3) Ventricular arrhythmias
(4) Sinus bradycardia

201. The actions of cocaine include which of the following?

(1) It potentiates sympathetic activity
(2) It blocks reuptake of cat-cholamines at nerve terminals
(3) It blocks nerve impulses with local application
(4) It desensitizes the emesis center in the brain

202. Plasmapheresis is useful in treating

(1) myasthenia gravis
(2) lupus cerebritis
(3) Guillian-Barré syndrome
(4) paraneoplastic peripheral neuro-pathies

203. An elderly man with Parkinson's disease and benign prostatic hypertrophy (BPH) suffers from urinary frequency. A trial of a low-dose anticholinergic drug results in urinary retention. True statements concerning a suggested trial of phenoxybenzamine include

(1) it would also induce urinary retention
(2) it would improve the problem if it were from BPH
(3) it could cause bladder-sphincter dyssynergia leading to renal failure
(4) it would increase frequency if the current problem was primarily due to a parkinsonian "spastic" bladder

204. Medications useful in the treatment of Parkinson's disease include which of the following?

(1) Benztropine
(2) Amantadine
(3) Pergolide
(4) Amitriptyline

205. True statements concerning the use of ergot alkaloids in the treatment of migraine include

(1) excessive use may lead to rebound migraines
(2) excessive use may cause retro-peritoneal fibrosis
(3) they are most useful during the aura
(4) they are useful in prophylaxis

NEUROPHARMACOLOGY

A N S W E R S

169. The answer is C. (Adams RD, 5/e, p 244.) Postganglionic lesions of the sympathetic chain produce denervation supersensitivity of the iris so that the pupil dilates more than normal to a sympathetic stimulus. Since it blocks the reuptake of norepinephrine, cocaine is not helpful in localizing a Horner's syndrome. Atropine will dilate all pupils that respond to cholinergic stimuli. Pilocarpine constricts both pupils. Timolol is a beta blocker that will not alter the pupil size. Hydroxyamphetamine 1% causes a release of sympathetic stores in the neuron innervating the pupil. If the lesion is postganglionic, the nerves to the iris are damaged and will have little or no norepinephrine to release, whereas the norepinephrine supply is normal if the lesion is preganglionic. Hydroxyamphetamine will therefore cause a marked dilatation in a preganglionic Horner's syndrome and little response in a postganglionic lesion.

170. The answer is C. (Lucas, N Engl J Med 333:201–205, 1995.) A double-blind study was performed on pre-eclamptic women to test whether magnesium sulfate or phenytoin was superior in preventing seizures. Ten of 1089 woman treated with phenytoin had seizures, whereas none of the 1049 women treated with magnesium did. This study resolved an old dispute because the use of magnesium had been based on anecdote only and not on data.

171. The answer is B. (Brust, p 91.) Chronic use of cocaine leads to an abstinence syndrome characterized by three phases. The first is a "crash" with depression, fatigue, anxiety, agitation, and drug craving, often associated with paranoia. This is followed by hypersomnolence lasting up to several days with REM rebound and frequent awakening. Phase two is a lengthy period of dysphoria and cocaine craving. In phase three the dysphoria clears but drug craving may continue.

86

172. The answer is D. (Brust, pp 187–188. Hardman, 9/e, pp 442–443.) The combination of delirium, pupillodilatation, dryness of skin and mucous membranes, tachycardia, and fever exhibited by the patient presented in the question suggests cholinergic (muscarinic) blockade, which most commonly would be due to ingestion of atropinelike drugs, including the tricyclic antidepressants. The drug of choice both for therapy and as a diagnostic aid is physostigmine, a potent peripheral and central anticholinesterase. Physostigmine, like many other anticholinesterases, penetrates the blood-brain barrier to counteract the central effects of the cholinergic blocking agents. It must be administered cautiously and the patient monitored in an intensive care unit (ICU) because of the tendency of this drug to cause cardiac arrhythmias and hypotension. Phenothiazines, which have cholinergic blocking action, would only worsen the patient's condition. Phenobarbital would further impair the patient's sensorium. A preferable anticonvulsant would be diazepam. Edrophonium would have muscarinic and cholinergic effects peripherally, but not centrally, and would act for too short a period of time. Metocurine iodide (Metubine) would block the nicotinic action of acetylcholine on skeletal muscle (which would not prove beneficial), and thiamine would be ineffective, although not harmful.

173. The answer is D. (Hardman, 9/e, pp 332–333.) Local anesthetics such as procaine appear to act by blocking the voltage-dependent transient rise in membrane permeability to sodium that accompanies the nerve impulse. As sodium exits from the cell during passage of the nerve impulse, the membrane shows an increasing conductance to sodium that is voltage-dependent. The anesthetic agent binds within the sodium channel in such a way as to block the inward flow of sodium with the passage of the impulse. The action appears to take place on the inner surface of the neuron membrane and raises the threshold for neuronal excitability. At higher concentrations potassium channels are also blocked.

174. The answer is A. (Bodner, Neurology 45:219–223, 1995.) The "serotonin syndrome" was first described in patients taking L-tryptophan and nonspecific monoamine oxidase (MAO) inhibitors for depression. Serotonin is metabolized via MAO-A; dopamine is metabolized via MAO-B. Several case reports have documented the occurrence of this syndrome with a variety of drugs, including the selective serotonin reuptake inhibitors (SSRI). The syndrome resembles the neuroleptic malignant syndrome (NMS) in that both generally consist of rigidity, altered mentation, and tremors. Myoclonus is seen with the serotonin syndrome, whereas very high fevers and CPK elevations are more likely with NMS. The serotonin syndrome resolves within several hours and is treated with hydration alone to prevent renal failure in case of myoglobinuria, whereas the NMS lasts much longer. There is some controversy over treatment of NMS, but most clinicians favor a dopamine agonist, such as bromocriptine. In cases where patients are taking an MAO inhibitor, an SSRI, and a neuroleptic, distinguishing the two diagnoses may be impossible.

175. The answer is A. (Jankovic, N Engl J Med 324:1186–1194, 1991.) Botulinum toxin A (Botox) is one of seven toxins produced by *Clostridium botulinum*. It produces weakness by blocking nerve release of acetylcholine and thus providing functional motor denervation of the injected muscles. It has proved extremely effective in the treatment of hemifacial spasm and blepharospasm and has been approved by the FDA for use in these conditions as well as for the treatment of strabismus. While Botox is also effective in other forms of dystonia and is recommended as the drug of first choice for torticollis, it has not yet been approved for use in these other conditions (as of 1996).

176. The answer is D. (Hardman, 9/e, pp 122–123.) *Tachyphylaxis* refers to the decreasing effect of repeated doses or repeated infusions of a drug. The usual explanation is that those drugs displaying tachyphylaxis act indirectly by releasing some of the natural neurotransmitter stored at the presynaptic nerve endings. Because only a limited amount of neurotransmitter is available for release, the repeated administration of the drug fails to produce any further release. The amount available for release by the drug is judged to be quite small because nerve stimulation will produce the expected response even though repeated drug administration becomes ineffective. The administration of the appropriate sympathomimetic drug also will elicit the response, which shows that the receptors remain functional.

177. The answer is A. (The European Atrial Fibrillation Trial Study Group, N Engl J Med 333:5–10, 1995.) There is a much lower incidence of stroke with nonrheumatic than rheumatic atrial fibrillation, and recent studies have addressed the question as to whether anticoagulation was worth the risk of the bleeding complications that always accompany use of warfarin. The European Atrial Fibrillation Trial Study Group found that an INR of 2.0 to 3.9 for the prothrombin time was most beneficial. They found no benefit below 2.0 and increased bleeding problems above 3.9. This group recommends an INR of about 3.0.

178. The answer is C. (Hardman, 9/e, p 391.) Disulfiram by itself is a relatively innocuous drug. It interferes with aldehyde dehydrogenase, an enzyme that oxidizes acetaldehyde. Since ethanol is oxidized to acetaldehyde by the liver's alcohol dehydrogenase, ingestion of as little as 7 mL of alcohol leads to a buildup of acetaldehyde, causing an "acetaldehyde syndrome." This unpleasant syndrome develops within 5 to 10 min and lasts 30 min to several hours. The person feels hot, flushes all over, and develops a throbbing headache, dyspnea, vomiting, hypotension, vertigo, blurred vision, and confusion. The same syndrome will occur if intravenous acetaldehyde is given.

179. The answer is E. (McLean, Neurology 44 (suppl. 5):S17–S22, 1994.) Gabapentin does not alter the pharmacokinetics of carbamazepine, phenytoin, phenobarbital, or valproic acid. In addition, it does not induce liver metabolism and, in small studies, it has been shown not to impair oral contraceptives. Gabapentin absorption can be reduced, however, by concomitant use of some antacids (magnesium hydroxide [Maalox TC]) and gastric acid inhibitors. Gabapentin's lack of effect on the four primary anticonvulsants listed above is not shared by the other new anticonvulsants, felbamate and lamotrigine, both of which have effects on these other, older anticonvulsants.

180. The answer is B. (Hardman, 9/e, p 188.) Malignant hyperthermia (MH) is distinguished clinically from malignant neuroleptic syndrome by its pharmacologic characteristics. MH is often familial, although this history is often lacking because family members with the predisposition may not have been exposed. It is precipitated by halothane, succinylcholine, and occasionally other general anesthetics or neuromuscular blockers. It is treated with dantrolene sodium, ventilation, and careful attention to acidosis from muscle contraction and renal function, which can be damaged by the myoglobin released from damaged muscles. MH may not occur on first exposure to the anesthetic.

181. The answer is A. (Hardman, 9/e, p 1158.) Isoniazid (INH), the single most important antituberculous drug, has a potent effect against vitamin B_6. It inhibits formation of the coenzyme form of the vitamin. Pyridoxine is one of three forms of vitamin B_6, the others being pyridoxal and pyridoxamine. Deficiency of vitamin B_6 may cause seizures in neonates. In adults the most common neurologic problem is a sensory neuropathy, a common problem with INH. INH is frequently given with pyridoxine supplements to prevent this.

182. The answer is A. (Hardman, 9/e, p 1089.) Although penicillin is generally a very benign drug in people who are not allergic to it, problems may occur in two unrelated settings. Intravenously administered penicillin G is mainly excreted by the kidney so that renal failure leads to toxicity if doses are not chosen judiciously. CNS toxicity produces confusion, lethargy, focal or generalized seizures, or multifocal myoclonus (recall that penicillin is used as a convulsant in animals by applying it directly to the cortex). Procaine penicillin, given intramuscularly in a large dose, may cause rapid liberation of the procaine, leading to an immediate reaction of headaches, tinnitus, hallucinations, and occasionally seizures.

183. The answer is B. (Adams RD, 5/e, p 1321.) The appearance of diarrhea, ataxia, fasciculations, overactive muscle stretch reflexes, and seizures in a patient who has been started on lithium therapy is entirely compatible with lithium toxicity. Since the usual therapeutic range for lithium is between 0.8 and 1.2 meq/L, the observed value of 1.5 meq/L would support a diagnosis of lithium toxicity. Moreover, since the patient recently began treatment, this blood level probably represents a fairly rapid climb of the lithium level. Such sudden changes are more likely to cause symptoms than very gradual changes. To invoke a coexistent disorder in this patient would violate the principle of diagnostic parsimony. Many of the symptoms of lithium overdosage imitate other states like delirium tremens, barbiturate withdrawal, or a thyroid storm—all of which may be associated with signs of overactivity of the nervous system in the form of tremors, increased stretch reflexes, and seizures. A thyroid crisis would be unlikely in this patient because the effect of lithium is to reduce thyroid function.

184. The answer is C. (Langston, Adv Neurol 9:485–507, 1986.) MPTP was discovered by an unfortunate accident followed by diligent detective work. It is a synthetic drug derived from meperidine and was sold to intravenous narcotics abusers without knowledge of its neurotoxicity. MPTP destroys nigral dopaminergic neurons in animals and had the same effect in the one human autopsied. In older animals it affects the locus ceruleus, a noradrenergic set of neurons, as well. The drug is itself nontoxic but is taken into glial cells where it is metabolized to MPP+. This then exits the glial cell and poisons the nigral neurons. MAO-B is required in this toxification process. Blocking MAO-B with inhibitors such as pargyline or deprenyl prevents MPTP from becoming toxic.

185. The answer is A. (Cooper, 7/e, p 308.) Usually, when a neuronal pathway ceases to function or becomes less active, the synthesis and metabolism of the neurotransmitter are reduced accordingly. The nigrostriatal dopaminergic pathway seems to be anomalous in this regard. When impulse flow in this pathway is interrupted by mechanical or pharmacologic lesions, the amount of dopamine in the axonal terminals in the striatum increases, and the activity of the rate-limiting enzyme tyrosine hydroxylase also increases. Just how this increased enzyme activity occurs is unclear. Similar increases in the activity of tyrosine hydroxylase fail to occur in central norepinephrinergic pathways when they are quiescent. In fact, the norepinephrinergic pathways respond in the opposite way.

186. The answer is D. (Adams RD, 5/e, p 282.) Infantile spasms are more likely to respond to ACTH (20 to 40 units daily) than to standard anticonvulsants. Drugs useful in myoclonus, such as clonazepam and valproic acid, may also be helpful. The ketogenic diet is another important approach to therapy.

187. The answer is B. (Plum, 3/e, pp 243–245.) Glutethimide intoxication can produce an unusual neurologic picture including midposition pupils that may be unreactive and unequal. Overwhelmingly high doses of barbiturates may also produce unreactive pupils but this is very uncommon. Glutethimide also produces a prolonged and fluctuating level of coma. Persistent noxious stimulation may transiently increase the patient's level of consciousness or responsiveness. The fixed and unequal pupils that may occur in glutethimide poisoning may mislead the examiner into diagnosing a structural lesion in the midbrain as the etiology of the coma.

188. The answer is A. (Parkinson Study Group, N Engl J Med 321:1364–1371, 1989.) Deprenyl (selegiline; Eldepryl) is a nonreversible inhibitor of the enzyme MAO-B. There are two forms of MAO. The A form is found in the gut and is important in metabolizing tyramine. Blockade of the A form, which occurs with the MAO-inhibiting antidepressants, subjects patients to tyramine-induced hypertensive crises. Blockade of the B form occurs in the brain and is quite safe. The DATATOP study, which followed 800 patients with Parkinson's disease, half treated and half not, showed that deprenyl slows progression of disability in Parkinson's disease without producing a significant symptomatic improvement in motor function, depression, or intellectual or memory function. It is not known, however, if the drug actually slows disease progression.

189. The answer is C. (Hardman, 9/e, p 470.) The pharmacokinetics of phenytoin must be understood to use the drug properly. It has a plasma half-life of 6 to 24 h in the subtherapeutic range, which is due to first-order (exponential) elimination characteristics. Above about 10 mg/mL, the elimination becomes dose-dependent, so that half-life increases with the plasma concentration. Most of the drug is bound to albumin and the rest is free. The free fraction equilibrates with the brain level of the drug so that the free drug level is a more accurate indicator of therapeutic range than is the total plasma concentration. When increasing doses in a patient, one must be careful of the increasing half-life to avoid toxicity.

190. The answer is D. (Hardman, 9/e, p 542.) Meperidine may cause respiratory depression or severe agitation with delirium, seizures, and high fevers when used in combination with an MAO antidepressant. This reaction is associated with the MAO-inhibiting drugs that block both forms of MAO and has yet to be associated with deprenyl, a drug that blocks only the B form of MAO. The interaction of meperidine and MAO inhibitors is potentially lethal. Interestingly, the same interaction has not been noted with other opiates.

191. The answer is D. (Adams RD, 5/e, pp 911–912.) Some chronic alcoholics develop a syndrome of auditory hallucinosis. The sounds are usually voices that say bad things about the subject. Initially the voices are thought to be real, and the subject behaves appropriately for that delusion. Generally the hallucinations resolve and the subject returns to normal, but occasionally alcoholics develop a chronic state in which they continue to suffer from the auditory hallucinations. In general the subject then is able to separate the false sounds from the real.

192. The answer is E. (Samuels, pp 633–637.) Levodopa has a large number of adverse behavioral effects, including confusion, delusions, paranoia, depression, mania, and psychoses. One of the more common psychiatric side effects is a syndrome of visual hallucinations, usually involving nonthreatening people, often children, who visit. These visions never make any sounds and are often perceived as illusions after a very brief period. Recognition of their illusory nature, however, does not prevent their recurrence. This is partly a dose-related phenomenon and is often due to the concomitant use of other antiparkinson drugs as well. Ethanol causes visual hallucinations only in the context of delirium tremens. Amphetamine may induce a schizophrenic-like psychosis, but hallucinations occur in an altered mental state. Methanol and cocaine do not cause visual hallucinations.

193. The answer is A. (Hardman, 9/e, pp 1246–1247.) The combination of altered mentation, multifocal lower motor neuron abnormalities, and a lymphocytic pleocytosis is classic for carcinomatous meningitis. The lack of malignant cells in the CSF is not uncommon and repeated studies may be required to identify the cancerous cells. The only medication of any use in treating this condition is intrathecal methotrexate, which may cause a chemical meningitis and increases the risk of white matter degeneration with radiation.

194. The answer is C (2, 4). (Hardman, 9/e, p 1481.) Steroids have been shown to be effective in reducing vasogenic edema, that is, the brain edema caused by abnormally permeable blood vessels. This condition occurs with inflammation around abscesses and also around neoplasms. Steroids have no demonstrated efficacy in brain swelling caused by cytotoxic edema, which is caused by cell swelling and cell death. They have been studied in both stroke and trauma without the demonstration of benefit. This is in contrast, however, to a recent study that shows significant benefit in the early use of large steroid boluses following severe injury to the spinal cord.

195. The answer is C (2, 4). (Adams RD, 5/e, pp 547–549.) Pseudotumor cerebri, by definition, is a syndrome due to increased intracranial pressure without apparent cause. Its clinical presentation typically is progressive headache or blurred vision and dizziness. It generally occurs in obese, young women. The elevated intracranial pressure results in papilledema, which, if severe and chronic, may lead to progressive visual loss. Sixth nerve palsies may also occur. While the syndrome has been occasionally associated with steroid withdrawal and various endocrine abnormalities, there is a clear association with excessive doses of vitamin A and tetracycline.

196. The answer is D (4). (Cooper, 7/e, pp 231–234.) Tyrosine hydroxylase converts tyrosine to dihydroxyphenylalanine on its way to norepinephrine and epinephrine. The activity of tyrosine hydroxylase undergoes a homeostatic adjustment to the need for catecholaminergic neurotransmitter, but pharmacologic manipulation can also alter its activity. Increased neuronal activity requires more neurotransmitter and activates or increases the action of the synthetic enzymes like tyrosine hydroxylase that produce the transmitter. Administration of an MAO inhibitor will increase the amount of intraneuronal catecholamine, resulting in a feedback inhibition of tyrosine hydroxylase. Administration of tyramine increases the amount of intracellular catecholamine and also produces a feedback inhibition of catecholamine synthesis. Administration of 6-hydroxydopamine selectively kills catecholaminergic neurons and thus results in an absence of their contained enzymes, including tyrosine hydroxylase. Many drugs, like α-methyl-ρ-tyrosine and other amino acid analogues, will inhibit tyrosine hydroxylase, and some may find clinical application for that reason.

197. The answer is B (1, 3). (Adams RD, 5/e, p 276.) Petit mal seizures respond equally well to valproic acid and ethosuximide. These seizures do not respond to antiepileptic drugs useful in other forms of epilepsy such as phenytoin, phenobarbital, and carbamazepine. When petit mal seizures are also associated with tonic clonic activity, then valproic acid is the drug of choice because it is effective in both seizure types.

198. The answer is C (2, 4). (Rowland, 9/e, pp 733–736.) Tardive dyskinesia (TD) is thought to be related to dopamine receptor supersensitivity that occurs as a result of chronic receptor blockade. This occurs with typical antipsychotic drugs as well as antiemetics such as prochlorperazine (Compazine) and gastric motility enhancers such as metoclopramide (Reglan). TD can be masked by increasing the dopamine blockade or by depleting dopamine (with drugs such as reserpine). Anticholinergics will often worsen TD. A general rule is that drugs that improve parkinsonism worsen TD (such as anticholinergics) and drugs that worsen parkinsonism improve the signs of TD (such as antipsychotics).

199. The answer is C (2,4). (Kaplan, Comprehensive Textbook, 7/e, p 985. Winker, JAMA 271:1023–1024, 1994.) Tacrine was approved by the FDA for symptomatic treatment of memory dysfunction in mildly to moderately demented patients with Alzheimer's disease. Not all patients respond and 50 percent develop elevations of transaminase. About 25 percent of patients receiving 160 mg/d develop values above three times the upper limits of normal. These elevations are asymptomatic and values decline to normal upon discontinuation of the drug. Ninety-five percent of the laboratory abnormalities occur in the first 18 weeks of drug use. Cholinergic problems of nausea, vomiting, and diarrhea are also common causes of drug intolerance.

200. The answer is A (1, 2, 3). (Hardman, 9/e, p 439.) The tricyclic antidepressants inhibit norepinephrine uptake and block muscarinic receptors; both actions produce a sinus tachycardia. The drugs also slow conduction velocity throughout the heart and flatten or invert T waves. Ventricular arrhythmias, particularly in the presence of conduction blocks, are the most serious side effects of these drugs.

201. The answer is A (1, 2, 3). (Hardman, 9/e, p 338.) Cocaine has systemic activity that is due to its blockade of the catecholamine reuptake mechanism. It thus acts to increase the activity of the sympathetic autonomic system, with such effects as increased heart rate and blood pressure and mydriasis. When applied locally it inhibits initiation and conduction of nerve impulses, thus accounting for its properties as a local anesthetic. Its main therapeutic uses are as an anesthetic in the eye and the nasal and sinus passages. It does not inhibit the vomit center and actually induces emesis in some.

202. The answer is B (1, 3). (Adams RD, 5/e, pp 1129, 1261.) Plasmapheresis is a process in which plasma is exchanged for albumin. In two separate studies, plasmapheresis has been shown to be helpful in treating Guillain-Barré syndrome if instituted within 2 weeks of onset of the disease. It is recommended for patients with respiratory or gait failure. Plasmapheresis has been used effectively in treating myasthenia gravis for several years; however, its role is less well defined in this very unpredictable disease. Although it is thought to act by reducing concentrations of a toxic substance, improvement in myasthenia does not parallel changes in anti-acetylcholine-receptor antibody.

203. The answer is C (2, 4). (Hardman, 9/e, p 228.) Phenoxybenzamine is an adrenergic antagonist that blocks alpha receptors in smooth muscle. Since trigone and sphincter muscles in the base of the bladder are sympathetically innervated, blocking the alpha receptors leads to relaxation of the sphincter. In the patient described, there may be increased bladder contractions from the Parkinson's disease as well as excess outflow pressure. The anticholinergic was given to decrease the bladder contractions but without benefit. The next approach would be to reduce outflow resistance with phenoxybenzamine. This drug is used to treat obstruction caused by BPH.

204. The answer is E (all). (Rowland, 9/e, p 772.) Although the mainstay of therapy for Parkinson's disease (PD) is levodopa, other agents are often useful adjuncts. Anticholinergics such as benztropine are helpful with tremor and rigidity. Amantadine appears to have an effect on increasing dopamine release. Dopamine agonists such as bromocriptine and pergolide act directly on the striatum and bypass the degenerated nigral neurons. Tricyclic antidepressants are often useful, especially amitriptyline, because of the antidepressant (depression is a common PD problem), anticholinergic, and soporific effects (sleep disturbance is also common in PD).

205. The answer is B (1, 3). (Hardman, 9/e, pp 491–496.) Ergot alkaloids are effective in the treatment of individual migraine attacks, particularly when used very early in the episode. They are especially useful during the aura. The mechanism of action is still not clear, although ergot alkaloids had been previously thought to act via vasoconstriction. They are not sedating and are not analgesic; hence the antimigraine properties are quite specific. Long-term or excessive use leads to an increasing requirement for benefit and to rebound migraines on withdrawal. Thus, they are not useful for prophylaxis. Unlike methysergide, ergots do not cause connective tissue problems.

NEURORADIOLOGY

Directions: Each item below contains five suggested responses. Select the **one best** response to each item.

206. In the radiograph below, the most likely interpretation is

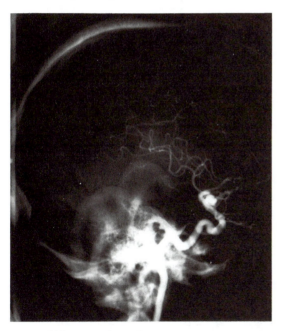

(A) normal angiogram
(B) hydrocephalus
(C) avascular anterior mass
(D) anterior cerebral aneurysm
(E) upward displacement of the first segment of the anterior cerebral artery

207. An AIDS patient has two intracranial masses, which enhance with contrast on CT scanning and have edema around them. The most appropriate treatment is

(A) oral pyrimethamine initially with sulfadiazine added 6 weeks later
(B) dexamethasone plus radiation therapy
(C) praziquantel plus dexamethasone
(D) zidovudine (AZT) plus pyrimethamine
(E) none of the above

208. The single most sensitive test for the demonstration of abnormalities associated with multiple sclerosis is

(A) spinal fluid analysis
(B) evoked response testing (all modalities combined)
(C) CT of the brain with a double dose of contrast and 4-h delayed scan
(D) MRI of the brain with and without enhancement
(E) positron emission tomography (PET) scan

209. The following brain CT scans (left is unenhanced, right enhanced) of a middle-aged man from central Africa is most consistent with which of the following?

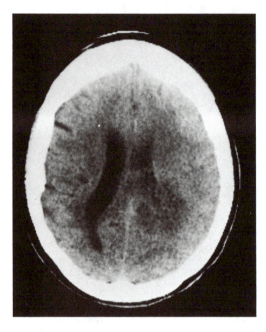 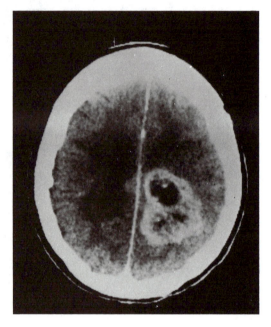

(A) Glioblastoma
(B) Tuberculoma
(C) Cysticercosis
(D) *Echinococcus* infection
(E) Lymphoma

210. A 30-year-old man with chronic pain and a neurogenic bladder had the MRI shown below. The diagnosis is

(A) tethered cord syndrome
(B) herniated disk
(C) spinal stenosis
(D) cord tumor
(E) cauda equina tumor

211. The CT scan of a teen-aged child below indicates which of the following disorders?

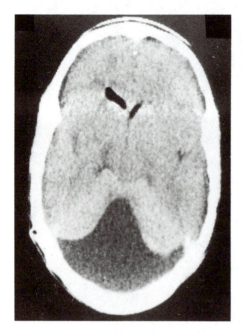

(A) Arnold-Chiari malformation
(B) Cystic astrocytoma
(C) Dandy-Walker syndrome
(D) Lissencephaly (agyria)
(E) Enlarged cisterna magna

212. The following unenhanced CT scan in a 54-year-old patient would be consistent with which of the following metabolic derangements?

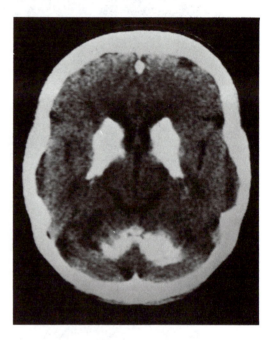

(A) Low serum calcium
(B) Elevated serum calcium
(C) Low serum copper
(D) High serum ceruloplasmin
(E) Cyanide intoxication

213. A 50-year-old single woman was brought to the doctor by her sister because of progressive depression and social isolation. Little was known about the patient, who had lived independently in another city. There were no known medical or psychiatric illnesses in the patient or her family. She had been self-supporting and was not known to abuse drugs. Examination revealed a woman who appeared depressed, followed some commands but not most, and occasionally answered questions, but mostly appeared self-absorbed and disinterested in events around her. Aside from her mental state, findings were normal. Her brain MRI scan (shown below), showing the T2-weighted sequence enhancement as the only abnormality, points to which diagnosis as the most likely? (Gadolinium did not produce enhancement.)

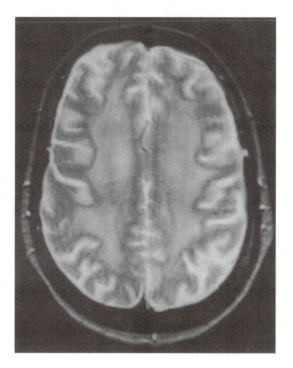

(A) Multiple sclerosis
(B) HIV encephalopathy
(C) Progressive multifocal leukoencephalopathy
(D) Adrenoleukodystrophy
(E) Psychiatric disorder (normal brain MRI)

214. A 45-year-old man was admitted to the hospital with fever and shoulder pain. Joint fluid contained *Staphylococcus aureus*. While on antibiotic treatment, he complained of numbness in both legs and unsteadiness in walking. Examination revealed mild punch tenderness over the spine at about T6, mild proximal leg weakness, and substantial residual urine after voiding. His emergency MRI (gadolinium-enhanced T1) is seen below. The next step in treatment should be

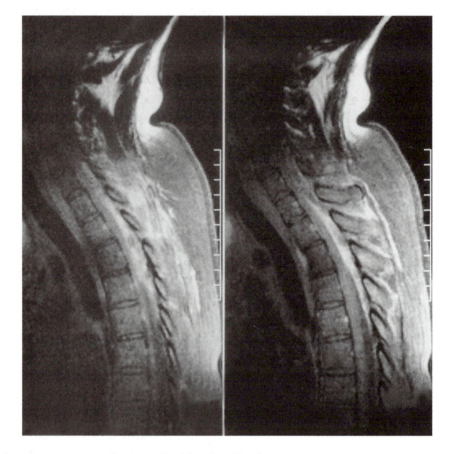

(A) percutaneous aspiration of epidural collection
(B) percutaneous biopsy of epidural mass
(C) addition of two antistaphylococcal antibiotics with good CSF penetrance
(D) emergency decompression of spine
(E) intravenous dexamethasone and emergency radiation followed by biopsy

215. The brain MRI scans below are from a 35-year-old man who has had seizures since childhood. He has mild right-sided weakness and a borderline low IQ. The most likely explanation for this lesion is

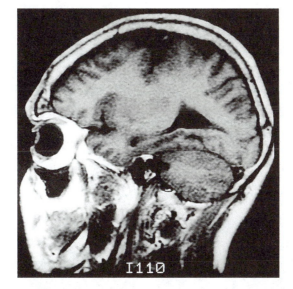

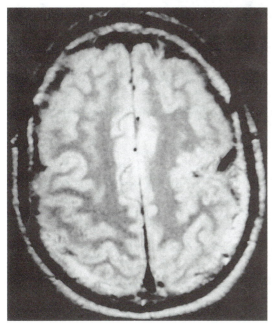
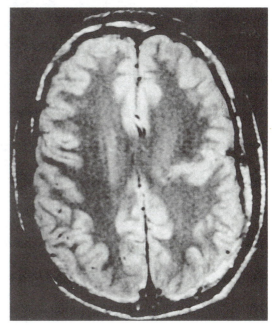

(A) herpes simplex encephalitis
(B) old contusion
(C) epilepsy surgery
(D) developmental anomaly
(E) normal variant

216. A patient with back pain has the MRI shown below. What neurologic problem is likely?

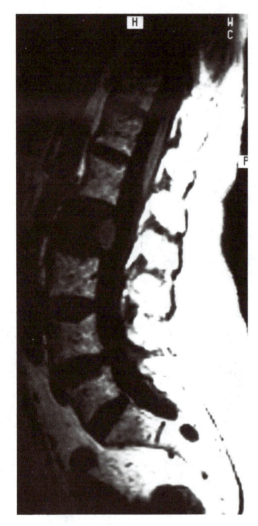

(A) Urinary incontinence
(B) Urinary retention
(C) Proximal leg weakness
(D) Distal leg weakness
(E) Paraplegia

217. In the radiograph below, the patient most likely suffers from

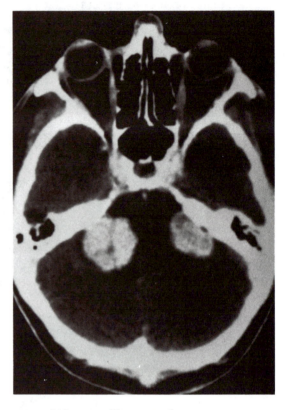

(A) neurofibromatosis
(B) tuberous sclerosis
(C) Paget's disease
(D) polycystic kidney disease
(E) Hand-Schüller-Christian disease

218. The most sensitive test for diagnosing the presence of subarachnoid blood following rupture of a berry aneurysm is

(A) CT scan without contrast
(B) CT scan with contrast
(C) spinal tap
(D) MRI of brain without contrast
(E) MRI of brain with contrast

219. In the radiograph below, the most likely diagnosis is

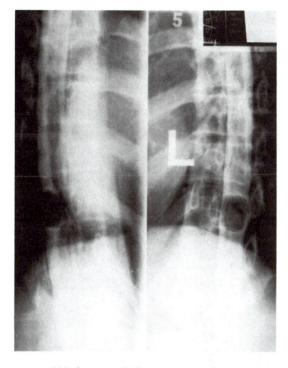

(A) intramedullary metastasis
(B) epidural hematoma
(C) astrocytoma
(D) disk herniation
(E) meningioma

220. In the unenhanced CT scan below, the most likely diagnosis is

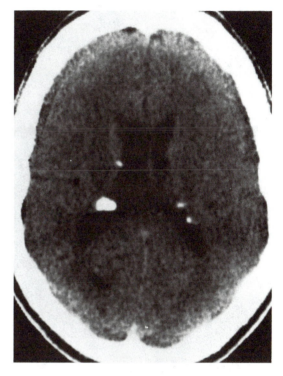

(A) metastatic disease
(B) polycystic kidney disease
(C) hypoparathyroidism
(D) tuberculosis
(E) tuberous sclerosis

221. In the radiograph below, the most likely diagnosis is

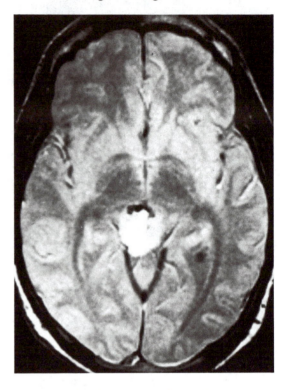

(A) middle cerebral artery infarct
(B) head trauma
(C) cysticercosis
(D) herpes simplex encephalitis
(E) Creutzfeldt-Jakob disease

222. A patient who has the MRI below is most likely to have which of the following neurologic abnormalities?

(A) Light-near pupillary dissociation and upgaze paresis
(B) Gait ataxia
(C) Bitemporal field cuts
(D) Binasal field cuts
(E) Alien hand syndrome

223. In the CT scans below, the left is unenhanced and the right is enhanced. The most likely diagnosis is

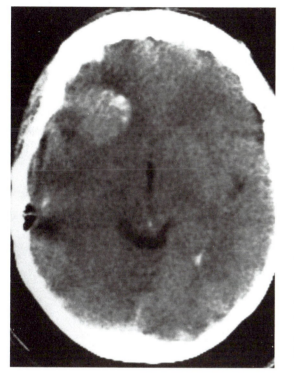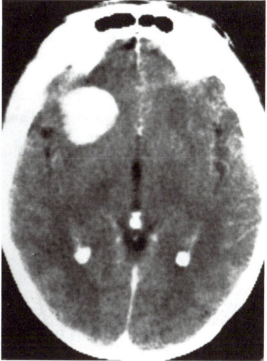

(A) abscess
(B) mycotic aneurysm
(C) glioma
(D) metastatic melanoma
(E) orbital roof meningioma

224. A patient with AIDS has the MRI below. All the following are diagnostic considerations EXCEPT

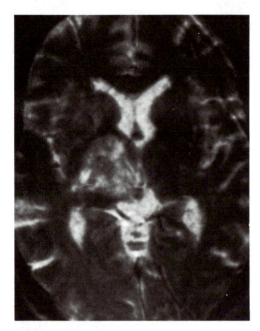

(A) lymphoma
(B) Kaposi's sarcoma
(C) toxoplasmosis
(D) progressive multifocal leuko-encephalopathy (PML)
(E) tuberculosis

225. A child develops premature closing of the sagittal suture. Which one of the following statements most accurately describes the resulting skull deformity?

(A) The whole head would be small (microcephaly)
(B) Diffuse enlargement due to secondary hydrocephalus would occur (macrocephaly)
(C) The head would be pointed (oxycephaly)
(D) The head would be wide and fore-shortened (brachycephaly)
(E) The head would be long and narrow (scaphocephaly)

226. An isolated tumor growing from the clivus would most likely be

(A) eosinophilic granuloma
(B) osteosarcoma
(C) chordoma
(D) osteoma
(E) Wegener's granulomatosis

227. Fibromuscular dysplasia is a disease primarily of renal arteries that may also affect the cerebral arteries. The most common cerebrovascular angiographic abnormality is

(A) aneurysm of the circle of Willis
(B) stenosis of the carotid bifurcation
(C) malformation of the vein of Galen
(D) "string of beads" sign in the vertebral arteries
(E) "string of beads" sign in an internal carotid artery

Directions: Each item below contains four suggested responses of which **one or more** is correct. Select:

A	if	**1, 2, and 3**	are correct
B	if	**1 and 3**	are correct
C	if	**2 and 4**	are correct
D	if	**4**	is correct
E	if	**1, 2, 3, and 4**	are correct

228. In the first 24 h of an ischemic stroke, which of the following imaging studies would be likely to reveal an abnormality?

(1) CT with and without contrast
(2) T1 MRI
(3) CT with double-dose contrast after 1 h
(4) T2 MRI

229. A 6-year-old American child develops headaches and ataxia. The CT scans with and without contrast are shown below. Other sections show no other abnormalities. The likely diagnoses include which of the following?

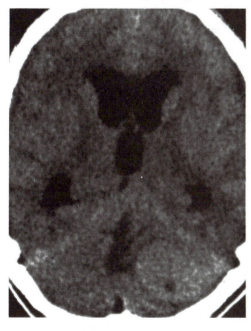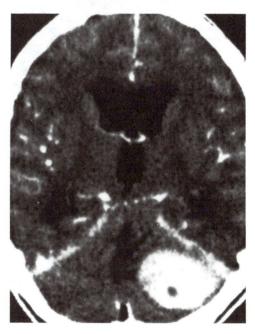

(1) Medulloblastoma
(2) Meningioma
(3) Astrocytoma
(4) Metastatic tumor

Directions: Each group of questions below consists of lettered options followed by a set of numbered items. For each numbered item, select the **one** lettered option with which it is **most** closely associated. Each lettered option may be used **once, more than once, or not at all.**

Items 230–233

Match the structures with the appropriate letter labels on this coronal section through a normal brain. Answer "(E) None of the above" if none of the labels apply.

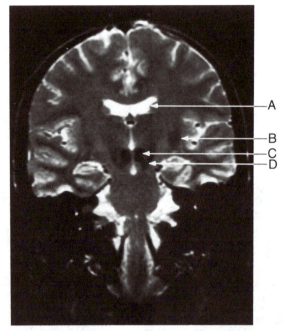

Adapted from Fischer and Ketonen, Fig. 2-43, with permission.

230. Head of caudate nucleus

231. Globus pallidus

232. Substantia nigra

233. Red nucleus

Items 234–238

For each cranial nerve listed below, choose the skull aperture through which it passes.

    (A) Foramen magnum
    (B) Superior orbital fissure
    (C) Jugular foramen
    (D) Stylomastoid foramen
    (E) Foramen lacerum

234. Xth cranial nerve

235. IIIrd cranial nerve

236. Ophthalmic division of the Vth cranial nerve

237. VIth cranial nerve

238. IXth cranial nerve

NEURORADIOLOGY

A N S W E R S

206. The answer is D. (Osborn, pp 257–266.) This angiogram shows an outpouching at the junction of the anterior cerebral and anterior communicating arteries. On a single projection, the exact location is difficult to identify, but the balloon-shaped structure is evident. In general it is important to have multiple views, both to identify the existence of the aneurysm and to localize its neck. The most common location for aneurysms is at the junction of these two vessels.

207. The answer is A. (Simpson, Ann Intern Med 121:769–785, 1994.) Since toxoplasmosis is the most common intracranial mass lesion in AIDS patients, the current approach to therapy is to treat even without proof of the diagnosis by biopsy. The treatment of choice is to load with oral pyrimethamine, 50 to 200 mg/d, followed by maintenance doses of 25 to 75 mg/d. Sulfadiazine, 4 to 8 g/d, is added 2 to 6 weeks later. If imaging or clinical assessment fails to show improvement within 1 to 2 weeks, a re-evaluation for an alternative diagnosis should be done.

208. The answer is D. (Osborn, p 757.) MRI of the brain is the most sensitive test for identifying abnormalities in multiple sclerosis. There are several problems, however, associated with the use of MRI. The findings can be nonspecific and may be difficult to distinguish from ischemic disease. Some patients with clinically definite multiple sclerosis have normal brain studies, either due to confinement of the disease to the spinal cord or to a certain degree of test insensitivity. Finally, there is little correlation between the lesions seen on MRI and the neurologic examination or prognosis. Gadolinium enhancement indicates a new plaque, hence active disease.

209. The answer is A. (Osborn, pp 541–543.) While a central African man must be considered at high risk for parasitic infections of the brain such as cysticercosis and infection with *Echinococcus*, tuberculomas, and AIDS-related diseases, this CT is most consistent with a diagnosis of glioblastoma. These tumors usually are hypodense on the unenhanced CT and usually, but not always, enhance with contrast. Unlike metastases and abscesses such as those of TB, they often have an irregular shape and are almost always solitary. CNS lymphoma is typically periventricular in location and generally enhances diffusely. The two parasitic infections usually show multiple, round cysts on CT; cysticercosis also often has a central calcified region corresponding to the scolex of the worm.

210. The answer is A. (Osborn, pp 807–808.) A tethered cord is a congenital abnormality that usually causes back pain, scoliosis, and bladder and bowel dysfunction and is frequently associated with other spine and spinal cord anomalies, such as lipoma or myelomeningocele. The conus medullaris often appears elongated and the distinction between the conus and the filum terminale is blurred. Because the cord is pulled down, some roots may travel upward instead of down.

211. The answer is C. (Adams RD, 5/e, p 1020.) The Dandy-Walker syndrome is caused by a developmental aberration in which the midline cerebellum fails to develop normally. This causes a huge cyst in place of the fourth ventricle. Other abnormalities of midline structures occur, including enlargement of the other ventricles and anomalies of the corpus callosum. The four Arnold-Chiari malformations are tonsillar herniation of the cerebellum, downward displacement of the medulla and fourth ventricle into the cervical canal, cervical meningomyelocele with cerebellar herniation, and cerebellar hypoplasia. Lissencephaly (agyria, or "smooth brain") refers to a small brain without sulci and gyri. An astrocytoma, although typically in the posterior fossa in a child, has a round shape and should show a rim of solid tissue. Similarly, an enlarged cisterna magna would not produce a midline indentation in a pattern similar to that of the fourth ventricle.

212. The answer is A. (Adams RD, 5/e, p 895.) Hypoparathyroidism results in low levels of serum calcium. In about half of cases there is deposition of calcium in the small blood vessels of the basal ganglia and the dentate nuclei of the cerebellum. While calcifications in these areas may occur on an idiopathic basis without deranged calcium metabolism, the occurrence of this type of CT scan abnormality in the setting of dementia, parkinsonism, chorea, or seizures should raise suspicion of hypoparathyroidism. Low serum calcium and parathormone levels confirm the diagnosis. Hyperparathyroidism with elevated calcium and Wilson's disease with low serum copper levels do not alter the brain CT scan. Cyanide poisoning on rare occasions has been reported to induce infarcts of the basal ganglia and a parkinsonian syndrome but does not cause calcifications.

213. The answer is B. (Osborn, pp 696–698.) This MRI shows T2 enhancement of virtually the entire white matter of both hemispheres. PML and MS are much more likely to show patchy demyelination and to be less symmetric. Although there is often a wide discrepancy between demyelinated lesions on MRI and the clinical picture, one would expect some physical signs. Adrenoleukodystrophy is a disorder of males. This patient was admitted to the hospital shortly after her initial medical encounter, before the brain MRI could be performed, with infection by *Pneumocystis carinii*. HIV testing was positive.

214. The answer is D. (Adams RD, 5/e, pp 1087–1089. Osborn, pp 824–825.) The diagnosis is epidural abscess. The scenario described is not uncommon as these abscesses may arise from hematogenous spread as well as from extension of a vertebral osteomyelitis. MRI revealed a soft tissue mass that frequently covers several spinal levels. The lesion is hypointense to spinal cord on T1 and hyperintense on proton density and T2; it may enhance diffusely or heterogenously with gadolinium or may reveal rim enhancement. The treatment of choice is emergency evacuation of the purulent material because the abscess can expand rapidly and unpredictably, potentially causing irreversible cord damage.

215. The answer is D. (Miller, Neurology 34:997–1001, 1984. Osborn, pp 52–55.) These MRI scans show a cleft in the hemisphere, with cortex lining the cavity. The smooth contour and the cortical lining indicate this must have been a developmental problem since injuries to the brain after birth would not cause cortex to line a cavity. This developmental disorder is called schizencephaly ("split brain"). It is uncertain if it is due to a vascular accident in the developing hemisphere or whether there is a problem in neuronal migration. In this case, the cleft is closed (type I). More commonly, the cleft is open (type II).

216. The answer is C. (Osborn, p 893.) The MRI shows severe destruction of the L2 vertebral body caused by multiple myeloma. The level of the lesion is below the caudal end of the spinal cord in most patients and in this particular case the cord's tip can be seen ending at the level of L1. Therefore one should not expect a cauda equina syndrome with urinary incontinence due to bladder atonicity, but rather a syndrome of root compression of L2 or L3. The patient is therefore most likely to have weakness in hip and quadriceps muscles and a diminished knee jerk.

217. The answer is A. (Osborn p 87.) The CT scan shows two large masses that emanate from the internal auditory canal. The differential diagnosis of the lesions would include meningiomas, metastatic tumors, and giant aneurysms. However, the symmetry of their location would argue strongly for an underlying illness such as neurofibromatosis type 2, which has a marked increased incidence of bilateral acoustic neuromas. This has been linked to a gene abnormality on chromosome 22. Patients would present with progressive deafness.

218. The answer is C. (Rowland, 9/e, p 277.) The diagnosis of subarachnoid hemorrhage is one of the few areas in which MRI is not of significant value. The CT scan without contrast is clearly a better test and is the first diagnostic test that should be performed. It confirms the diagnosis in most cases, showing blood outside the brain, but it is also sensitive to the presence of blood in the ventricles and parenchyma. Occasionally it will reveal the aneurysm as well. The CT scan is helpful in predicting vasospasm, as the location and size of the blood clot is useful for this. However, if the blood volume is small and dispersed, the CT will not visualize it. It is thought that a spinal tap will yield the diagnosis in virtually all cases if a few hours elapses between the ictus and the tap in order to allow the blood time to diffuse into the lumbar sac.

219. The answer is E. (Osborn, p 899.) This myelogram is clearly of the thoracic region, as the ribs are easily seen. The large segment that blocks the dye is clearly not at disk level, which eliminates the diagnosis of disk herniation. Since there is not a complete blockage of the canal, the upper and lower limits of the lesion are seen. One can see the cord pushed to the right (in the radiograph on the left), away from the thecal sac, which implies an intradural but extramedullary lesion. Intradural extramedullary lesions are most likely neurofibromas or meningiomas.

220. The answer is E. (Adams RD, 5/e, pp 1029–1030.) The CT shows calcifications extending into the lateral ventricles, a classic radiologic sign for tuberous sclerosis. The lateral ventricles contain masses that look like candle drippings. When these calcify, the CT looks like the one shown. Patients with this inherited disorder are at increased risk for malignant degeneration of their abnormal glial cells and develop large cell astrocytomas that tend to occur near the lateral ventricle.

221. The answer is D. (Osborn, pp 695–696.) The CT shows a large, hypodense region in the left frontal and temporal lobes. The abnormality spares large areas of cortex in both these lobes. In addition the lesion extends medially into the anterior cerebral territory as well as laterally into the middle cerebral artery territory, yet spares parts of both. There is effacement of the gyral pattern on the left, which indicates that the pathology is acute. Head trauma is an unlikely cause of such a large lesion because no blood is evident. CMV does not usually cause CT abnormalities, and cysticercosis causes relatively round, discrete lesions often with a central calcified scolex. Herpes simplex enters the brain via the inferior surface of the frontal and temporal lobes and typically causes a necrotizing encephalitis affecting the frontal and temporal lobes.

222. The answer is A. (Rowland, 9/e, pp 576–580.) This MRI shows a large mass of the pineal region. The differential diagnosis for tumors in this area includes pinealoma, dysgerminoma, glioma, and meningioma. Clinically one would expect a Parinaud's syndrome: light-near pupillary dissociation, upgaze paralysis, and convergence or retraction nystagmus.

223. The answer is E. (Osborn, p 593.) The unenhanced CT shows a large right frontal mass that is clearly seen without contrast enhancement. The stippled nature and the density in one area suggest this represents calcification rather than blood. The enhanced study shows that the mass enhances diffusely. These findings are most consistent with a meningioma. Lower planes of section would reveal an attachment to the meninges not seen here. An abscess would not enhance diffusely. Mycotic aneurysms are intraparenchymal but do not become this large. Gliomas generally do not calcify. Melanoma does tend to bleed but is usually smaller and not solitary.

224. The answer is D. (Rowland, 9/e, pp 664–665.) There is a large mass in the right basal ganglia. While this is most likely to be toxoplasmosis, other possibilities include any of the causes of masses in AIDS patients. These include all the other entities except PML, which causes white matter disease and has no mass effect.

225. The answer is E. (Adams RD, 5/e, p 1013.) Skull growth occurs perpendicular to the suture line. New bone is laid down along the suture line so that as the bone grows, the two opposing plates push against each other. When the suture closes, the bone growth along the suture line stops. When the sagittal suture closes, the remainder of the skull continues growing, largely perpendicular to the frontal occipital sutures, that is, parallel to the sagittal suture. This produces a long, narrow skull known as *scaphocephaly*.

226. The answer is C. (Osborn, pp 506–507.) Chordomas are notochordal in origin and characteristically arise in the sacrococcygeal spine, the skull, or the vertebral spine in descending order. In the skull they originate in the clivus, where they cause bone destruction, but they may extend in any direction and cause CNS dysfunction. Eosinophilic granuloma most commonly involves the outer skull. Osteosarcoma does not arise from the skull. Osteomas generally occur in the sinuses. Wegener's granulomatosis primarily involves sinuses and extends from there.

227. The answer is E. (Adams RD, 5/e, pp 714–715.) Originally described as a renal arterial disease, fibromuscular dysplasia also may affect the cerebral arterial tree. While often associated with cerebral aneurysms, the most common cerebrovascular abnormality occurs in the internal carotid artery. Several areas of dilatation alternating with areas of stenosis cause a "beaded string" appearance. Two-thirds of cases have bilateral involvement. One-third of cases have aneurysms. The common carotid and the carotid bifurcation are spared in this disease. Clinical manifestations include TIA, CVA, and subarachnoid hemorrhage.

228. The answer is C (2, 4). (Osborn, p 349.) In the first 24 h of an ischemic stroke the CT scan is often negative. It often takes 24 h or longer for the decreased attenuation on unenhanced CT and the irregular enhancement on contrast CT to appear. T1 MRI is usually negative in the earliest stage of stroke but reveals decreasing signal and increasing distinctness of the lesion over time. The T2 MRI tends to be positive early and to produce a bright signal (T1 produces a dark image of the lesion) that initially has indistinct margins due to the irregularity of the edema surrounding the early infarct. In the first few hours T1 and T2 may both be negative but are always more likely to reveal the stroke before the CT.

229. The answer is B (1, 3). (Osborn, p 407.) Childhood brain tumors, both primary and metastatic, tend to occur equally often in the supratentorial and infratentorial regions. This is true for metastatic brain abscesses as well. Therefore, the location of this mass and the secondary hydrocephalus are not unexpected. The most common childhood brain tumors are primary, with medulloblastomas and astrocytomas most common. Meningiomas do not occur in children and metastatic disease is rare.

230–233. The answers are 230-A, 231-B, 232-D, 233-C. (Fischer, p 97.) The head of the caudate creates the comma shape in the frontal horns of the lateral ventricles. The other basal ganglia structures are generally seen in the usual CT planes of sections that do not include portions of the midbrain. In the coronal sections, one gets an appreciation of the proximity of the substantia nigra to the putamen and globus pallidus and of the substantia nigra to the red nucleus. The red nucleus and the substantia nigra are located at midbrain levels. The globus pallidus is separated into external and internal segments; the external segment is contiguous with the putamen. Together the putamen and globus pallidus make up the lentiform nucleus, so called because of its lenslike shape.

234–238. The answers are 234-C, 235-B, 236-B, 237-B, 238-C. (Osborn, p 487. Rowland, 9/e, pp 470–471.) All the cranial nerves pass through apertures in the base of the skull. Some apertures transmit more than one nerve. Characteristic syndromes occur when a lesion affects the conjunction of nerves at particular sites of exit from the skull.

Cranial nerves III, IV, VI, and the ophthalmic division of V run through the superior orbital fissure. The VIth cranial nerve runs through Dorello's canal at the medial tip of the petrous part of the temporal bone, in company with the inferior petrosal sinus. Both nerve and vessel then enter the cavernous sinus. Inflammation of the petrous bone involves the VIth nerve at the canal of Dorello and the nearby Vth nerve, producing Gradenigo's syndrome.

The IXth, Xth, and XIth cranial nerves all run through the jugular foramen in the posterior fossa. A lesion at this site, such as a tumor of the glomus jugulare, involves all three nerves (syndrome of Vernet).

In contrast to these apertures that transmit multiple cranial nerves, other apertures such as the optic canal and the hypoglossal canal transmit only one cranial nerve. The arteries traverse the apertures as follows: carotid arteries through the foramen lacerum, ophthalmic arteries through the optic canal, vertebral arteries through the foramen magnum, and the middle meningeal arteries through the foramen spinosum.

OPHTHALMOLOGY, ENT, CSF, MICROBIOLOGY, ENDOCRINOLOGY, AND IMMUNOLOGY

Directions: Each item below contains five suggested responses. Select the **one best** response to each item.

239. Which of the following statements is true of Leigh's disease (subacute necrotizing encephalitis)?

(A) The biochemical abnormality is a deficiency of thiamine

(B) A biochemical abnormality of the pyruvate dehydrogenase complex is thought to result in lesions similar to those of Wernicke syndrome, except for sparing of mamillary bodies

(C) A biochemical abnormality leads to extensive cerebral demyelination

(D) The pathologic lesions of spongiform degeneration, focal necrosis, and vascular proliferation affect the brainstem and cortex equally

(E) The brainstem abnormality that causes respiratory dysfunction results in hypoxic brain changes such as the loss of neurons in Sommer's sector

240. The fast (kickback) phase of caloric or optokinetic nystagmus is thought to depend on

(A) efferent brainstem connections from the frontal eye fields

(B) ascending connections from the proprioceptors in the neck

(C) integrity of the cerebellar vermis

(D) impulses originating in the retina

(E) the dorsal longitudinal fasciculus

241. All the following statements concerning the Adie's (tonic) pupil are correct EXCEPT

(A) there is light-near dissociation

(B) the pupil contracts very slowly

(C) the knee jerk is absent

(D) there may be mild adduction weakness

(E) vision may be blurred

242. A patient with a polyneuropathy that has developed over several weeks has anemia, white transverse bands across the nails, jaundice, and brownish cutaneous pigmentation. The most likely explanation is

(A) porphyria
(B) lead poisoning
(C) arsenic poisoning
(D) INH (isoniazid) neuropathy
(E) a paraneoplastic syndrome

243. Patients with carbon dioxide narcosis from respiratory failure in the setting of chronic obstructive pulmonary disease (COPD) commonly exhibit

(A) seizures
(B) ophthalmoparesis
(C) asterixis or myoclonus
(D) increased sensitivity to pain
(E) respiratory rates increased from baseline

244. Downbeating nystagmus localizes the lesion to which one of the following?

(A) Thalami
(B) Cervicomedullary junction
(C) Edinger-Westphal nucleus
(D) Lateral geniculate body
(E) Cerebellar vermis

245. An enlarged head with normal ventricles (macrocephaly) is commonly seen in children as a result of all the following conditions EXCEPT

(A) Tay-Sachs disease
(B) Alexander's disease
(C) spongy degeneration of infancy (Canavan-van Bogaert-Bertrand disease)
(D) subdural hematomas
(E) Menke's disease

246. The EMG finding that is most characteristic of chronic denervation and most reliably distinguishes it from other neuromuscular diseases is

(A) fibrillations
(B) giant polyphasic motor units
(C) low-amplitude motor units
(D) electrical silence during rest
(E) myotonia

247. A full interference pattern with low-amplitude potentials in the EMG is most characteristic of

(A) McArdle's disease
(B) muscular dystrophy
(C) myasthenia gravis
(D) acute denervation
(E) chronic denervation

248. All the following statements about neurologic manifestations of Lyme disease are true EXCEPT

(A) most patients have a history of erythema chronicum migrans (ECM)

(B) facial weakness is an early occurrence (within 2 months of the appearance of the lesion)

(C) most patients have a history of arthritis

(D) the second most common cranial neuropathy is of the VIIIth nerve

(E) nerve conduction studies are usually normal in Lyme neuropathy

249. The most common cranial neuropathy seen in Lyme disease is

(A) an Argyll Robertson pupillary defect

(B) facial weakness

(C) facial numbness

(D) acoustic nerve dysfunction

(E) VIth nerve palsies

250. Which one of the following statements concerning the genetic concept of anticipation is true in Huntington's disease?

(A) There is no evidence of anticipation

(B) Anticipation occurs in affected male children

(C) Anticipation occurs in affected children of affected men

(D) Anticipation is an artifact of better detection

(E) Anticipation occurs in homozygotes only

251. The typical hemorrhages that occur in the retina secondary to acute increased intracranial pressure occupy the

(A) choroid

(B) nerve fiber layer

(C) subhyaloid space

(D) vitreous body

(E) anterior chamber

252. The site of a restricted lesion that would selectively impair vertical gaze is the

(A) collicular plate

(B) cerebellar vermis

(C) region dorsomedial to the red nuclei

(D) bioccipital region

(E) internal capsule

253. A patient presents with a fever, painful ear, facial pain, facial weakness, and a VIth nerve palsy. The most likely explanation is

(A) acoustic neuroma with hemorrhage

(B) basilar aneurysmal rupture

(C) inflammation of the apex of the petrous pyramid

(D) vasculitis

(E) external otitis

254. A patient has difficulty seeing to the left with the left eye and to a lesser degree to the right with the right eye. Visual acuity and the remainder of the neurologic examination are normal. The most likely diagnosis is

(A) lesion of the optic chiasm

(B) lesion of the left lateral geniculate body

(C) lesion of both optic nerves

(D) vascular retinal disease

(E) psychogenic disorder

255. A 30-year-old man begins having persistent horizontal diplopia on looking only to the left. His neurologic examination is normal except for eye movements. The most lateral image disappears when the right eye is covered. What is the most likely diagnosis?

(A) Conversion
(B) Myasthenia
(C) Stroke
(D) Multiple sclerosis
(E) Graves' disease

256. A patient has diplopia on left lateral gaze. Examination shows slight weakness of abduction of the left eye, but the right eye hyperadducts when the patient looks to the left. In this case, hyperadduction of the right eye is best explained by

(A) a lesion of the ipsilateral medial longitudinal fasciculus
(B) a supranuclear palsy of gaze from interruption of frontobulbar pathways
(C) preexisting ocular malalignment
(D) Hering's law of equal supranuclear innervation of yoke muscles
(E) a malingering patient

257. To test for the integrity of the IVth cranial nerve in a patient with a IIIrd nerve palsy, the examiner asks the patient to look in which of the following directions?

(A) To the side opposite the IIIrd nerve palsy and down
(B) To the side ipsilateral to the IIIrd nerve palsy and up
(C) To the midline and up
(D) To the midline
(E) Upward

Items 258–259

A previously well, male patient has been experiencing a gradual onset of weakness for 2 days, with some vague tingling in the extremities but no incontinence. He has generalized flaccid muscle weakness, perhaps worse proximally. Ocular movements, speaking, and swallowing are normal, but facial movements are questionably weak. On percussing the tendons, the examiner elicits no response. Sensory examination discloses questionable loss of vibratory sensation in the toes. Serum electrolytes (meq/L) are Na^+ 137, K^+ 3.4, Cl^- 100, Ca^{2+} 7; CPK is normal.

258. The most likely diagnosis is

(A) electrolyte imbalance

(B) acute myelitis

(C) acute polymyositis

(D) acute polyradiculitis (Landry-Guillain-Barré syndrome)

(E) familial periodic paralysis

259. On the third day of illness of the patient described, a lumbar puncture is performed. Analysis of the CSF discloses these findings: WBCs $5/mm^3$; glucose 65 mg/dL; protein 35 mg/dL; immunoelectrophoretic profile normal. The best interpretation of these results is which of the following?

(A) They argue most strongly for acute myelitis

(B) They are most compatible with electrolyte imbalance

(C) They argue against polymyositis

(D) They exclude the Landry-Guillain-Barré syndrome

(E) They are compatible with acute myelitis, electrolyte imbalance, polymyositis, and Landry-Guillain-Barré syndrome

260. At what age should a normal child be able to start using grammar to create true, although simple, sentences?

(A) 12 to 18 months
(B) 18 to 24 months
(C) 24 to 36 months
(D) 36 to 48 months
(E) 48 to 60 months

261. Patients affected with the medial longitudinal fasciculus (MLF) syndrome, when attempting to look to one side, display

(A) nystagmus of the adducting eye and paresis of the abducting eye, with normal convergence during accommodation
(B) nystagmus of the abducting eye with paresis of the adducting eye, and adductor paresis during accommodation
(C) nystagmus of the abducting eye with paresis of the adducting eye, but adduction of the eyes during accommodation
(D) nystagmus of both adducting and abducting eyes, with paresis of vertical movements
(E) paresis of the abducting and adducting eyes, but adduction of the eyes during accommodation

262. Neurologic complications of adult myxedema include all the following EXCEPT

(A) decreased CSF protein
(B) facial weakness
(C) vertigo
(D) hearing loss
(E) delirium

263. An abnormal IgM spike found on a serum protein electrophoresis that is not associated with a plasma cell dyscrasia would most likely be associated with which one of the following neurologic syndromes?

(A) Peripheral neuropathy
(B) Cerebellar degeneration
(C) Limbic encephalitis
(D) Optic neuritis
(E) Guillain-Barré syndrome

264. Opsoclonus in children and infants is mainly associated with

(A) small cell carcinoma of the lung
(B) Sydenham's chorea
(C) neuroblastoma
(D) Wilms' tumor
(E) acute lymphocytic leukemia

265. The true vestibular component of caloric nystagmus is

(A) the slow deviation phase
(B) the quick kickback phase
(C) both quick and slow horizontal phases
(D) the vertical quick phase only
(E) both quick and slow vertical phases

266. The muscles most likely to be weakened by trichinosis are the

(A) facial
(B) proximal arm and leg
(C) diaphragmatic
(D) posterior cervical
(E) distal limb

267. In performing a cold caloric irrigation of the ear of a patient sitting upright, an examiner should position the patient by

(A) leaving the patient's head vertical
(B) inclining the patient's head 60 degrees backward
(C) inclining the patient's head 30 degrees forward
(D) tilting the patient's head to the side of the irrigation
(E) bending the patient's trunk forward

268. A 65-year-old hypertensive man develops painless loss of vision in one eye over several hours. The eye and neurologic examination are normal aside from one eye having light perception only and an afferent pupillary defect. No funduscopic abnormalities are noted. An erythrocyte sedimentation rate is 20. The most likely diagnosis is

(A) retinal infarct
(B) temporal arteritis
(C) infarct of the lateral geniculate body
(D) infarct of the posterior cerebral artery
(E) ischemic infarction of the optic nerve

Directions: Each item below contains four suggested responses of which **one or more** is correct. Select:

A	if	**1, 2, and 3**	are correct
B	if	**1 and 3**	are correct
C	if	**2 and 4**	are correct
D	if	**4**	is correct
E	if	**1, 2, 3, and 4**	are correct

269. Lead poisoning in children may cause

(1) ataxia
(2) hemiplegia
(3) seizures
(4) lethargy

270. True statements regarding syphilis in an HIV-positive patient include which of the following?

(1) The delay between primary infection and neurologic involvement is reduced
(2) The CSF VDRL test may be negative
(3) Strokes due to meningovascular involvement are extremely rare
(4) Intravenous rather than intramuscular penicillin is the treatment of choice

271. Diagnostic features that distinguish nonparalytic (concomitant) heterotropia from paralytic heterotropia include which of the following?

(1) The angle of the ocular malalignment remains the same during all directions of movement when both eyes are used
(2) Each eye shows a full range of movements when the other is covered
(3) Opacity of the media or severe refractive error may be present in one eye
(4) The patient complains of diplopia

272. Clinical characteristics of Adie's pupil include

(1) anisocoria
(2) irregular pupillary margin
(3) slow constriction and dilation
(4) frequent association with hyperactive stretch reflexes

273. An examiner places strong positive lenses (Frenzel lenses) over a patient's eyes to inspect for positional or caloric-induced nystagmus in order to

(1) produce pupilloconstriction
(2) occlude visual fixation
(3) prevent vertigo
(4) magnify the eye movements

274. Ragged red fibers are associated with which of the following?

(1) Myoclonus and ataxia
(2) Cardiac arrhythmias
(3) Diplopia
(4) Paroxysmal ataxia

275. Hyperthyroidism is frequently accompanied by which of the following motor system syndromes?

(1) Myasthenia gravis
(2) Periodic weakness with hypokalemia
(3) Ophthalmoplegia
(4) Enlarged, firm muscles

276. Correct statements concerning the syndrome of progressive ophthalmoplegia include which of the following?

   (1) Historically, opinions have differed concerning its classification as a myopathic or a neurogenic disease
   (2) It is frequently associated with retinitis pigmentosa
   (3) It is characterized by ptosis and weakness of eye closing as well as by ophthalmoplegia
   (4) Affected patients frequently present with diplopia

277. Which of the following will cause xanthochromia?

   (1) Jaundice
   (2) Elevated CSF protein
   (3) Hypercarotenemia
   (4) Rifampin

278. With closed head injuries, commonly affected brain sites include

   (1) frontal
   (2) brainstem
   (3) temporal
   (4) occipital

279. True statements concerning primary CNS lymphomas include

   (1) they diffusely enhance with contrast
   (2) they almost always are surrounded by significant edema
   (3) they are usually periventricular
   (4) the contrast enhancement is exquisitely sensitive to steroid but the tumor itself rarely shrinks

280. Myotonia may be identified by which of the following features?

   (1) It increases with increasing contractions of the muscle
   (2) It is demonstrable by percussion
   (3) It is electrically silent in EMG
   (4) It occurs after a single strong contraction

281. Diabetes is associated with which of the following neurologic problems?

   (1) Bell's palsy
   (2) Subacute proximal leg weakness
   (3) Impotence
   (4) Complete third nerve palsy

Directions: Each group of questions below consists of lettered options followed by a set of numbered items. For each numbered item select the **one** lettered option with which it is most closely associated. Each lettered option may be used **once**, **more than once**, **or not at all**.

Items 282–285

Match the eye movement response to the correct maneuver in a patient with progressive supranuclear palsy (PSP). The patient is lying supine with the head inclined at 30 degrees to the horizontal.

    (A) Warm water instilled into both ears
    (B) Cold water instilled into both ears
    (C) Warm water instilled into right ear
    (D) Cold water instilled into right ear
    (E) None of the above

282. Both eyes move up in midline

283. Both eyes move down in midline

284. Both eyes move to the left along the equator

285. The left eye moves to the left

Items 286–289

Match each description with the correct disorder.

    (A) Polymyositis
    (B) Trichinosis
    (C) Carnitine palmitoyl transferase (CPT) deficiency
    (D) Limb girdle dystrophy
    (E) Myotonic dystrophy

286. This muscle disorder usually begins in the third decade and is associated with a peculiar facial appearance due to masseter atrophy, ptosis, and frontal baldness

287. This disorder affects women more than men and generally begins in middle age with subacute, painless, symmetric, proximal weakness

288. Patients with this disorder usually have extraocular muscle and tongue involvement

289. This disorder, primarily of males, causes recurrent episodes of myoglobinuria

Items 290–293

For each disorder listed below, choose the chromosomal condition with which it is most closely associated.

    (A) 5 Deletion
    (B) Trisomy 21
    (C) Trisomy 13
    (D) XXY
    (E) No deletion or error of chromosome number is found

290. Holoprosencephaly/arhinencephalia

291. Cri du chat (cat's cry syndrome)

292. Neurofibromatosis

293. Klinefelter's syndrome

OPHTHALMOLOGY, ENT, CSF, MICROBIOLOGY, ENDOCRINOLOGY, AND IMMUNOLOGY

239. The answer is B. (Adams RD, 5/e, pp 812–813.) Leigh's disease is an autosomal recessive disorder that generally has its onset in the first few years of life. It has a variable clinical presentation dependent in part on the age of onset. One of the characteristic features that occurs in some children is a markedly abnormal respiratory pattern. Although multiple biochemical abnormalities have been found, none has yet been proved to be universally present. It is generally agreed that the central problem occurs in the pyruvate dehydrogenase complex. The pathologic features are similar to those of Wernicke's disease except for sparing of the mamillary bodies. Spongiform degeneration, necrosis, vascular proliferation, and gliosis occur in the thalamus, brainstem, and spinal cord.

240. The answer is A. (Adams RD, 5/e, p 2398.) The fast, or kickback, phase of caloric nystagmus depends in large part on the integrity of the efferent pathway from the frontal eye fields. Large hemispheric lesions that destroy the cortical projection system to the brainstem will abolish the kickback phase of nystagmus. In patients thus afflicted, the slow deviation phase (the vestibular, or optokinetic, phase) remains. Absence of the cerebral efferent pathway converts the response to merely deviation rather than to an organized nystagmus. Retinal receptors play no part in producing the fast phase of caloric nystagmus. In fact, voluntary fixation tends to inhibit caloric nystagmus. Integrity of the retinal receptors would be necessary for the pursuit phase of optokinetic nystagmus, but the kickback phase is related to the integrity of the pathway from the frontal eye fields to the brainstem.

241. The answer is D. (Adams RD, 5/e, p 243.) The Adie's, or tonic, pupil refers to a pupillary abnormality thought to be due to deterioration of the ciliary ganglion and the postganglionic parasympathetic fibers, which control pupillary contraction and, to a lesser extent, accommodation. The patient may notice anisocoria or blurred vision. Cursory examination reveals a fixed, dilated pupil, but with continued bright illumination the pupil slowly constricts.

The accommodation response is much quicker, inducing a light-near dissociation similar to that seen with neurosyphilis. With neurosyphilis, however, the pupils are generally small. The diminished accommodation causes blurring. The disorder affects more women than men and frequently is associated with absent knee and ankle jerks. Extraocular movement disorders are not known to occur.

242. The answer is C. (Adams RD, 5/e, p 1133.) Arsenic can cause a polyneuropathy evolving over days after acute poisoning or over weeks to months with chronic poisoning. The neuropathy is axonal and is associated with anemia, jaundice, hyperkeratosis of the palmar surfaces, brownish cutaneous pigmentation, and Mees' lines (white transverse bands across the nails). Diagnosis can be made definitively with measurement of arsenic in urine or hair.

243. The answer is C. (Plum, 3/e, p 231.) Patients with COPD who develop respiratory failure with hypercarbia also develop many brain changes. Increased intracranial pressure from the elevated CO_2 may cause optic disk swelling. Anesthesia may develop along with a dull, diffuse headache, lethargy, or coma. Asterixis and myoclonus are extremely common, whereas seizures are rare.

244. The answer is B. (Adams RD, 5/e, p 239.) Downbeat nystagmus localizes the lesion to the cervicomedullary junction. While it is associated with a number of structural abnormalities, such as basilar invagination, syringobulbia, and most commonly an Arnold-Chiari malformation, it may also be present in the Wernicke-Korsakoff syndrome, with lithium use, or in cerebellar degenerations. Its pathophysiology is not understood and many cases have no identifiable cause. Its presence, however, whether symptomatic with oscillopsia or not, should precipitate an evaluation for an etiology.

245. The answer is E. (Adams RD, 5/e, p 1013.) Statistically most enlarged heads in children are due either to hydrocephalus or to a nonpathologic familial hereditary pattern of large heads. However, there are certain conditions in which a large head without significantly enlarged ventricles occurs in the setting of serious neurologic abnormalities. Most degenerative neurologic disorders of children cause small heads. The only three degenerative conditions causing macrocephaly are Tay-Sachs disease, Alexander's disease, and spongy degeneration of infancy. Subdural hematomas in infants should be symptomatic.

246. The answer is B. (Adams RD, 5/e, p 1071.) The EMG finding most indicative of chronic denervation is giant polyphasic motor units. These units are virtually pathognomonic and are absent in normal persons or in patients with dystrophy. They are thought to represent enlargement of the motor units from regenerating nerve sprouts. In many disorders involved in the differential diagnosis of chronic denervation, the EMG will show fibrillations or low-amplitude motor units. Characteristically, patients with chronic denervation show fibrillations and slow positive waves in addition to the giant polyphasic units, but fibrillations also can occur in polymyositis and some dystrophies and lack the pathognomonic significance of the giant polyphasic units. Patients with muscular dystrophy and normal persons show no electrical activity with the muscle at rest.

247. The answer is B. (Adams RD, 5/e, p 1072.) The characteristic EMG pattern of muscular dystrophy is a full interference pattern with low-amplitude potentials. The interference pattern depends on the number of motor units contracting and the number of muscle fibers responding. In dystrophies, the number of motor units remains the same, but the number of muscle fibers available to respond decreases as the disease advances. The reduced number of responding muscle fibers leads to the reduction in amplitude of the interference pattern. The full interference pattern with low-amplitude potentials, in combination with the absence of any of the EMG changes such as fibrillations and giant polyphasic units, lends support to a diagnosis of a primary muscle disease rather than neuronal disease.

248. The answer is E. (Logigian, N Engl J Med 323:1438–1443, 1990.) The spectrum of neurologic disorders reported with Lyme disease is large and the clinical course is not yet fully understood. Diagnosis is not always clear-cut, as most, but not all patients have a history of erythema chronicum migrans (ECM) and arthritis. The history of a tick bite is more difficult to ascertain because the tick vector is the size of the period at the end of this sentence. Facial and VIIIth nerve lesions occur early, often within a month of the ECM. Polyneuropathy is a common long-term problem, with abnormalities evident on electrophysiologic studies. Improvement in symptoms parallels improvement in electrical studies.

249. The answer is B. (Rowland, 9/e, pp 209–211.) Facial weakness, often bilateral, is probably the most common cranial neuropathy; however, the neurologic manifestations of Lyme disease include aseptic meningitis, encephalitis, dementia, myelitis, and peripheral nerve problems. The neurologic literature is somewhat hazy because of the frequent difficulty in making the diagnosis if the erythema chronicum migrans or the arthritis was not observed by physicians. No test currently exists to point to active Lyme infection in the CNS other than a finding of pleocytosis, so that the meaning of a positive Lyme titer is not always clear.

250. The answer is C. (Rowland, 9/e, p 696.) The concept of anticipation refers to the earlier onset of an inherited disorder in the children of the affected parent. Huntington's disease is caused by an excess number of CAG repeats in the "Huntington" protein gene. In general the disease occurs earlier the greater the number of repeats. For reasons not yet clear, men generally amplify the number of repeats while the number remains steady in women. Hence the children (both male and female) of affected men, inheriting an increased number of repeats, in general, are more likely to develop the disease earlier than the father, thus displaying anticipation. This does not appear to hold true for all CAG-repeat disorders.

251. The answer is C. (Adams RD, 5/e, p 214.) The retinal hemorrhage typical of acute increased intracranial pressure occupies the space between the internal limiting membrane of the retina and the hyaloid membrane. Therefore, it is a subhyaloid or preretinal hemorrhage. The blood apparently comes from rupture of the retinal arterioles. The ophthalmoscopic appearance of the various types of hemorrhage depends on the space into which the hemorrhage ruptures or upon the retinal layer into which it ruptures. Common conditions associated with subhyaloid hemorrhages include ruptured intracranial aneurysms and head injuries, often with acute epidural or acute subdural hemorrhage. Occasionally, severe coughing may induce a subhyaloid hemorrhage. The presence of subhyaloid hemorrhages, at least in a comatose patient, requires immediate investigation by CT scan or angiography.

252. **The answer is A.** (Adams RD, 5/e, p 229.) The clinical importance of a vertical gaze palsy lies partly in the localization of mass lesions to the region of the superior colliculus, particularly of the pineal gland, causing Parinaud's syndrome (loss of convergence, light-near pupillary dissociation, retraction nystagmus). The loss of vertical gaze is important in distinguishing progressive supranuclear palsy (PSP) from Parkinson's disease. The superior colliculus is important in initiating saccadic movements only. Clinically, lesions of the superior colliculus affect upgaze, while lesions slightly lower affect only downgaze.

253. **The answer is C.** (Adams RD, 5/e, p 1372.) The syndrome of purulent otitis, ipsilateral facial pain, and Vth, VIth, and VIIth nerve palsies is called *Gradenigo's syndrome*. It occurs with extension of the inflammation from the middle ear to the apex of the petrous pyramids over which course the involved nerves. Appropriately placed neoplasms, such as nasopharyngeal carcinoma, can cause a similar syndrome but without the fever.

254. **The answer is A.** (Adams RD, 5/e, pp 220–221.) Bitemporal field cuts are the hallmark of optic chiasm syndromes. Most commonly these do not affect both eyes equally. Pituitary tumors are the most common etiology but other tumors and aneurysms are also in the differential diagnosis. Because the progression is insidious, patients are often unaware of the severity of their deficit.

255. **The answer is D.** (Adams RD, 5/e, p 235.) Horizontal diplopia indicates that the lateral eye muscles, the lateral and medial rectus muscles, are unyoked. The fact that this occurs only on looking to the left indicates the problem must be in the left lateral rectus or right medial rectus muscles. The image furthest from the center arises from the eye with the weakened muscle, thereby implying a medial rectus problem since the patient has no diplopia in the other fields of gaze. He does not have a third nerve palsy; hence he most likely has an internuclear ophthalmoplegia (INO). An INO is almost diagnostic of MS in a young adult. The other conditions are either unlikely at the age of 30 or are more likely to cause diplopia in multiple fields or ptosis.

256. **The answer is D.** (Newell, 7/e, p 96.) Excessive action of an intact ocular muscle of one eye that normally is yoked to a paretic muscle of the opposite eye is explained by Hering's law. Hering's law states that the yoke muscles receive equal supranuclear innervation. A patient affected with a weak lateral rectus muscle overinnervates in an effort to activate the paretic muscle. The central connections of the nervous system, in obedience to Hering's law, send an equally strong innervation to the intact medial rectus. The paretic lateral rectus muscle underacts, and the intact medial rectus overacts, causing hyperadduction. The reverse occurs with a medial rectus palsy. When a patient with this deficit attempts to look to the side opposite the medial rectus palsy, the overaction of the intact lateral rectus muscles hyperabducts the eyeball.

257. The answer is A. (Adams RD, 5/e, p 314.) To test for an intact IVth nerve when the patient has a IIIrd nerve palsy, the examiner asks the patient to look to the side opposite the palsy and down. The examiner then watches for rotation of one of the conjunctival vessels. If the IVth nerve and superior oblique muscle are intact, the examiner will observe intorsion of the eye, although it will fail to adduct. With the eye laterally rotated from the pull of the intact VIth nerve and lateral rectus muscle, the eye is in the position in which the superior oblique muscle has its maximum strength as an intorter. The effort to look medially and down will activate the superior oblique muscle, but it will mainly display its action as an intorter of the eye.

258. The answer is D. (Adams RD, 5/e, pp 1126–1130.) The patient described in the question has an acutely evolving, flaccid paralysis with areflexia and retention of percussive irritability of muscle. Sensation is only questionably involved, and the patient retains sphincter control. These features argue strongly against myelitis, which would manifest sensory loss and incontinence, even though flaccid paralysis may be present early in the course of the myelitis. Polymyositis usually has a much more indolent onset than occurred in this patient and would not cause acute flaccid paralysis. The electrolyte values are slightly low, but not low enough to cause flaccid paralysis. Familial periodic paralysis of normokalemic type remains a possibility but in terms of probability is much rarer and thus much less likely than the Landry-Guillain-Barré syndrome.

259. The answer is E. (Adams RD, 5/e, pp 1126–1130.) Normal spinal fluid is compatible with any of the four diagnoses mentioned in the question. Acute myelitis may or may not show a significant change in the CSF; but very mild, acute electrolyte disturbances, polymyositis, and periodic paralysis characteristically would fail to show changes in the components ordinarily measured in a routine CSF examination. In Landry-Guillain-Barré syndrome, the protein level does increase, but occasionally the initial tap may show a normal protein content. The protein level then will increase, usually reaching a peak several weeks after the onset of the illness. Thus, a normal CSF during the acute stage of the illness does not exclude the Landry-Guillain-Barré syndrome.

260. The answer is C. (Kaplan, Synopsis, 7/e, p 41.) In the third year of life children begin having conversations with other children and start putting together grammatically correct sentences. They begin to comprehend family name categories (e.g., grandma, grandpa, baby), size, and the names of body parts not commonly used. Vocabulary begins to increase dramatically and speech becomes much more intelligible.

261. The answer is C. (Adams, 5/e, pp 226–227.) In the medial longitudinal fasciculus (MLF) syndrome, the patient shows nystagmus of the *ab*ducting eye and paresis of the *ad*ducting eye. Both eyes adduct during accommodation. The medial longitudinal fasciculus conveys fibers from the region of the contralateral abducens nucleus to the lower motor neurons of the medial rectus muscle in the IIIrd nerve nucleus. These MLF fibers yoke the medial rectus of one eye with the lateral rectus of the opposite eye to mediate conjugate lateral gaze.

Interruption of these MLF fibers causes paresis of adduction of the eye ipsilateral to the MLF lesion. During accommodation, the medial rectus is activated by pathways that run directly into the midbrain without traveling down into the pons and back through the MLF. The normal medial rectus action during convergence proves that the lower motor neurons of the medial rectus muscle remain intact in the MLF syndrome.

262. The answer is A. (Rowland, 9/e, p 892.) Severe hypothyroidism in adults may cause a large number of neurologic complications. These include cranial neuropathies such as unilateral or bilateral facial weakness, decreased hearing, tinnitus, and vertigo. Delirium, agitation, and psychosis (myxedema madness) may occur as well as acute coma. Myopathy and sensory neuropathy are other rare complications. Laboratory abnormalities in myxedema include low thyroid hormones, elevated TSH, elevated CSF protein, and elevated cholesterol.

263. The answer is A. (Kelly, Arch Neurol 45:1355–1359, 1988.) The laboratory evaluation of peripheral neuropathies should include a protein electrophoresis to look for immune abnormalities. Some of these antibodies have been clearly shown to cross-react with peripheral nerve and are thought to be causal in disease progression and not simply representative of a systemic response to nerve degeneration. The other disorders are also thought to be due to autoimmune dysfunction but have not been linked with benign IgM spikes.

264. The answer is C. (Rowland, 9/e, p 942.) More than 50 percent of infants and children who develop opsoclonus have an associated neuroblastoma, usually in the chest. In adults the most commonly associated malignancy is a small cell cancer of the lung. Opsoclonus may also develop with encephalitis or metabolic and toxic states. In children with a neuroblastoma, opsoclonus is a good prognostic sign. The opsoclonus responds to ACTH.

265. The answer is A. (Adams RD, 5/e, p 226.) The vestibular component of caloric nystagmus is the slow deviation phase and the nonvestibular component is the quick kickback phase. The quick phase depends, in large part, on the cortical efferent system from the frontal eye fields. Interruption of this system will result in loss of the quick phase, but the slow deviation phase in response to caloric irrigation remains. The direction of vestibular or caloric nystagmus unfortunately is named by the direction of the fast component, which is not the primary vestibular action.

266. The answer is C. (Adams RD, 5/e, p 634.) Trichinosis is caused by ingestion of undercooked pork. The first manifestation is gastroenteritis due to larvae invading the intestinal mucosa. About a week later the larvae invade muscles, causing conjunctival and eyelid swelling, low-grade fever, fatigue, pain, and muscle tenderness. Muscle weakness may be severe and diffuse, but certain muscles are more likely to be affected. The diaphragm is the most common, followed by the extraocular and lingual muscles. Usually muscle symptoms remit. With severe infection, the brain may be infected, causing seizures, delirium, or focal neurologic signs with abnormal spinal fluid.

267. The answer is B. (Adams RD, 5/e, p 263.) Before performing a caloric irrigation test, an examiner has the patient sit erect, tilting the patient's head 60 degrees backward. The purpose of this maneuver is to place the lateral canal in the exact vertical plane. The lateral canal inclines 30 degrees above the horizontal, and the additional 60 degrees of inclination places it in a vertical position. With the lateral canal in the vertical plane, the effect of gravity plus the temperature effect of the irrigating fluid stimulates circulation of the fluid in the lateral semicircular canal, which in turn stimulates the vestibular receptors.

268. The answer is E. (Adams RD, 5/e, p 218.) Anterior ischemic optic neuropathy is a syndrome of blindness that occurs in older patients in a painless manner. The pathogenesis is believed to be from atherosclerotic changes in the posterior ciliary artery. Depending on how close to the optic nerve head the ischemia occurs, the funduscopic examination may reveal disk swelling and flame-shaped hemorrhages, but it may also look completely normal. Temporal arteritis would be extremely unlikely with a normal ESR and no symptoms. A retinal infarct should be apparent on funduscopic examination. The brain syndromes mentioned should cause homonymous field cuts.

269. The answer is E (all). (Rowland, 9/e, pp 990–991.) Lead poisoning is more common in children than adults. The latter generally have occupational exposure to lead paint or old car radiators and develop autonomic or motor neuropathies. Children may eat lead paint chips in old houses and develop acute encephalopathies. The signs may include generalized or focal seizures, ataxia, hemiplegia, decerebrate rigidity, lethargy, delirium, or coma.

270. The answer is E (all). (Musher, Ann Intern Med 113:872–881, 1990.) Tertiary syphilis, unlike secondary syphilis, is increased in HIV-positive patients because of the immunodeficiency. The CSF VDRL test is often negative in HIV-negative as well as HIV-positive patients (30 of 37 HIV-positive patients with neurosyphilis had a negative VDRL test in one study), which makes diagnosis difficult. In the HIV-positive patient, treatment with intravenous penicillin G, 2 to 4 million units every 4 h, is recommended, and on this regimen there are no known failures. The typical delay between primary and tertiary infection appears to be markedly reduced as evidenced by the increasing frequency of young people with tertiary syphilis. Neurosyphilis causes neuroretinitis, deafness, stroke, and acute meningitis. Meningovascular syphilis causes ischemic events and does occur in HIV patients. With syphilitic meningitis, patients present with typical meningitic complaints. Cranial nerve involvement also occurs; the IIIrd and VIIIth nerves are most commonly involved.

271. The answer is A (1, 2, 3). (Adams RD, 5/e, pp 232–233.) Diagnostic features of non-paralytic (concomitant) heterotropia include the following: (1) the degree of deviation remains the same throughout all directions of movement when both eyes are used; (2) each eye shows a full range of movement when the other is covered; (3) one eye frequently will show an opacity of the media or a severe refractive error; and (4) the patient does not complain of diplopia. In contrast, in paralytic heterotropia from a nerve lesion, the degree of deviation of the eyes increases as the eyes move in the direction of pull of the paretic muscle; the affected eye shows the same restriction of movement when used alone as when both eyes are used together; and the patient *will* complain of diplopia (at least if the nerve lesion occurred after infancy and the patient does not have suppression amblyopia).

272. The answer is B (1, 3). (Adams RD, 5/e, p 243.) Adie's syndrome consists of anisocoria, myotonic constriction following response to light accommodation, regular pupillary margin, normal response to mydriatics, and frequent association with hypoactive or absent muscle stretch reflexes. This benign, fairly common syndrome is to be distinguished from other causes of anisocoria, especially the pupillary abnormalities in syphilis in which the Argyll Robertson pupil may be associated with tabes dorsalis and absence of the muscle stretch reflexes. Usually Adie's syndrome is discovered incidentally during an examination for some other complaint. Patients with this syndrome are free of symptoms or complaints despite the pupillary abnormality and hypoactive muscle stretch reflexes.

273. The answer is C (2, 4). (Adams, 5/e, p 238.) Frenzel lenses (strong positive lenses) are placed over a patient's eyes during caloric irrigation in order to occlude visual fixation and to magnify the eye movements for ease of inspection. The strong lenses abolish visual acuity and prevent visual fixation, which inhibits nystagmus. Blocking of fixation by the Frenzel lenses permits faint nystagmus to appear. The strong lenses magnify the eye movements, making it possible to observe faint, low-amplitude nystagmus. The lenses neither produce pupilloconstriction nor abolish the vertigo that may accompany caloric nystagmus.

274. The answer is A (1, 2, 3). (Rowland, 9/e, pp 615–629.) Ragged red fibers are found in mitochondrial disorders. The abnormal mitochondria make muscle sections look like ragged red fibers on the Gomori trichrome stain. Mitochondrial disorders cause a wide spectrum of CNS and peripheral abnormalities. The MERRF (myoclonic epilepsy ragged red fibers) syndromes include ataxia. Kearns-Sayre syndrome is a progressive external ophthalmoplegia with cardiac conduction disturbances. Paroxysmal ataxia has no known physiologic, histologic, or biochemical marker.

275. The answer is A (1, 2, 3). (Rowland, 9/e, pp 891–894.) Patients with hyperthyroidism may have myasthenic weakness with pathologic fatigability, periodic weakness with low blood levels of potassium, and ophthalmoplegia. Enlarged, firm muscles occur in *hypo*thyroidism. The possibility of thyroid dysfunction should be considered if a patient displays any of these four types of muscle disorders. Enlarged, firm muscles may occur prior to the stage of atrophy in several disorders, including Duchenne's dystrophy, some muscle disorders with myotonia, and glycogen storage disease. The variety of muscle disorders found in association with thyroid disease indicates the importance of testing for thyroid dysfunction in patients who have muscle disorders of obscure origin.

276. The answer is A (1, 2, 3). (Rowland, 9/e, pp 618–621.) Progressive external ophthalmoplegia has been the subject of controversy for many years. At one time, it was considered to be an ocular form of progressive motor neuron degeneration, but now it is usually classified as a myopathy. The problem lies in interpreting neurogenic and myopathic changes in eye muscle biopsies. The disease does have an association with retinitis pigmentosa, far more so than do other forms of muscular dystrophy. Patients with progressive external ophthalmoplegia do not characteristically complain of, or present with, diplopia. The eyes may become completely immobile but generally remain in the primary position because all muscles are equally involved. This fact, in conjunction with the extremely gradual evolution of the disease, makes diplopia an uncommon complaint.

277. The answer is E (all). (Adams RD, 5/e, p 113.) It is well known that the bilirubin pigment from hemoglobin breakdown colors the CSF yellow. This occurs after blood enters the CSF. When protein levels exceed 150 to 200 mg/dL, a yellowish tint appears so that CSF below a spinal canal block from any cause may yield xanthochromic fluid. Less well known but occasionally of clinical importance is the fact that certain pigments in blood cross the blood-brain barrier and color the CSF. Hypercarotenemia (e.g., from ingestion of large amounts of carrots), marked jaundice, and rifampin all cause yellowing of the CSF.

278. The answer is B (1, 3). (Adams RD, 5/e, p 755.) The severity of the brain lesions caused by closed head injuries varies not only with the force but also with the location of impact and the direction. Linear impacts cause significantly less damage than those with an angular direction. Frontal impacts tend to cause injury mainly at the coup site, whereas posterior impacts tend to cause both coup and contrecoup injuries. Regardless of the site or direction of impact, however, most injuries occur in the frontal and temporal regions probably because the inferior surfaces of these regions slide along the irregularities of the skull.

279. The answer is B (1, 3). (DeAngelis, Neurology 41:619–621, 1991.) Primary central nervous system lymphomas are increasing in immunocompetent hosts. They are almost always periventricular and frequently involve the basal ganglia. They enhance diffusely with contrast and have little or no edema surrounding them. The tumors may be single or multiple and in 40 percent of cases lyse with steroids, which makes diagnosis impossible. Diagnosis requires a biopsy, which is best performed stereotactically since debulking of lymphomas does not enhance survival, unlike the case with gliomas.

280. The answer is C (2, 4). (Adams RD, 5/e, pp 1276–1277.) Myotonia usually decreases with increasing use of the involved muscle, is demonstrable by percussion, causes a distinctive EMG pattern, and occurs after a single contraction. These criteria serve to differentiate it from other types of cramps and contractures of the muscle. It is important to have positive criteria by which to identify myotonia because there are many other causes of muscle cramps. In addition, myotonia may be associated with weak muscles (as in myotonia dystrophica) or with strong muscles (as in myotonia congenita).

281. The answer is A (1, 2, 3). (Adams RD, 5/e, p 1136.) Diabetes is associated with an increased risk of all neuropathic conditions such as Bell's palsy and carpal tunnel syndromes. In addition to an axonal, primarily sensory neuropathy, diabetic men are commonly afflicted with impotence on a neurogenic or vascular basis. Diabetic amyotrophy is a particularly disabling problem with back pain, proximal leg weakness leading to atrophy, and a variable degree of sensory deficit. Diabetic third nerve palsies spare the pupils.

282–285. The answers are 282-A, 283-B, 284-C, 285-E. (Glaser, 2/e, pp 306–307.) The mnemonic for eye movements in response to caloric stimulation is "cows," meaning "cold opposite, warm same." The movements of the eyes refer to the direction of the nystagmus, labeled, by convention, for the direction of the fast phase. The fast phase is the nonvestibular phase and requires consciousness and an intact saccadic system. In PSP the saccadic system, which is the nonpursuit voluntary movement system, is nonfunctional. Eyes are maintained in the midline as the result, in part, of tonic firing of the vestibular apparatus. With cold water stimulation in the left ear, the nerve fires less and the eyes deviate conjugately to the left. The kickback phase, which is nonvestibular, is nonfunctional, so the eyes do not suddenly jerk back to primary position as occurs in an awake, intact patient. Warm water instilled in the right ear causes increased right nerve firing, which in turn causes the eyes to deviate to the left. Bilateral ear stimulation causes vertical movements, up for warm water and down for cold. The response to vestibular caloric stimulation in PSP is the same as the response in a comatose patient with intact brainstem reflexes.

286–289. The answers are 286-E, 287-A, 288-B, 289-C. (Adams RD, 5/e, pp 634–635, 1202–1209, 1220–1223.) Myotonic dystrophy is an autosomal dominantly inherited disorder that causes progressive weakness and myotonia. Tapping on muscle, particularly the tongue, causes the muscle to painlessly contract. It is often difficult for patients to relax muscles after prolonged contraction. The abnormal gene is located on chromosome 19 and causes widespread systemic abnormalities in the lens, endocrine glands, and skin as well as cardiac rhythm disturbances. The peculiar muscle wasting distribution causes a hatchetlike face due to masseter wasting. Ptosis, frontal baldness, wrinkled forehead, and slender mandible complete the facial changes.

Women develop polymyositis at twice the rate of men. It is a subacute progressive syndrome of weakness that causes pain in only about 15 percent of cases. Polymyositis generally develops in the age range of 30 to 60 but may occur outside of this. It can sometimes be difficult to distinguish clinically from limb girdle dystrophy when family history is lacking. Polymyositis is sometimes associated with systemic autoimmune disorders.

Trichinosis is a parasitic disease that, in the acute stage, affects muscles; it shows a predilection for the tongue, masseter, extraocular, and pharyngeal muscles. Involvement is initially painful and affected muscles are swollen. At presentation the face may be swollen as well. In addition the blood often reveals an eosinophilia. Generally the parasites become encysted and calcify and leave the patient asymptomatic.

The enzyme CPT is important in regulating long-chain fatty acids and its absence leads to deposition of lipid vacuoles in muscle fibers. Patients develop recurrent bouts of myoglobinuria starting in the first or second decades, precipitated by cold or a high-fat, low-carbohydrate diet. Between attacks of myoglobinuria the patients are normal, although exercise will cause elevated blood CPK levels.

290–293. The answers are 290-C, 291-A, 292-E, 293-D. (Adams RD, 5/e, pp 1015, 1025, 1030–1031.) Some disorders have well-established chromosomal anomalies and others, although unquestionably hereditary, have no obvious disorders in chromosome number or size. Trisomies and deletions are common disorders of chromosome number or size; of these, trisomies 13 and 21, XXY syndrome, and the 5 deletion syndrome (cri du chat) constitute some of the best known. Neurofibromatosis fails to show a gross disturbance of chromosomal morphology. It has, however, been classified into two forms. In type 1, the defect is on chromosome 17. This is the peripheral form with skin changes and subcutaneous tumors. Type 2, due to a defect on chromosome 22, is the central form and associated with acoustic neuromas. Holoprosencephaly may occur with a normal karyotype, but when a karyotype abnormality exists, it is usually trisomy 13 (although other errors also occur).

By knowing which disorders have gross chromosomal errors, a clinician can offer amniocentesis to mothers at risk for producing infants with that disorder, which allows elective abortion with an identifiable clinical syndrome of malformations. Not only do the affected persons exhibit a clinically recognizable set of external malformations, they often have visceral malformations as well. The majority of patients with gross abnormalities of chromosome number or morphology have some degree of mental deficiency. Thus, a chromosomal deviation may produce a defective brain, but no chromosomal abnormalities are known to be associated with superior intelligence.

PSYCHIATRY QUESTIONS FOR NEUROLOGISTS

Directions: Each item below contains five suggested responses. Select the **one best** response to each item.

294. The sudden onset of a confusional disorder, without language dysfunction and with minimal focal findings, may be seen with infarctions of the

(A) right occipital lobe
(B) right parietal lobe
(C) left parietal lobe
(D) left occipital lobe
(E) anterior cerebral artery

295. The production of motor stereotypies by chronic amphetamine use in humans and animals is thought to involve which of the following mechanisms?

(A) Stimulation of the cholinergic mechanism of the reticular activating system
(B) Inhibition of the inhibitory outflow from the Purkinje cells to the dentate nuclei
(C) Direct stimulation of neurons in the motor cortex
(D) Activation of the substantia nigra neurons
(E) Activation of the dopaminergic systems

296. All the following are useful in distinguishing psychogenic unresponsiveness from true coma EXCEPT

(A) roving eye movements
(B) absent reflexes
(C) cold caloric induced nystagmus
(D) eyelid closure after passive eyelid opening
(E) EEG

297. The most common psychiatric presentation for the AIDS-dementia complex is

(A) confabulation
(B) mania
(C) depression
(D) delirium
(E) focal abnormalities such as aphasia, denial, or neglect

298. According to current knowledge, the effect of bifrontal lesions (sparing the motor cortex) on human behavior is best described by which of the following statements?

(A) Bifrontal lesions are characterized by excessive eating, altered sleep cycles, and hypersexuality
(B) Bifrontal lesions may cause profound effects on behavior or personality, frequently with little effect on standard IQ tests
(C) Bifrontal lesions produce behavioral and personality alterations that cannot be produced by lesions elsewhere in the cerebrum
(D) Bifrontal lesions heighten self-awareness of bodily dysfunction
(E) A specific frontal lobe syndrome exists that can be recognized by characteristic neurologic signs

299. The most common mental abnormality on presentation with the Wernicke-Korsakoff syndrome is

(A) a global confusional state
(B) delirium with hallucinations
(C) impaired recent memory without confusion
(D) coma
(E) stupor

300. Which one of the following tricyclic antidepressant drugs has the greatest anticholinergic adverse effects?

(A) Desipramine
(B) Amitriptyline
(C) Clomipramine
(D) Maprotiline
(E) Amoxapine

301. Culture-bound psychiatric syndromes are disorders that are found in particular cultures. Which one of the following is an example of a culture-bound disorder in North America?

(A) Schizophrenia
(B) Posttraumatic stress disorder
(C) Autism
(D) Bulimia
(E) Conversion reactions

302. Light therapy has demonstrable efficacy in treating which one of the following disorders?

(A) "Sundowning"
(B) Melatonin-secreting pineal tumors
(C) The "vampire" schizophrenia syndrome
(D) Sleep fragmentation in Parkinson's disease
(E) Seasonal depression

303. Levodopa-induced hallucinations are usually

(A) auditory
(B) visual and threatening
(C) visual and nonthreatening
(D) auditory and visual
(E) highly idiosyncratic

304. The transient global amnesia syndrome may be explained on which of the following pathoanatomic bases?

(A) Infarction of the dentate gyrus
(B) Destruction of the mamillary bodies
(C) Lacunar state of the thalamus
(D) Degeneration of the hippocampal pyramidal cells
(E) None of the above

305. Fluent aphasic patients lose the ability to

(A) correct their own speech errors
(B) speak with prosody
(C) communicate by gesturing
(D) understand pantomime or gesture
(E) understand any spoken or written commands

306. The so-called paradoxical effect of medication in hyperactive children refers to which one of the following responses?

(A) Calming effect of drugs classed as stimulants
(B) Calming effect of phenobarbital
(C) Reduction in hyperactivity from benzodiazepines
(D) Proven adverse response to salicylates and red dyes
(E) Minimal response to alcohol as adults

307. The psychosis associated with chronic use of amphetamines resembles naturally occurring schizophrenia. Which of the following, however, is absent in the former?

(A) Paranoia
(B) Hallucinations
(C) Withdrawal and apathy
(D) Affective flattening and disordered thought associations
(E) Stereotyped movements, repetitive behaviors, and grimacing

308. A brief, counterproductive response to a stressful situation, such as a move or the loss of a job, would be classified as

(A) a brief psychotic episode
(B) an impulse dyscontrol
(C) an adjustment disorder
(D) an antisocial behavior disorder
(E) narcissism

309. A 30-year-old woman is referred for evaluation of "spells" during which she typically takes short trips and "awakens," hours later, amnestic for what has transpired. She has had many such episodes and has never been injured or gotten into trouble. She cannot identify precipitating factors. Findings with neurologic examination, brain CT, and EEG are normal. There is no history of substance abuse. The most pertinent historical data would most likely concern

(A) bed wetting
(B) a family history of similar behavior
(C) sleep disorders
(D) childhood sexual abuse
(E) seizure disorder

310. A 65-year-old man, while traveling on an overnight train trip, is arrested for fighting with another passenger late at night. This passenger, a stranger, reported that the man left his bunk, where he had apparently been sleeping, came over to the passenger, and began to hit him for no apparent reason. The 65-year-old man was wrestled to the ground, held for a minute or two, and then profusely apologized. He claimed to occasionally injure himself when he slept at night. Findings on EEG, brain imaging, and blood studies are normal. The most likely diagnosis is

(A) REM sleep disorder
(B) fugue states
(C) complex partial epilepsy
(D) substance abuse
(E) temporal lobe sclerosis

311. Of the five axes in the fourth edition of *Diagnostic and Statistical Manual of Mental Disorders* (*DSM IV*), the mental disorders are classified by

(A) I alone
(B) I and II
(C) II alone
(D) I, II, and III
(E) all five

312. Dissociative states and panic attacks are frequently seen in which of the following psychiatric disorders?

(A) Depression
(B) Mania
(C) Conversion reactions
(D) Posttraumatic stress disorder
(E) Gilles de la Tourette syndrome

313. A 50-year-old patient complains of increasing weakness of extremity and trunk muscles of several months' duration, with sparing of the cranial nerve muscles. Examination reveals proximal weakness and possibly atrophy, with preserved muscle stretch reflexes. EMG and muscle biopsy are normal. Screening tests for collagen-vascular disease are negative. Serum enzyme levels are normal. Results of a toxicology screen for heavy metals are negative. These findings warrant which of the following conclusions?

(A) Organic disease of the neuro-muscular system is excluded
(B) A lumbar puncture should be performed
(C) A myelogram should be performed
(D) A psychiatric consultation is required
(E) Thyroid function tests should be performed

314. An accurate description of stuttering is that

(A) it often begins in the first year of life
(B) there are usually other associated language disorders
(C) it usually is a manifestation of a neurotic or anxiety disorder
(D) it is a manifestation of a stressful upbringing
(E) true stuttering varies over time

315. A 25-year-old woman is brought to the ER for evaluation of a "spell" in which she suddenly, without apparent precipitating factors, felt fearful and expressed a feeling to her friend that she was about to die. Her pulse reportedly increased to 120 beats per minute as she became diaphoretic and dyspneic. Her friend reports that the patient had trouble talking during the spell, which lasted about 20 min. Findings in the ER examination are normal. The patient can only describe an overwhelming sense of imminent death associated with chest pressure. The most likely explanation is

(A) a psychomotor seizure
(B) a fugue state
(C) angina and possible myocardial infarct
(D) a drug high
(E) a panic attack

316. A 30-year-old woman reports developing progressive problems writing because her hand cramps. The results of her neurologic examination are normal, but you confirm that when she attempts to write, her hand cramps. She can use knives, forks, screwdrivers, and hairbrushes appropriately and has no difficulty performing delicate tasks. Your leading diagnosis would be

(A) malingering
(B) hysteria
(C) writer's cramp
(D) Hallervorden-Spatz disease
(E) reflex epilepsy

317. *DSM IV* defined all the currently known mental disorders. Since several are also considered neurologic, there is a possible discrepancy in diagnosis. For Gilles de la Tourette syndrome, what distinctions, if any, are there between the neurologic and psychiatric diagnoses?

(A) *DSM IV* requires vocal and motor tics; neurologists require only one type
(B) *DSM IV* requires presence of tics for longer than 1 year; neurologists do not
(C) *DSM IV* requires "marked distress or significant impairment" in social or other important areas of function; neurologists do not
(D) *DSM IV* requires concomitant attention-deficit or obsessive-compulsive disorder; neurologists do not
(E) There are no differences

318. A previously normal elderly man is brought to the emergency room for presumed intoxication. He denies all problems and wants to go home. Unfortunately he appears to be blind and bumps into objects and walls when allowed to walk alone. Otherwise his examination is normal, including that of his pupils and eye movements. Your leading diagnosis would be which one of the following?

(A) Posterior cerebral artery infarction
(B) Right parietal infarction
(C) Conversion reaction
(D) Glutethimide intoxication
(E) Methanol poisoning

319. A patient in a chronic care hospital was normal until middle age, when an acute but unknown illness caused him to become apathetic, hypersexual, aphasic, and amnestic. In addition he appeared to have difficulty interpreting how to use various objects, so that he needed to touch them and sometimes to put them into his mouth. The most likely cause of this syndrome is

    (A) schizophrenia
    (B) amphetamine use
    (C) MPTP
    (D) herpes simplex encephalitis
    (E) brain tumor

320. A teenaged boy has a violent temper that has gotten him arrested on several occasions. In each episode, he has abruptly assaulted his stepfather with seemingly little provocation. He has never assaulted anyone else. After the episodes he is sometimes amnestic and sometimes contrite. The likely explanation is

    (A) temporal lobe epilepsy
    (B) frontal lobe epilepsy
    (C) temporal lobe damage without seizures
    (D) bifrontal disease
    (E) none of the above

321. A 40-year-old man with a family history of Huntington's disease has become depressed. He had no children and wanted none. Evaluations by a psychiatrist and a neurologist find no evidence of Huntington's disease, and the depression appears to be reactive. The patient noted that his mother had developed the illness at his current age. The patient wanted to know if he carried the gene. The most appropriate step at this point is to

    (A) send his blood for gene testing
    (B) discourage him from testing since there is no risk of transmitting the disease
    (C) refer him to an approved genetic counseling program
    (D) treat his depression and re-evaluate
    (E) obtain an EEG to assess organicity

322. Which of the following disorders has the highest suicide rate?

    (A) Alzheimer's disease
    (B) Parkinson's disease
    (C) Amyotrophic lateral sclerosis (ALS)
    (D) Huntington's disease
    (E) Wernicke-Korsakoff syndrome (WKS)

323. Autism is a behavioral syndrome that

    (A) begins with a marked dissociation between motor skills and those of emotion and language
    (B) is seen in schizophrenia
    (C) is one aspect of catatonia
    (D) is a symptom of bifrontal disease
    (E) usually appears after age 2

324. A patient who has a basilar skull fracture complains that sounds seem uncomfortably loud. This symptom most probably represents

(A) a conversion reaction
(B) a partial lesion of the VIIIth cranial nerve
(C) a lesion of the transverse temporal gyri
(D) interruption of the lateral lemniscus
(E) paralysis of the stapedius muscle

325. A patient appears to have a right field cut. Despite being unable to read, she can write sentences, though minutes later she cannot read these sentences. The most likely explanation for this is

(A) hysteria
(B) a stroke or tumor in the left occiput
(C) conversion
(D) multiple lesions, either tumors or strokes, in both hemispheres
(E) a dominant thalamic infarct

326. A 4-year-old previously normal girl begins to display personality changes. Her parents feel that she does not walk as well as previously. The examination discloses slight clumsiness without overt motor signs. Stretch reflexes are somewhat hypoactive. The history and examination are otherwise noncontributory. The procedure most likely to yield a specific diagnosis is which of the following?

(A) CT scan with contrast
(B) Neuropsychological test battery
(C) Determination of karyotype
(D) Lysosomal enzyme battery
(E) Urinary amino acid screen

327. A *folie à deux* refers to which of the following?

(A) Close friendship between two actively psychotic persons
(B) Marriage between two manic-depressive persons when both are out of phase
(C) Poorly thought-out plan by two schizophrenic persons to accomplish a distinct goal
(D) Mutually self-destructive word contest engaged in by two schizophrenics
(E) Psychotic delusional system shared by two people

328. Which of the following is a defense process common in obsessive compulsive disorder and in which unacceptable impulses are transformed into their opposites?

(A) Intellectualization
(B) Displacement
(C) Reaction formation
(D) Sublimation
(E) Dissociation

Directions: Each item below contains four suggested responses of which **one or more** is correct. Select:

A   if   **1, 2, and 3**   are correct
B   if   **1 and 3**   are correct
C   if   **2 and 4**   are correct
D   if   **4**   is correct
E   if   **1, 2, 3, and 4**   are correct

329. Patients who are very likely to produce excessive countertransference in male physicians include which of the following?

(1) Patients with manic-depressive personalities
(2) Patients with antisocial personality disorders
(3) Middle-aged, overweight women who are given to complaining
(4) Attractive young women

330. The neuroleptic malignant syndrome should be treated with which of the following drugs?

(1) Benztropine
(2) Bromocriptine
(3) Valproic acid
(4) Dantrolene

331. Advantages of benzodiazepines as anti-anxiety agents include which of the following?

(1) Wide gap between effective doses and lethal doses
(2) Relatively low activation of hepatic microsomal enzymes
(3) Long duration of action
(4) Relatively low risk of producing physical tolerance

332. "Negative symptoms" in reference to schizophrenia include

(1) anhedonia
(2) obstinate and obstructive behavior
(3) poverty of thought
(4) refusal to acknowledge one's illness

333. Characteristic sleep disorders present in depression are

(1) increased sleep latency
(2) early morning awakening
(3) repeated awakening
(4) excessive sleep

334. A 60-year-old, previously healthy woman with no history of substance abuse, psychiatric problems, or family history of psychiatric dysfunction is brought to the emergency room because of abnormal behavior. She is agitated and acting in a bizarre manner but not hallucinating. Her vital signs and findings on physical examination are normal and she is fully oriented. The diagnosis is unlikely to be schizophrenia because of which of the following?

(1) Negative family history
(2) Absence of hallucination
(3) Good orientation
(4) Age

335. Correct statements concerning behavior modification therapy include which of the following?

(1) It regards behavior disorders as maladaptive learning
(2) It excludes the use of extinction techniques
(3) It ignores psychodynamic formulations
(4) It dispenses with desensitization techniques

336. Anticholinergic medications often cause which of the following side effects?

(1) Dry mouth
(2) Urinary retention
(3) Confusion
(4) Memory dysfunction

337. Gilles de la Tourette syndrome (GTS) is associated with which of the following neuropsychiatric disorders?

(1) Attention-deficit disorder
(2) Depression
(3) Obsessive-compulsive disorder
(4) Encopresis

338. Delusions of grandeur are frequently associated with

(1) mania
(2) L-dopa psychosis
(3) general paresis (neurosyphilis)
(4) lead encephalopathy

339. Rapid eye movement (REM) sleep has which of the following characteristics?

(1) It occurs cyclically throughout the night
(2) It exhibits low-voltage fast activity in the EEG
(3) It is associated with dreaming states
(4) It is useful in studying causes of impotence

340. Profound memory loss with little involvement of other mental functions is produced by bilateral damage to which of the following structures?

(1) Dorsomedial nuclei of the thalamus
(2) Ammon's horn and dentate gyrus
(3) Parahippocampal gyrus
(4) Fornix

341. Sleep paralysis is associated with which of the following characteristics?

(1) It occurs most commonly during transition to or from sleep
(2) It is initially associated with a strong feeling of fear
(3) It disappears when a person is called or touched
(4) It is associated with a shift of potassium into muscle

342. Statements that correctly describe the sexual consequences of neuroanatomic lesions include which of the following?

(1) Bilateral ventrolateral chordotomy usually causes loss of erection and ejaculation in males
(2) Destruction of the lumbar sympathetic ganglia causes loss of ejaculation but retention of erectile capacity
(3) Paraplegic males with complete cord transections may have intercourse and father children
(4) Destruction of the vulva or amputation of the penis prevents orgasm

SUMMARY OF DIRECTIONS

A	B	C	D	E
1,2,3	1,3	2,4	4	All are
only	only	only	only	correct

343. The ego, as defined by classical psychoanalytic formulations, is described as

(1) incorporating the reality-testing and cognitive functions

(2) incorporating the solution-forming, defense-creating aspects of the personality

(3) bringing about a *modus operandi* for perceiving and relating to other persons

(4) containing the internalized ideal of what the person should be like

344. The narcolepsy syndrome typically includes which of the following?

(1) Irresistible sleep under inappropriate circumstances

(2) Cataplexy

(3) Hypnagogic hallucinations and sleep paralysis

(4) Episodic automatic behavior with amnesia

345. Statements that correctly describe the characteristics of the amnesia associated with head trauma and a period of unconsciousness include which of the following?

(1) The period of retrograde amnesia is usually shorter than the anterograde amnesia

(2) After recovering consciousness, a patient may seem rational and coherent for days or weeks yet fail to remember the period of unconsciousness

(3) Frequently, the period of retrograde amnesia shrinks during recovery

(4) The retrograde and anterograde aspects of amnesia differ greatly in comparing posttraumatic amnesia with amnesia associated with psychomotor seizures

346. Clinical features that help to establish a diagnosis of pseudodementia in elderly patients include a tendency on the part of such patients to

(1) complain greatly about loss of mental faculties

(2) exhibit low attention span and concentration

(3) exert little effort to perform on formal tests

(4) display behavior that is poor relative to mental function

347. As classically defined, Gerstmann's syndrome includes

(1) right-left disorientation
(2) digital agnosia
(3) acalculia
(4) agraphia

348. Visual hallucinations in an otherwise neurologically intact person can be induced by diseases affecting

(1) both retinas
(2) the bilateral vitreous humor
(3) the optic tract
(4) the occipital cortex

349. Psychedelic or hallucinogenic drugs are characterized by which of the following features?

(1) They produce heightened awareness of sensory input
(2) They have a strong tendency to cause addiction and continued use
(3) They are generally classified as indoleamines or phenyethylamines
(4) They are a common cause of auditory hallucinations

350. A 30-year-old man was involved in a minor car accident in which he struck his head and seemed transiently stunned. He did not lose consciousness and was able to get out of his car within seconds according to reliable observers. When the police arrived at the scene, the man could not recall the accident and did not know where he was or what his name was. He seemed otherwise normal. Likely diagnoses include

(1) postictal confusional state
(2) malingering
(3) postconcussive syndrome
(4) fugue state

Directions: Each group of questions below consists of lettered options followed by a set of numbered items. For each numbered item, select the **one** lettered option with which it is **most** closely associated. Each lettered option may be used **once, more than once, or not at all.**

Items 351–354

Match each description with the appropriate personality disorder.

    (A) Passive-aggressive
    (B) Inadequate
    (C) Antisocial
    (D) Obsessive-compulsive
    (E) Schizoid

351. Isolated and secretive; few friends; aloof with diminished emotional responsiveness

352. Meticulous; perfectionist; excessive concern about self-image and standards; inflexible

353. Dependent; unable to meet deadlines or responsibilities; always "falling apart"

354. Impulsive; relatively guilt-free; tendency to blame others; unwilling to obey social rules and conventions

Items 355–358

For each example of a mental defense mechanism, choose the term with which it is most closely associated.

(A) Fixation
(B) Regression
(C) Identification
(D) Projection
(E) Rationalization

355. A shy young man, formerly only moderately interested in athletics, begins to practice throwing a football and frequently organizes touch football games among acquaintances who then become friends. He has his hair cut in the style of Joe Namath and assumes that athlete's mannerisms. When he has a T-shirt imprinted with the great quarterback's number, his new friends nickname him Junior Joe

356. A young woman with a large sexual appetite is married to a man whom she loves and with whom she feels basically compatible. While he is struggling to make a success of a business, she engages in a series of affairs with a variety of men. By most criteria, the husband does not neglect his wife, who nevertheless believes that her husband is more interested in his business than in her. She ascribes her many sexual affairs to traits in her husband rather than in herself

357. A soldier inflicts a wound on himself to escape front-line duty during a war. Later he feels guilty. To ward off the painful resultant anxiety, the soldier blames his physician for neglecting to treat the wound (which is slow to heal) and tries to kill him. The soldier is not consciously aware that, in trying to kill his physician, he is attempting to destroy his own actual deficiencies

358. A 3-year-old child is fully toilet-trained until a sibling is born, whereupon he starts to have toileting accidents and to wet the bed at night

Items 359–362

For each definition below, choose the term with which it is most closely associated.

(A) Palinopsia
(B) Visual allesthesia
(C) Micropsia
(D) Simultagnosia
(E) Dyschromatopsia

359. Any defect in the perception of color

360. The persistence or recurrence of visual images after the stimulus object has been removed

361. Inability to organize a series of related pictures into the correct sequence or to understand the full meaning of a series of perceived parts

362. The displacement of a visual image from the visual field of perception into the opposite visual field

Items 363–366

For each clinical description below, choose the term with which it is most closely identified.

(A) Broca's aphasia
(B) Conduction aphasia
(C) Transcortical motor aphasia
(D) Anomic aphasia
(E) Transcortical sensory aphasia

363. Nonfluent spontaneous speech; good repetition and comprehension but poor naming

364. Fluent spontaneous speech; good repetition and comprehension but poor naming

365. Nonfluent spontaneous speech; good comprehension but poor repetition and variable naming

366. Fluent spontaneous speech; good comprehension, variable naming, and poor repetition

Items 367–370

For each clinical description given below, choose the term with which it is most closely associated.

    (A) Negativism
    (B) Catalepsy
    (C) Gegenhalten
    (D) Rigidity
    (E) Catatonia

367. A patient sits quietly, mute and motionless, making no movement of body or face and showing little reaction to environmental events or stimuli, while the eyes remain fixed on a distant point; this behavior alternates with periods of overactivity

368. A patient shows slight resistance to movement but then maintains the body parts in any new position the examiner places them in

369. A patient shows plastic resistance to movement of the body parts in any direction, as if automatically resisting whatever movement the examiner imposes

370. A patient actively resists any effort to be moved or to move in response to command

Items 371–374

For each clinical feature described below, choose the speech disorder with which it is most closely associated.

    (A) Elective mutism
    (B) Palilalia
    (C) Cluttering
    (D) Aphemia
    (E) Perseveration

371. A patient repeats the last syllable of words or the last phrase

372. A patient runs words together, omitting sounds or entire words

373. A patient talks to selected persons but, under certain circumstances, may fail to speak at all to others

374. A patient suddenly loses the ability to say any words but remains alert and able to understand, read, and write

Items 375–380

For each stage of sleep or wakefulness listed, choose the EEG pattern with which it most nearly corresponds.

sponds.

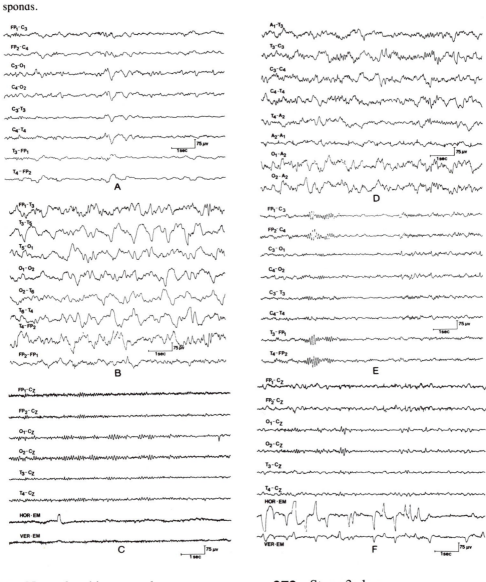

375. Normal waking record

376. Stage 1 sleep

377. Stage 2 sleep

378. Stage 3 sleep

379. Stage 4 sleep

380. REM sleep

PSYCHIATRY QUESTIONS FOR NEUROLOGISTS

ANSWERS

294. The answer is B. (Mesulam, J Neurol Neurosurg Psychiatry 39:84–89, 1976.) Right parietal infarctions may present with confusional syndromes and little in the way of focal weakness or obvious signs of neglect and denial. Sometimes testing of these patients is incomplete because of their poor level of cooperation, but even after resolution of the acute state, patients often do not reveal clear signs of laterality on examination. The acute onset of confusional states in the elderly should always raise the possibility of a new infarction.

295. The answer is E. (Hardman, 9/e, pp 219–221.) Chronic use of amphetamines in humans or experimental animals results in a motor syndrome characterized by repetitive, stereotyped behaviors. The production of stereotyped behaviors in this situation is believed to result from activation of the dopaminergic systems. These systems arise in either the zona compacta of the substantia nigra where they end in the striatum, or in the interpeduncular region where they play upon the medial basal olfactory and limbic structures. The amphetamine appears to act by increasing the release of dopamine and blocking its reuptake, making more of it available at the postsynaptic ending. L-Dopa and methylphenidate produce a similar movement disorder.

296. The answer is B. (Plum, 3/e, pp 306–308.) Psychogenic unresponsiveness can be documented using several tests. If the patient is truly awake, the EEG should show normal awake activity, although rarely, an EEG may be normal in coma (alpha coma). In awake patients cold water in the ear produces nystagmus with the fast component away from the ear, whereas coma patients either do not react or one or both eyes slowly deviate to the cold water in a smooth fashion. Roving eye movements cannot be simulated by awake persons as voluntary nonpursuit eye movements are saccadic. Eyelid closure in comatose patients occurs in a slow, steady fashion that awake patients cannot mimic. Deep tendon reflexes can be suppressed and can even be absent or asymmetric.

297. The answer is C. (Simpson. Ann Intern Med 121:769–785, 1994.) It is common early in the development of the AIDS-dementia complex for patients to be depressed. It can be impossible to distinguish a reactive depression due to the presence of the disease itself from an "organic" depression due to HIV infection in the brain. Although the presence of dementia may be a helpful diagnostic clue, this may be very mild and difficult to distinguish from pseudodementia due to the depression. MRI may be helpful in making the diagnosis, whereas spinal fluid analysis may not because the HIV antigen may be present in the CSF of AIDS patients without the AIDS-dementia complex.

298. The answer is B. (Adams RD, 5/e, pp 386–390.) While it has long been recognized that bifrontal lesions may profoundly alter behavior and personality, the type and specificity of change remain in question. Similar changes may follow diffuse brain disease or diencephalic lesions. Patients with bifrontal lesions tend to exhibit a syndrome of apathy and indifference that reduces their regard for and concern about bodily dysfunctions. Thus, after a prefrontal lobotomy, chronic cancer patients still report pain but seem to have an attitude of indifference toward it. Yet the results are not always predictable. Some patients with bifrontal lesions become hypomanic or even have a transient state of compulsive walking and may become sexually overactive. In spite of the obvious clinical changes in behavior, patients with bifrontal lesions may score normally on IQ tests; indeed, the failure of routine IQ tests to show the specific effects of frontal lesions and frontal lobotomies was one of the historical reasons for the development of neuropsychology.

299. The answer is A. (Victor, 2/e, pp 17, 39–52.) Wernicke-Korsakoff syndrome is a clinical triad consisting of ataxia, oculomotor abnormalities, and mental status impairment, though all three signs may not be present. In 229 patients with the Wernicke-Korsakoff syndrome, 56 percent had a global confusional state at the time of presentation compared with 16 percent with delirium tremens, 5 percent with stupor or coma, and 10 percent without mental abnormality. Although 57 percent had a prominent memory impairment, many of these patients were also confused. Upon resolution of the acute syndrome, some patients return to normal but most evolve into a Korsakoff syndrome, characterized by a retrograde memory loss for months or years prior to onset of the illness and anterograde amnesia.

300. The answer is B. (Kaplan, Synopsis, 7/e, p 992.) Amitripytline has more muscarinic anticholinergic effects than any other available tricyclic antidepressant. As such, it is often used for treating depression in Parkinson's disease, where the anticholinergic effects are mildly helpful for treating the tremor, drooling, and hyperactive bladder often present. Amoxapine is the only tricyclic that also has antidopaminergic effects.

301. The answer is D. (Kaplan, Synopsis, 7/e, pp 189–191.) There are multiple psychiatric disorders that appear to be restricted to a single culture or a few related cultures. Eating disorders such as bulimia and anorexia are very much Western-oriented problems related to Western values of body image and striving towards thinness. Other cultures have syndromes virtually unknown in most Western cultures, such as *amok*, a sudden rampage that occurs in Malaysia, or *koro*, an Asian fear that the penis will withdraw into the abdomen and cause death. A condition such as *nervios*, seen in Latin America, is also common in North America; this manifests as anxiety and depression.

302. The answer is E. (Kaplan, Synopsis, 7/e, p 1011.) Seasonal affective disorder (SAD) is a depressive syndrome occurring predominantly in women with median age of onset of 40. The depression correlates with winter's onset and is associated with fatigue, hypersomnia, hyperphagia, carbohydrate craving, and irritability. Many published studies attest to the benefits of light therapy. The light must be bright and should simulate natural sunlight. Standard indoor lights, even when very bright, have no effect.

303. The answer is C. (Goetz, Am J Psychiatry 139:494–497, 1982.) Levodopa hallucinations are fairly common but occur mainly in older patients with some degree of cognitive dysfunction, although this is not always the case. The hallucinations may be threatening, but this is extremely uncommon; they are mainly nonthreatening and visual. It is common to hallucinate about children, friendly strangers, or occasionally relatives. The hallucinations may occur in a clear or clouded sensorium and may or may not be recognized as hallucinatory in origin by the patient.

304. The answer is E. (Adams RD, 5/e, pp 373–374.) Transient global amnesia occurs in middle-aged and elderly persons. The patient loses memory for a period of several hours but retains consciousness and many cognitive abilities. Although the differential diagnosis of this condition includes psychomotor seizures, the pathologic substrate remains to be identified. The best surmise is that the syndrome represents a type of transient ischemic attack involving territories irrigated by the posterior cerebral artery, which supplies the inferomedial aspect of the temporal lobes and sends arcades to the hippocampus. The syndrome usually does not recur and does not increase the risk for stroke.

305. The answer is A. (Adams RD, 5/e, pp 418–419.) Among other speech deficits experienced by fluent aphasic patients is the inability to correct their own speech errors and, frequently, the failure even to perceive them. Such patients produce an excess of words that are often composed of unrelated syllables (a word salad). The fluent aphasic patient retains the ability to speak with prosody (the normal inflections and rhythms) but loses the faculty to control *content* of speech. Also retained are the ability to understand certain written or spoken commands and a limited ability to communicate by gestures.

306. The answer is A. (Adams RD, 5/e, p 521.) A paradox about hyperactive children (as has been stated in the past) is the observation that drugs classed as stimulants seemed to improve the cardinal symptoms of hyperactivity, impulsiveness, short attention span, and hyperexcitability. Contrarily, drugs that should have sedative action, such as the barbiturates, frequently worsen the target symptoms. One resolution of the paradox lies in the interpretation of the state of arousal. The hyperactivity might be interpreted as a reaction to a *hypo*aroused nervous system. The stimulant drug normalizes the arousal and eliminates the compensating overactive behavior. Barbiturates would further reduce the state of arousal and cause the target symptoms to become correspondingly worse. This formulation might aid in selecting children who could benefit from stimulant medication by subjecting them to tests for hypoarousal.

307. The answer is D. (Kaplan, Synopsis, 7/e pp 413–414.) The chronic abuse of amphetamines may produce a paranoid psychosis that very closely resembles the naturally occurring disease. This psychosis is characterized by paranoid ideation, many stereotypies and mannerisms, hallucinations, and, in the later stages, withdrawal and apathy. Affective flattening and disorders of thought association, which characterize the naturally occurring disease, are absent with the amphetamine-associated psychosis. Amphetamine administration to other primates produces the same motor disturbances seen in humans.

308. The answer is C. (Kaplan, Synopsis, 7/e, p 727.) Adjustment disorders, which are very common, are seen more in females and teenagers than in others. Precipitating stresses include problems with socialization at school, academics, divorce, and drug abuse. Business setbacks, particularly the loss of a job, are common precipitants. The adjustment disorders are classified by the nature of the main maladaptive symptom, such as adjustment disorder with depression, with anxiety, with disturbance of content, and so on. The reaction usually resolves within 3 months.

309. The answer is D. (Kaplan, Synopsis, 7/e, p 789.) The most likely diagnosis of these spells is fugue, a dissociative state. This is much more common in women and is frequently associated with a childhood history of sexual abuse. Sleep disorders such as REM behavioral disorder are much shorter and do not involve sophisticated behaviors. Bed wetting could be a seizure phenomenon. Seizures do not last long enough to cause the picture described aside from the rarely encountered psychomotor status epilepticus with primarily psychiatric signs.

310. The answer is A. (Daly, 2/e, pp 587–588.) REM sleep disorder is a relatively recently described syndrome in which the affected person is not paralyzed during the dreaming portion (REM) of sleep, as is normal. As a result, these people will act out portions of their dreams and tend to injure themselves by getting out of bed or hitting furniture adjacent to the bed. Fugue states are dissociative states that occur while the person is awake and tend to be prolonged. Complex partial seizures tend to be brief and rarely, if ever, cause directed violence. Temporal lobe scarring can produce a host of abnormal behaviors, but all while the person is awake. Substance abuse usually causes a more prolonged behavioral change. REM behavior disorder typically affects men over the age of 60 who have no prior psychiatric or neurologic problems. It occurs in the last third of the night and involves "wild dream enactments" that are frequently violent.

311. The answer is B. (Kaplan, Synopsis, 7/e, pp 315–316.) *DSM IV* classifies all known psychiatric disorders based on purely descriptive rather than theoretical terms. It contains five axes. Axis I contains the clinical syndromes while axis II describes the developmental and personality disorders. Axis III lists all physical disorders whether related or not, axis IV rates psychosocial stressors, and axis V is a global assessment of the patient's highest level of function during the preceding year. Thus axes I and II are the only ones that list psychiatric diagnoses.

312. The answer is D. (Kaplan, Synopsis, 7/e, pp 609–610.) Posttraumatic stress disorder covers a wide range of problems that occur after severe psychological trauma. It was called "shell shock" during World War I but not adequately studied until the Vietnam War. The abnormality extends to all traumatizing events "outside the range of usual human experience, that would be markedly distressing to almost anyone," such as incest, rape, seeing a murder, and so on. The subject often re-experiences the event and undergoes a process of numbing. Dissociative episodes, in which patients experience fugue states, may occur, as well as panic, guilt, humiliation, illusions, and delusions. Sometimes the dissociative episodes may be described in ways that suggest complex partial seizures.

313. The answer is E. (Adams, 5/e, pp 1233–1234.) Thyrotoxic myopathy may present with weakness but few other physical or laboratory signs. The affected patient may have none of the classic historical or physical findings of hyperthyroidism. Standard laboratory tests such as EMG and muscle biopsy may fail to show distinct abnormalities. All patients with chronic unexplained weakness should have thyroid function studies. This diagnosable and potentially treatable cause of weakness should not be overlooked. The blood tests for thyroid function are very inexpensive and carry no risk for the patient other than those associated with venipunctures. Since the threat to life arises from involvement of cardiac or respiratory muscles, the affected patient should be carefully followed by clinical examination and laboratory tests for cardiac and pulmonary complications of the disease.

314. The answer is E. (Kaplan, Synopsis, 7/e, p 1097.) There are no data to connect stuttering with any psychiatric disorder, except secondarily; that is, stuttering is not the result of a stressful upbringing or a manifestation of anxiety or neurosis. Anxiety may, however, worsen stuttering, and stutterers, like others with language disorders, have an increased incidence of depression and anxiety. Stuttering generally begins between 18 months and 9 years of age with peaks at 2, 3, 5, and 5 to 7 years. Ambidextrous and left-handed persons are at greater risk for the development of stuttering.

315. The answer is E. (Kaplan, Synopsis, 7/e, p 586.) Panic attacks, by *DSM IV* definition, initially appear in an unprovoked manner. The attacks may take on a pattern. At the onset there is a sense of fear and imminent death, lasting about 10 min. Hyperventilation, perceived by the patient as shortness of breath, is frequently associated with chest pressure, tachycardia, and diaphoresis. The patient has impaired memory and difficulty communicating, probably due in large part to the limited ability to concentrate. Attacks generally last 20 to 30 min but may last for an hour. Syncope may occur during a panic attack.

316. The answer is C. (Adams RD, 5/e, p 96.) Writer's cramp is a form of focal dystonia in which the hand involuntarily cramps when writing. There are two forms of this condition. In simple writer's cramp, the dystonia occurs with writing but with no other maneuvers. In the other form, various activities will induce the dystonia. Similar conditions occur in skilled workers who perform repetitive maneuvers, such as musicians. Of note in writer's cramp is the fact that it transfers sides in a significant percentage of those persons who learn to write using their unaffected hand.

317. The answer is C. (APA, DSM IV, 307.23. Erenberg, Arch Neurol 53:588, 1996.) Although there is no "bible" or diagnostic criteria comparable to *DSM IV* for neurologists, many syndromes have "generally accepted" criteria. For Tourette syndrome, both neurologists and psychiatrists require both motor and vocal tics, present for a year or more without other apparent cause (e.g., tardive tics). *DSM IV* does not require concomitant psychiatric problems but does require onset before age 18 and the presence of "marked distress or significant impairment" in some sphere of activity as a result of the tics. This concept has been rejected by neurologic experts, who point out that Tourette syndrome is often hereditary and that one frequently finds family members with marked differences in severity of disease, some suffering marked distress and others not, though they clearly share the same gene. Arbitrary classification of some affected persons as having Tourette syndrome and others as not, based on severity of tics and secondary psychological problems, runs counter to most modern concepts of disease.

318. The answer is A. (Adams RD, 5/e, p 400.) This patient clearly suffers from a visual anosognosia. The occurrence of cortical blindness (normal pupils) with denial of the problem is the syndrome of Anton, due to posterior cerebral infarction involving the occipital cortex and the visual association cortex as well. The denial is very similar to that seen with right middle cerebral artery infarcts in which patients deny their weakness and occasionally even deny body parts.

319. The answer is D. (Kaplan, Synopsis, 7/e, pp 106–107.) The syndrome described is the human analogue to the Klüver-Bucy syndrome in primates. If both medial temporal lobes are resected in a primate, it becomes apathetic and hypersexual and develops agnosias, so that the animal mouths every object. In humans the syndrome is somewhat different and includes aphasia, dementia, and bulimia without the constant mouthing of objects. A bilateral medial temporal lobe deficit in humans is most likely to occur with herpes simplex encephalitis.

320. The answer is E. (Weiger, J Psychiatr Res 22:85–98, 1988.) Directed rage attacks are not a feature of epilepsy. While rare convulsions involve violence, these are typically undirected attacks. In patients with interictal violent behavior, there tends to be a strong emotional feeling attached, either justification or remorse, whereas this patient was only sometimes remorseful. He always attacked a single person, which suggests an emotional problem rather than a nonspecific convulsive attack. After episodic rage attacks, patients may have variable degrees of amnesia.

321. The answer is C. (Bird, Ann Neurol 38:141–146, 1995.) Although this patient is depressed and at risk for Huntington's disease (HD), he has none of the stigmata of the disease. Only patients with signs of HD can be tested directly. Patients who are at risk without clear evidence of psychosis, dementia, chorea, personality change, or some other tangible sign must undergo genetic counseling before having their test performed. The decision to undergo testing in a symptomatic patient is entirely the patient's, so long as the patient understands the risks of learning of a positive result.

322. The answer is D. (Adams RD, 5/e, p 971.) Although Parkinson's disease and early Alzheimer's disease are frequently associated with depression, there is not a known increased rate of suicide. In patients with Huntington's disease, however, there is a very high suicide rate, possibly due to the combination of depression and impulsivity. ALS patients are not similarly afflicted. WKS patients are not particularly depressed, but rather apathetic and unlikely to be suicidal.

323. The answer is A. (Adams, 5/e, p 519.) Although the pathology is not defined, autism is undoubtedly an organic developmental disorder. It has two peaks of onset (or recognition): one noted soon after birth and one at about 18 months. Children have normal motor skills, but language use is minimal and emotional attachments are seemingly nonexistent. Self-stimulatory, stereotypic behaviors, sometimes self-injurious, are common. While schizophrenics and catatonics may display behavioral abnormalities similar to those seen in autism, they are not autistic.

324. The answer is E. (Adams RD, 5/e, p 1174.) A patient who complains of uncomfortable loudness of sounds (hyperacusis) may have paralysis of the stapedius muscle. This tiny muscle dampens the vibrations of the ossicles and may act as a protective mechanism or modulator of the amplitude of vibrations transmitted to the inner ear. The stapedius muscle receives its innervation from the VIIth nerve. Either the VIIth nerve or its stapedius branch may be damaged by a basilar skull fracture. Trauma may also affect hearing by disarticulating the ossicles; this results in fuzzing or duplication of sound (diplacusis), which may also reflect damage to the inner ear.

325. The answer is B. (Adams, 5/e, p 421.) Alexia without agraphia describes a so-called disconnection syndrome in which one language function, in this case reading, is disconnected from the expressive speech centers. The lesions are usually in the left occipital lobe, interrupting the connections of the left visual cortex and deeper white matter tracts that interrupt the connections of the right visual cortex with the left-sided language centers.

326. The answer is D. (Adams RD, 5/e, pp 558–561.) A child with personality changes, gait disturbance, and hypoactive stretch reflexes may be showing signs of a progressive degenerative disease. The combination of a possible central and peripheral nervous system disorder as evidenced by these clinical findings should, first of all, suggest metachromatic leukodystrophy. Because the child described in the question is a girl, Pelizaeus-Merzbacher disease and adrenoleukodystrophy are virtually excluded because both have a sex-linked recessive inheritance pattern. The child's age of 4 years excludes Krabbe's globoid leukodystrophy, and her normal somatotype virtually rules out a mucopolysaccharidosis. The normal physical appearance of the child and the absence of malformations, along with the normal period of development, all virtually exclude the possibility of a chromosomal error. The normal retina argues against cerebromacular degeneration. Her previously normal mental state and lack of seizures exclude the usual amino acid disorders. The lysosomal enzyme battery will include tests for deficiency of aryl sulfatase A, which will lead to the specific diagnosis of metachromatic leukodystrophy.

327. The answer is E. (Kaplan, Synopsis, 7/e, pp 491–492.) *Folie à deux* is a rare disorder that is usually restricted to two people but can involve more. Typically, in a long-standing relationship one person, the more dominant one, becomes psychotic and gradually brings the more submissive person into the psychosis so that the two share the same delusional system. This has been called "infectious insanity." In some cases the shared psychosis develops simultaneously in two closely associated persons.

328. The answer is C. (Kaplan, Synopsis, 7/e, pp 250–251.) Displacement refers to a process in which an emotion related to one idea or object is shifted to another that bears some resemblance to the original. Sublimation is a defense process that allows one to achieve gratification through achievement of more acceptable goals than those actually desired. Dissociation is a major alteration of a person's character to avoid emotional distress, often without memory for the alteration, as with fugue states. Intellectualization is a defense process in which emotions are avoided through a highly rationalized and intellectual interpretation of events.

329. The answer is E (all). (Kaplan, Synopsis, 7/e, p 7.) Many patients will incite an excessive emotional response—*countertransference*, as Freud called it—in their physicians. The intensity of the response may then interfere with the physician's objectivity, professional judgment, and ability to treat the patient. Among these patients are those who suffer from manic-depressive psychosis. When manic, they may focus with unremitting zeal on generating antagonisms and difficulties. When depressed, they become mute and withdrawn, manifesting tenacious expressions of pain and anguish, powerless to help themselves or others. For male physicians, the nonpsychotic, overweight, complaining, pain-ridden woman in her forties offers a similar challenge because she is almost invariably depressed. A different problem is presented by the young, physically attractive sociopathic woman who, seemingly cheerful, rational, contrite, and cooperative while hospitalized, may excite the rescue fantasies of the physician who feels he has finally found a responsive patient. Deceived into placing undue trust in his patient, the physician unwisely grants her a week-end pass from the hospital, whereupon she resumes her sociopathic behavior. A similar countertransference may occur on the part of a physician for the attractive young woman who may excite his sexual fantasies, causing the physician to become entrapped in her seductive behavior.

330. The answer is C (2, 4). (Adams, 5/e, p 1339.) The neuroleptic malignant syndrome is a life-threatening complication of dopamine-blocking drugs and is also sometimes seen with abrupt withdrawal of L-dopa in Parkinson's disease. It is characterized by high fevers without other explanation, extrapyramidal signs (usually rigidity), autonomic instability, and mental status changes, usually obtundation. The object of treatment is to offset the dopamine deficiency, which is most readily done with a direct dopamine agonist. Dantrolene acts peripherally to loosen the muscles and thereby reduce the fever and the often massive elevations of CPK. Because dantrolene does not act on the brain, where the problem is, it is a second-line drug after bromocriptine or one to be used in concert with bromocriptine.

331. The answer is E (all). (Kaplan, Synopsis, 7/e, pp 906–914.) Benzodiazepines have become the most frequently prescribed antianxiety medication. Although overused, they do have specific advantages when they are indicated. These advantages include a wide gap between the effective and lethal doses, low activation of hepatic microsomal enzymes, long duration of action (around 24 h), and relatively low production of physical tolerance. The low activation of hepatic microsomal enzymes means that the benzodiazepines produce little alteration in the metabolism of drugs such as coumarin, antipsychotic agents, tricyclic antidepressants, and certain anticonvulsants, all of which are acted on by these enzymes. The benzodiazepines will, however, add to the pharmacologic effects of other medications, such as increasing the sedation caused by anticonvulsants or alcohol.

332. The answer is B (1,3). (APA, DSM IV, 295.XX.) Schizophrenia is characterized by major problems in interaction with the real external world. Patients have positive symptoms, which are symptoms "added" to normal function, such as excessive and uncontrollable thoughts, hallucinations, grandiose delusions, paranoid delusions, and excess energy and activity. They also have negative symptoms, such as lack of energy, pleasure (anhedonia), emotions, and thoughts. Loss of insight is not generally considered a negative symptom because a patient may, out of grandiosity, be convinced that he is simply an unrecognized genius or God incarnate. Obstinate behavior is called *negativism*.

333. The answer is A (1, 2, 3). (Kaplan, Synopsis, 7/e, p 520.) Mood disorders are frequently associated with sleep disorders. The severity of the sleep disorder frequently parallels that of the mood disorder. Depression is associated with normal or increased latency of falling asleep, repeated awakenings during the night, and early morning awakenings. Patients also have shorter-than-normal latencies for developing REM sleep.

334. The answer is D (4). (Kaplan, Synopsis, 7/e, p 461.) Schizophrenia typically occurs in the late teens or early twenties. Onset after age 50 is very rare. Primary psychotic patients are usually completely oriented and, if their attention can be engaged long enough, can score perfectly on a mini-mental status examination. This is one of the distinguishing points between encephalopathic or delirious states and psychosis. Secondary psychoses (e.g., drug-induced as with LSD, PCP) generally have visual hallucinations rather than auditory, although chronic alcoholism may induce auditory hallucinations. Family history is frequently not positive in schizophrenia, and hallucinations are not required for diagnosis. In this patient, a secondary psychosis or manic depression, not schizophrenia, must be considered.

335. The answer is B (1, 3). (Kaplan, Synopsis, 7/e, pp 852–856.) Behavior modification is a system of therapy that regards maladaptive behavior as a type of learning disorder. It is assumed that the behavior is perpetuated by environmental contingencies that should be investigated. Behavior therapists attempt neither to formulate the psychodynamics of the behavior nor to rely on insight techniques. They do use extinction techniques (the ignoring by staff and family of unwanted behavior), although there is disagreement about their role. Behavior modification therapists also have tried to treat phobias by desensitization. After a therapist has determined the stimuli that elicit the unwanted behavior, patient and therapist construct a series of scenes that recapitulate the precipitating stimuli. After the patient has been taught deep muscular relaxation, the offending stimulus is conjured by means of mental images. The muscular relaxation is considered to be the means for deconditioning the anxiety initiated by the stimulus.

336. The answer is E (all). (Kaplan, Synopsis, 7/e, p 898.) Acetylcholine receptors are nicotinic (found in skeletal muscle) and muscarinic (central and peripheral). Anticholinergic drugs are antimuscarinic and have a plethora of side effects. They block innervation of the salivary glands and thus cause dryness of the mouth. They inhibit the brain's cholinergic system, which is important in memory, so that memory impairment is relatively common among the elderly. Antimuscarinic drugs inhibit detrusor muscle contraction, thereby increasing the possibility of urinary retention. The drugs also may produce confusion and hallucinations.

337. The answer is B (1, 3). (Rowlands, 9/e, pp 704–705.) Approximately half the children diagnosed with GTS also suffer from attention-deficit and hyperactivity disorder. About 40 percent suffer from obsessive-compulsive disorder. These neuropsychiatric disorders need not be present in a person with motor and vocal tics and may be inherited independently of the tics themselves. Although GTS patients may become depressed, depression is neither inherited nor a particularly common element of the syndrome. Encopresis is a psychiatric disorder in which children defecate inappropriately and is not a feature of GTS. Coprolalia, the involuntary use of obscenities, is occasionally present with GTS.

338. The answer is B (1, 3). (Adams RD, 5/e, pp 624, 1317.) Mania is associated with feelings of unbounded energy and frequently with delusions of omnipotence or omniscience. General paresis of the insane was a common cause of chronic psychiatric hospitalization in the preantibiotic era, and these patients frequently developed, in addition to a slowly progressive dementia, a delusional system in which they were kings or presidents with great powers. L-Dopa produces a wide variety of psychoses, but the most common are paranoid. Lead causes apathy and irritability.

339. The answer is E (all). (Rowland, 9/e, p 875.) Rapid eye movement (REM) sleep occurs in cycles of about 90 min throughout the night. Besides rapid eye movements, this state of sleep is characterized by a low-voltage, fast EEG pattern; irregular breathing and pulse; blood pressure elevation; and diminished muscle tone. Penile erection occurs automatically, a fact that can be used to distinguish functional from organic impotence by demonstrating the integrity of the neural and vascular apparatus for erection. When awakened from REM sleep, a person usually reports dreaming; however, those awakened from non-REM sleep do not. REM sleep occupies a much greater percentage of sleep time in young infants than in adults. From the age of 3 to 5 years to senility, it occupies about 20 percent of sleep time. However, whether or not young infants dream remains a matter of conjecture.

340. The answer is A (1, 2, 3). (Adams RD, 5/e, p 372.) Bilateral destruction of several sites in the cerebrum produces a relatively pure loss of memory but leaves cognitive functions relatively intact, including an ability to score in the normal range on IQ tests. Lesion sites that produce an amnestic syndrome include the dorsomedial nuclei of the thalamus, Ammon's horn and dentate gyrus, and the parahippocampal gyrus. Unilateral lesions cause only small or transient memory deficits. Since the fornix is an essential part of the circuitry connecting these structures, it is surprising that transection of the fornices, as has been performed in humans in an attempt to treat epilepsy, does not produce the amnestic syndrome. Although widespread bilateral loss of neurons in the cerebral cortex also causes memory loss, the affected patient will show overt signs of dementia in other areas of mental function. Thus, diffuse cerebral disease does not produce the relatively pure amnestic syndrome equated with lesions in the medial temporal lobes, hippocampal formation, or thalami.

341. The answer is A (1, 2, 3). (Adams, 5/e, p 341.) Sleep paralysis occurs most commonly in the narcolepsy tetrad. It appears during the transition phases of wakefulness-to-sleep and of sleep-to-wakefulness. At the onset it frequently creates fear in the subject, but with repeated episodes patients learn to deal with the phenomenon. It is most frequent when a patient is falling asleep and may be accompanied by dreams, the so-called hypnagogic hallucinations. The striking feature of sleep paralysis is its instantaneous disappearance when the patient is touched or hears a sound. This fact indicates that the disorder is related to a disturbance in the CNS rather than to a sudden potassium shift in muscle, which would be too slow to explain so rapid an arousal from sleep paralysis. However, patients with periodic paralysis who have a disturbance in potassium balance also may experience severe fright and anxiety because of a similar feeling of helplessness during their muscular paralysis.

342. The answer is A (1, 2, 3). (Adams RD, 5/e, pp 476–478.) In the male, bilateral destruction of the lumbar sympathetic ganglia, particularly the second one, leads to loss of ejaculation but retention of erectile capacity. Erectile capacity requires the integrity of the parasympathetic fibers that travel from the sacral cord to dilate the arterioles of the penis, which allow the penis to fill with blood. In addition, the axons of the pudendal nerve innervate the periurethral muscles, which compress the draining veins of the penis. The fibers that convey sexual sensation and the suprasegmental fibers, which mediate the psychic and brain influences on the genitalia, travel in the ventrolateral quadrant of the spinal cord. Thus, ventrolateral chordotomy causes loss of erection and ejaculation in males and loss of orgasmic capacity in females. Even after vulvectomy or loss of the penis, patients may still experience sexual sensation and even orgasm. A different situation prevails following *complete* cord transection with paraplegia. As part of the exaggeration of certain reflexes after cord transection, erection may be produced by stimulation of the penis and, in fact, priapism may occur as a troublesome complication. Once the paraplegic patient has achieved erection, intercourse and ejaculation can take place.

343. The answer is A (1, 2, 3). (Kaplan, Comprehensive Textbook, 6/e, pp 247–248.) Freud, upon whose work much of classical psychoanalytic theory rests, divided the personality into the id, ego, and superego. The id consists of the instinctual drives (which reflect primary biologic needs for food, sexuality, sleep) and the vegetative, homeostatic, and visceral functions. The primitive drives related to these functions produce states of emotion, aggression, fear, pleasure, and satisfaction. The ego is the reality-testing self that deals with the environment through conscious, cognitive processes. It brings about a modus operandi for psychosocial adaptation that establishes the manner in which persons both perceive themselves in relation to other persons and relate toward them. The superego, on the other hand, incorporates the ego ideal, which is the internalized model of what persons think they should be like, as established by childhood perceptions of the kind of person they perceive authority figures wanted them to be.

344. The answer is E (all). (Adams, 5/e, pp 345–347.) In addition to the well-known narcolepsy tetrad of symptoms including pathologic sleep, cataplexy, hypnagogic hallucinations, and sleep paralysis, narcoleptic persons often may exhibit episodes of automatic behavior. These episodes might be interpreted as daytime somnambulism. Such persons may remember the beginning of such an attack, then gradually lose awareness of surroundings but continue to perform routine tasks. They may answer simple questions or may burst out with a series of irrelevant words or phrases. These episodes should be distinguished from fugue states, psychomotor seizures, and psychotic intervals. Such attacks of clouding of the sensorium, occurring in more than half of the affected patients, are more common than the better-known episodes of sleep paralysis and hypnagogic hallucinations. Moreover, the classic features of narcolepsy may appear asynchronously over a period of several years, which makes a diagnosis very difficult in patients with only partial expressions of the syndrome. The full expression of the four classic features occurs in only about 10 percent of narcoleptic patients.

345. The answer is A (1, 2, 3). (Rowland, 9/e, p 425.) Amnesia following head injuries and amnesia following psychomotor seizures closely resemble each other in a qualitative sense.

In either instance, patients show a period of ictal amnesia with retrograde and anterograde components. The retrograde amnesia is shorter than the anterograde and tends to shrink as the patient recovers. During the recovery phase, the patient will display a period of seemingly rational, responsive behavior and consciousness but later may be unable to recall this period of time. For the posttraumatic patient, this period may last days or weeks, but lasts only briefly after the usual psychomotor seizure. The patient who has suffered epileptic status will have a memory deficit quantitatively and qualitatively like that of a posttraumatic patient.

346. The answer is B (1, 3). (Kaplan, Synopsis, 7/e, p 354.) Patients with pseudodementia may manifest many features that suggest an organic brain disorder, although their disorder is actually functional. While no absolute distinction can be made, several features suggest pseudodementia. These include a tendency of such patients to dwell upon their seeming mental incapacity, whereas the organic patient often lacks an appreciation of the degree of disability. The patient with pseudodementia displays little effort or interest in formal testing, preferring to respond with "I don't know," whereas the organic patient usually tries to perform well. In addition, patients with pseudodementia will have normal attention span and ability to concentrate and will retain a high level of successful general behavior in relation to the apparent loss of intellectual function.

347. The answer is E (all). (Adams RD, 5/e, p 398.) The symptoms of Gerstmann's syndrome are the result of a left, or dominant, parietal lesion. This syndrome is characterized by a disorientation as to left and right and an inability to designate fingers (digital agnosia), calculate (acalculia), or write (agraphia). Word blindness and homonymous hemianopia or a lower quadrantanopia may also be present.

348. The answer is E (all). (Adams RD, 5/e, pp 222–223, 392, 400–402. Cogan, Graefes Arch Clin Exp Ophthalmol 188:139–150, 1973.) Loss of vision occurs with lesions in any of the listed regions. Visual hallucinations may occur in any patient who is blind. If hallucinations are sudden in onset, one should suspect a brain process, typically in the occipital lobe. These are generally elementary hallucinations such as colors and geometric forms. Hallucinations arising from the visual association cortex are complex; for example, they may involve people and landscapes. With progressive blindness, anywhere in the visual system, one may experience purely visual hallucinations of elementary or complex types. These occur in the blind regions, however, so that a patient with a homonymous hemianopia experiences hallucinations only in the affected field, whereas patients with macular disease see hallucinations in all quadrants.

349. The answer is B (1, 3). (Kaplan, Synopsis, 7/e, pp 429–433.) Although the psychedelic drugs are difficult to define, they all act to produce a heightened awareness of sensory input; in many instances they cause hallucinations that affect various senses. However, auditory hallucinations are rare in contrast to the state of auditory hallucinosis that follows prolonged use of alcohol. The psychedelic drugs, which, in general, are indoleamines or phenylethylamines, lack strong addictive properties, and recreational users eventually tend to lose interest in them. A high degree of tolerance develops for lysergic acid diethylamide (LSD). Withdrawal symptoms are absent or slight, and fatal intoxication is rare, although severe hallucinations while under the influence of LSD may lead to suicide.

350. **The answer is C (2,4).** (Kaplan, Synopsis, 7/e, p 361.) Aside from profound dementia, no neurologic syndrome induces amnesia so profound that identity is lost. Postictal states, whether from trauma or seizure, produce global confusional states with diffuse behavioral abnormalities. Patients with acute remote memory deficits have nonphysiologic derangements that range from malingering to dissociative or fugue states ("split personalities").

351–354. **The answers are 351-E, 352-D, 353-B, 354-C.** (Adams, 5/e, p 1293.) Personality represents the totality of an individual's personal characteristics. Personality disorders are "pervasive and enduring" character traits that are far enough from normal that they are considered pathologic. Yet they are not, like psychoses, amenable to drug therapy. Approximately 15 percent of the population suffers from these disorders, although it is clear that what is pathologic and what is not varies over time and place. A large number of personality disorders exist and they are not to be confused with psychoses with similar names. Schizoid personality describes a set of characteristics that are in keeping with schizophrenia but without psychotic features. People with personality disorders don't "fit in" but do not lose touch with reality and do not hallucinate.

355–358. **The answers are 355-C, 356-E, 357-D, 358-B.** (Kaplan, Synopsis, 7/e, pp 250–251.) In 1896, Freud published his first work on defense mechanisms. Since that time, many other authors, chiefly psychoanalysts, have added to the literature. Kolb has listed 21 basic mental mechanisms and defensive processes. While all can be found in both mentally healthy and mentally ill persons, some mechanisms are more commonly used by mentally ill people, e.g., unrealistic projection, denial, symbolization, and the acting out of conflicts. Also, the mentally ill person uses only a few defenses in a stereotyped nonadaptive way and possesses relatively few appropriately adaptive mechanisms. These include sublimation (the transfer of psychic energy to behavior beneficial to the self or society), altruism, conscious control, and ego-strengthening identification, as exemplified by the Joe Namath admirer described in the question.

In contrast, the soldier described in the question, who blamed the physician for his own defection from duty, was using a highly maladaptive, unrealistic projection to save himself from his own painful guilt. Such a projection can lead to murder and other dangerous and self-defeating behavior.

Rationalization is a common mental mechanism used by nearly everyone at some time or another. Frequently, the strongest motives for our behavior are based on greed, gluttony, anger, or other self-centered urges. We like to think, however, that we are rational and fair; therefore, we hide from ourselves the selfish nature of many of our acts and focus on a partial truth (or the semblance of truth) in a situation as the main reason for our behavior. Saving our self-image may cause more trouble than it is worth, for we fail to appreciate where our best interests lie. The young wife described in the question, who rationalized her promiscuity, failed to fully acknowledge a trait she felt guilty about and blamed her husband. This failure, in turn, blocked her search for other solutions that might have strengthened rather than jeopardized her marriage.

Regression is another common defense mechanism of everyday life and frequently occurs during stress. Reverting to a behavior pattern of an earlier developmental period represents an unconscious bid for another person to take care of the sufferer as a young child or infant. The regression, if temporary, can be used to gather strength to fight the battles of the real world on a later occasion. However, continued neglect of developmental problems will, in due course, lead to mental illness.

Mechanisms of defense are subjects for scrutiny in patients undergoing psychoanalysis or dynamic psychotherapy. The rationale behind such exploration is that patients will be able to bring their intelligence to bear on their problems rather than mindlessly engaging in repetitive, destructive behavior whose sole legacy is unhappiness and failure.

359–362. The answers are 359-E, 360-A, 361-D, 362-B. (Adams RD, 5/e, pp 222–223.) Dyschromatopsia refers to any disturbance in the perception of color. A defect in color perception will accompany virtually any defect of visual perception due to a cerebral lesion. Thus, color testing is a very sensitive test of visual function. The disorders in color perception may take the form of achromatopsia (lack of color vision), metachromatopsia (change in color perception so that green, for example, may appear as brown), and monochromatopsia (perception of all visual objects as having one color—for example cyanopsia, or blue vision).

Palinopsia refers to the persistence of visual images after removal of the visual stimulus. The object previously seen will persist, often in very vivid form, for minutes or hours. A single object may appear as a chain of many objects (polyopsia). The palinoptic image usually appears in visual fields that are only partially affected rather than completely blind. The causative brain lesions usually are severely destructive, such as infarcts or neoplasms, and will cause other visual and neurologic manifestations as well.

Simultagnosia refers to the inability to organize a series of related pictures into the correct sequence or to understand the meaning of a series of related parts. If given a series of pictures that tells a story, an affected patient is unable to order them into the story-telling sequence but tends to perceive them as a series of independent events. In a series of dots that forms a letter, the patient may see the dots but fail to perceive them as forming a letter. In other words, the patient fails to see the simultaneous relationship of visual sequences.

Visual allesthesia refers to the displacement of a visual image from the visual field of perception into the opposite field. The displacement occurs from the affected to the non-affected field. Allesthesia also occurs in other sensory modalities, such as in the displacement of tactile stimuli.

363–366. The answers are 363-C, 364-D, 365-A, 366-B. (Adams RD, 5/e, pp 416–424.) Aphasias can be characterized in several ways. The current standard format is to categorize language disorders by fluency, auditory comprehension, repetition, naming, reading, and writing. Since many aphasias occur in connection with visual or motor dysfunctions, testing has to take this into account. For example, a patient should attempt to write using the unaffected hand, which will affect penmanship but not spelling or syntax. Broca's aphasia is a paradigmatic, nonfluent aphasia in which comprehension is preserved but patients are unable to speak fluently on command, although they can utter standard phrases fluently when they are frustrated. Because of their inability to speak fluently, they cannot repeat and may have problems naming. Generally they can select the correct name for an object when given choices.

Conduction aphasia is a type in which the arcuate fasciculus is interrupted, which causes a disruption in the pathway connecting Wernicke's and Broca's areas. Speech is fluent but subject to paraphasias. Comprehension for spoken and written words is good but naming is variably affected.

The transcortical aphasias are characterized by the preservation of repetition. There are three types of transcortical aphasias: motor, sensory, and mixed. Anomic aphasia, which is not of the transcortical type, also has preserved repetition. The transcortical motor is a Broca's type of aphasia but with preserved repetition; that is, it is nonfluent with good comprehension for spoken and written words. Transcortical sensory is a Wernicke's type with preserved repetition; the patient is fluent but with impaired comprehension. Anomic aphasia is a fluent aphasia with preserved repetition, auditory comprehension, and impaired naming.

367–370. The answers are 367-E, 368-B, 369-C, 370-A. (Adams RD, 5/e, pp 65–66. Kaplan, Synopsis, 7/e, p 304.) Many terms are available to describe states of immobility or resistance to movement. The patient with catatonia remains mute and still, showing little reaction to the usual environmental stimuli. Catatonia was described by Kahlbaum in 1874 as a component of the disorder newly termed *dementia praecox*, later to be supplanted by Bleuler's term *schizophrenia*. He noted that it was frequently associated with flexibilitas cerea, or catalepsy.

Catalepsy refers to the condition in which patients maintain their body or limbs in whatever position, however uncomfortable, the examiner places them. While this feature is classically associated with schizophrenia, it also occurs in dementia and in the twilight states of disturbed consciousness of any origin, including seizures. Catatonia as such seems today to be a much less frequent finding in schizophrenia than formerly, judging by the older literature on the subject.

In gegenhalten (paratonia or motor negativism), patients show plastic resistance to any movement the examiner seeks to impose. The resistance, while relatively slight, remains nearly constant throughout the course of movement and will remain so regardless of where the movement starts or stops. The resistance will increase if the examiner tries to move the part too quickly, or will nearly disappear if the examiner moves the part very slowly. It may be unilateral. Gegenhalten occurs in the intact limbs of stroke victims while these patients have obtundation of consciousness and under a variety of other conditions associated with altered consciousness.

Negativism is a general term for resistance by patients to any effort to move body parts, either passively by the examiner or in response to the examiner's command. This feature, often seen in the disturbed or retarded child, may totally defeat the parent when it pervades the whole behavior of the child. It may have partial expression in mutism and refusal to eat or dress or to go to school. The active opposition to the parental goal and the preservation of consciousness readily distinguish negativism from other resistances.

371–374. The answers are 371-B, 372-C, 373-A, 374-D. (Adams RD, 5/e, pp 415–417. Kaplan, Synopsis,7/e, pp 304–306.) Disorders of verbal expression take many forms. One method of classifying them is to recognize the differences between disorders of speech, of language, and of thought. Among the disorders of speech are stuttering, cluttering, palilalia, and several varieties of mutism. Disorders of language include the aphasias, echolalia, and perseveration.

Among the speech disorders, palilalia consists of the repetition of the final word or phrase. There is an increased speed of repetition but loss in volume of voice until the sound and lip movements fade away, with a patient then making only lip movements (aphonic palilalia). Sometimes, in exasperation at the repetitions, the patient may interrupt them by an expletive. Palilalia stands in contrast to stuttering, which involves the first sound of the word.

Cluttering consists of very rapid speech with the omission of entire sounds or words, resulting in incomprehensible speech in severe cases. Patients will say something like, "torow go toping" for "Tomorrow I want to go shopping." Asked to repeat the phrase, the patient says the same incomprehensible thing but, if cautioned to slow down, can produce the words individually. Nevertheless, the patient will revert to the cluttering upon making the next statement.

Among the many forms of mutism is elective mutism. In this disorder, a patient (usually a young child) consistently fails to speak to some persons or under certain conditions but can talk normally or almost normally under other conditions. The child may fail to speak when introduced to anyone new or strange or may not speak in the presence of a particular family member or other familiar person. Particular forms of mutism include akinetic mutism, due to a lesion of the brainstem or septal region, and aphemia.

Aphemia, or pure word mutism, is a particular type of aphasia. The patient suddenly loses all speech because of a lesion in the posterior inferior frontal region (Broca's area) but remains alert and able to write, read, and behave normally. Other terms for aphemia are *pure word dumbness, cortical anarthria,* and *subcortical motor aphasia.*

375–380. The answers are 375-C, 376-A, 377-E, 378-D, 379-B, 380-F. (Adams RD, 5/e, pp 333–334.) The stages of normal sleep, while continuous, exhibit fairly characteristic EEG patterns that must be recognized and distinguished from patterns of abnormal sleep. It is particularly important not to interpret early drowsiness as pathologic slowing, or vertex sharp waves as spikes. The EEG of the normal, awake person shows an occipitally dominant alpha rhythm of 8 to 12 cps and low-voltage, mixed-frequency activity. As drowsiness evolves, the EEG shows some activity in the theta range, and in stage 1, the lightest stage of sleep, it shows low-voltage desynchronized activity and low-to-moderate amplitude waves in the theta range (4 to 6 cps). Such a person displays slow, roving eye movements during stage 1 sleep. The EEG pattern is similar during rapid eye movement (REM) sleep.

Stage 2 sleep features 12 to 15 cps sleep spindles and K-complexes. K-complexes consist of high-amplitude, mixed sharp-slow waves, usually with a central or frontal dominance and often followed by sleep spindles. K-complexes will appear during attempts to arouse a sleeping person, as well as spontaneously. The spindles and K-complexes appear against a background of low-voltage, mixed-frequency waves.

Stage 3 sleep displays moderate amounts of high-amplitude, slow-wave activity. Some waves in the delta range (0.5 to 3 cps) appear. In stage 4 sleep, delta waves dominate the record.

The various stages of sleep alternate in cycles during the night, and although transitions occur between stages, the records can be scored as to how much of the night is spent in each stage. In young adults, stage 1 occupies 3 to 5 percent of the night; stage 2, 50 to 60 percent; stages 3 and 4, 10 to 20 percent; and REM, about 20 to 25 percent. The amount of time spent in the various stages of sleep varies with age. REM sleep occupies about 50 percent of the cycle in young infants. The elderly have very little stage 3 and 4 sleep.

The delta stage, stage 4, is generally interpreted as the deepest stage of sleep, in the sense that the person is least arousable during this stage. All the first four stages taken together occupy the first 70 to 120 min of the night's sleep. Then, the first cycle of REM sleep occurs. The EEG resembles that of stage 1 sleep, but the person now undergoes a phase of dreaming. Although the REM stage is often thought of as a lighter stage of sleep, the person is not necessarily easier to arouse. It is also called *paradoxical sleep* because of the dreaming in conjunction with profound loss of muscle tone. It is not readily categorized as light or deep sleep, rather as a different *kind* of sleep. Repeat REM cycles occur at intervals of 90 to 100 min throughout the night. REM stages of sleep appear in all mammals and even in birds and thus have some profound biologic significance. Daytime napping is associated with REM sleep that appears earlier and is of greater duration than in nocturnal sleep.

PSYCHIATRY

BIOLOGIC DIMENSIONS OF PSYCHIATRY

Directions: Each item below contains five suggested responses. Select the **one best** response to each item.

381. Each of the following is a true statement about the dopaminergic system in the brain EXCEPT

(A) brain dopamine circuits are organized into four main components

(B) the mesolimbic dopamine circuitry includes the ventral tegmental area, nucleus accumbens, and cingulate cortex

(C) D_2 receptors are distributed primarily in the basal ganglia

(D) the D_2 receptor has a high affinity for antipsychotic medications

(E) the A_9 dopaminergic neurons are located in the ventral tegmental area

382. True statements regarding serotoninergic neurons include all the following EXCEPT

(A) they are restricted to midline regions in the pons and brainstem

(B) they exhibit maximum firing during periods of sleep

(C) they are capable of autoregulation

(D) they have widespread projection to virtually all parts of the CNS

(E) they modulate neuronal excitability in diverse regions of the CNS

383. Identified risk factors in schizophrenia include all the following EXCEPT

(A) having a dizygotic twin with schizophrenia
(B) male sex
(C) a history of perinatal birth injury
(D) being born in winter
(E) having a first-degree relative who suffers from schizophrenia

384. Each of the following statements regarding G proteins is correct EXCEPT

(A) the G protein binds guanine nucleotide and mediates signal transduction
(B) G proteins allow a mechanism for signal amplification
(C) G proteins modulate adenylate cyclase-linked transduction
(D) G proteins exhibit stringent trans-mitter specificity
(E) abnormalities of G proteins have been reported in several psychi-atric disorders

385. All the following statements regarding dopaminergic neurons in the brain are correct EXCEPT

(A) D_1 neurons are distributed primar-ily in the substantia nigra
(B) D_4 neurons are located primarily in the the cortex, hypothalamus, hippocampus, and olfactory bulb
(C) different subtypes of dopamine receptor are frequently found in the same brain region
(D) D_2 receptors may have both pre-synaptic and postsynaptic functions
(E) D_2 receptors have a high affinity for haloperidol

386. Drugs that are metabolized via the 2D6 cytochrome P-450 system include each of the following EXCEPT

(A) nifedipine
(B) nortriptyline
(C) propranolol
(D) desipramine
(E) codeine

387. Which of the following medications is contraindicated with the use of fluvoxamine?

(A) Phenytoin
(B) Penicillin
(C) Terfenadine
(D) Alprazolam
(E) Clonazepam

388. True statements about the limbic system include all the following EXCEPT

(A) the term refers to those neural structures primarily involved in the pursuit of innate biologic drives
(B) the medial temporal cortex forms a significant portion of the limbic system
(C) the limbic system has clearly defined neuroanatomic boundaries
(D) the hypothalamus represents an integral part of the system
(E) the fornix forms the largest out-flow tract from the hippocampus

389. Each of the following is a true statement about benzodiazepines EXCEPT

(A) the major effects of benzodiazepines are produced secondary to their binding at $GABA_A$ receptors in the brain
(B) benzodiazepines increase the frequency of chloride channel openings on the cell membrane
(C) benzodiazepines enhance cellular excitability
(D) there are several subtypes of benzodiazepine receptor
(E) benzodiazepines are metabolized primarily by the liver

390. A destructive lesion involving both anterior temporal lobes would produce which of the following clinical syndromes?

(A) Bizarre repetitive automatisms with repeated lip smacking
(B) An inability to distinguish left from right, finger agnosia, and acalculia
(C) Hyposexuality, perseveration, distractibility, and poor impulse control
(D) Hyperorality, hypersexuality, placidity, visual agnosia, and amnesia
(E) Alexia without agraphia

391. Computed tomography (CT) is a more sensitive investigation than magnetic resonance imaging (MRI) for which of the following?

(A) A posterior fossa tumor
(B) A calcified parasagittal meningioma
(C) Multiple sclerosis
(D) Medial temporal sclerosis
(E) Binswanger's disease

392. All the following statements about evoked potentials are correct EXCEPT

(A) they may be used to determine the prognosis in coma
(B) the procedure may be useful in the evaluation of multiple sclerosis
(C) evoked potentials are not specific to any particular sensory modality
(D) evoked potentials may be helpful in diagnosing conversion disorders
(E) the technique is helpful in diagnosing deafness in newborns

393. Animal models of depression include each of the following EXCEPT

(A) learned helplessness
(B) exhaustion stress
(C) conditioned avoidance response
(D) isolation/separation paradigms
(E) kindling

394. The normal resting EEG in a healthy young adult is characterized by

(A) an evoked response in the frontal lobes with stroboscopic stimulation
(B) increasing frequency of the background rhythm during stages 1 through 4 sleep
(C) a background of 4 to 7 Hz alpha rhythm
(D) alpha rhythms predominantly over the frontal lobes when the eyes are closed
(E) attenuation of the background alpha rhythm and the appearance of beta waves in the frontal regions symmetrically when the eyes are opened

Directions: Each item below contains four suggested responses of which **one or more** is correct. Select:

A	if	**1, 2, and 3**	are correct
B	if	**1 and 3**	are correct
C	if	**2 and 4**	are correct
D	if	**4**	is correct
E	if	**1, 2, 3, and 4**	are correct

395. The activation of adenylate cyclase

(1) may result in either an inhibitory or stimulatory response
(2) may be triggered by more than one neurotransmitter
(3) is an example of a second messenger system
(4) facilitates the opening of chloride channels

396. The activation of a dopamine autoreceptor

(1) increases the release of dopamine at the synapse
(2) produces an inhibitory feedback loop
(3) occurs at the postsynaptic membrane
(4) results in decreased dopamine synthesis

397. The catabolism of dopamine involves which of the following enzymes?

(1) Monoamine oxidase
(2) Tyrosine hydroxylase
(3) Catechol-*O*-methyltransferase
(4) Dopa decarboxylase

398. Inhibitory neurotransmitters include which of the following?

(1) Glutamate
(2) Glycine
(3) Aspartate
(4) γ-Aminobutyric acid (GABA)

399. Prolactin secretion is correctly characterized by which of the following statements?

(1) It is stimulated by dopamine secretion in the hypothalamus
(2) It is increased by a generalized tonic clonic convulsion
(3) It is diminished by the administration of neuroleptics
(4) It occurs in the anterior pituitary

400. Which of the following statements regarding *N*-methyl-D-aspartate is true?

(1) It is an excitatory amino acid
(2) It may cause convulsions if injected intracerebrally
(3) It may cause neuronal damage
(4) It produces depolarization at the synapse

401. Serotoninergic 5-HT2 receptors are the probable site of action of

(1) buspirone
(2) fluoxetine
(3) haloperidol
(4) hallucinogens

402. Increased serum levels of endogenous opioids have been reported in

(1) exercise
(2) starvation
(3) stress
(4) pain

403. True statements about neurotransmitters include

(1) they are released into the synaptic cleft when repolarization occurs at the presynaptic terminal
(2) they influence the electrical and biochemical properties of the post-synaptic membrane
(3) they are resistant to catabolism
(4) they are found in highest concentration in the presynaptic terminal

404. The production of melatonin

(1) requires tryptophan as a precursor
(2) takes place in the pineal gland
(3) is decreased by light stimulation
(4) is increased by noradrenaline (norepinephrine)

405. Monoamine oxidase A is correctly described by which of the following?

(1) It selectively deaminates serotonin and noradrenaline (norepinephrine)
(2) It is reversibly inhibited by phenelzine
(3) It is selectively inhibited by clorgiline
(4) It increases intracellular levels of noradrenaline (norepinephrine)

406. Second messengers include

(1) calcium
(2) acetylcholine
(3) protein kinases
(4) dopamine

407. Dopamine D_1 receptors are

(1) situated on the presynaptic membrane
(2) autoreceptors
(3) selectively blocked by haloperidol
(4) located primarily in the parathyroid gland

408. Venlafaxine is accurately characterized by which of the following statements?

(1) It is chemically related to the tricyclic antidepressants
(2) It is extensively metabolized by the liver
(3) It has protein binding in excess of 80 percent
(4) It does not have significant affinity for histamine receptors

409. The sleep pattern in patients with the recurrence of a major depressive episode is characterized by

(1) decreased rapid eye movement (REM) latency
(2) decreased stages 3 and 4 sleep
(3) prolonged first REM period
(4) early morning awakening

410. Normal changes in sleep architecture that occur with aging include

(1) increased slow-wave sleep
(2) increased REM sleep
(3) decreased awakenings
(4) decreased total sleep time

SUMMARY OF DIRECTIONS

A	B	C	D	E
1,2,3	1,3	2,4	4	All are
only	only	only	only	correct

411. Chronic alcohol abuse produces which of the following changes in sleep architecture?

(1) Decreased stages 3 and 4 sleep
(2) Increased REM sleep
(3) Decreased total sleep time
(4) Decreased awakenings

412. Clinical features of narcolepsy include

(1) sleep paralysis
(2) increased REM latency
(3) cataplexy
(4) myoclonic jerks

413. The "dopamine hypothesis" of schizophrenia is supported by

(1) the emergence of psychosis following the chronic administration of amphetamine
(2) reduced concentrations of homo-vanillic acid in the CSF of schizophrenic patients
(3) an increase in D_2 receptors found in the postmortem studies of schizophrenic brains
(4) the therapeutic efficacy of D_1 receptor agonists in schizophrenia

414. A middle-aged man presents with the complaint of daytime drowsiness. Possible etiologies include

(1) a major depressive disorder
(2) alcoholic dependency
(3) sleep apnea
(4) restless legs syndrome

Directions: Each group of questions below consists of lettered options followed by a set of numbered items. For each numbered item, select the **one** lettered option with which it is most closely associated. Each lettered option may be used **once, more than once, or not at all**.

Items 415–418

Select the EEG recording that would be most likely in each of the following clinical vignettes.

    (A) EEG A
    (B) EEG B
    (C) EEG C
    (D) EEG D
    (E) EEG E

415. A young woman is brought to the emergency room in a semicomatose state. She says that she ingested a large number of "sleeping pills" 1 h prior to her arrival at the hospital

416. A 60-year-old man is accompanied by his wife to the emergency room. She states that her husband is unable to speak and has developed shaking of his right arm and leg

417. A 40-year-old alcoholic is brought to the emergency room confused and belligerent

418. A normal young male falls asleep while having a routine EEG as part of a research protocol

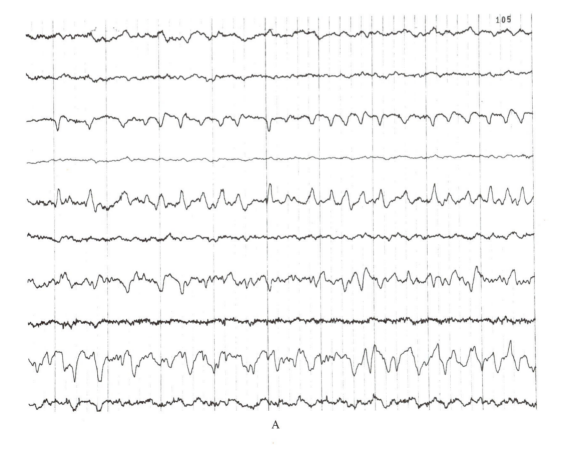

A

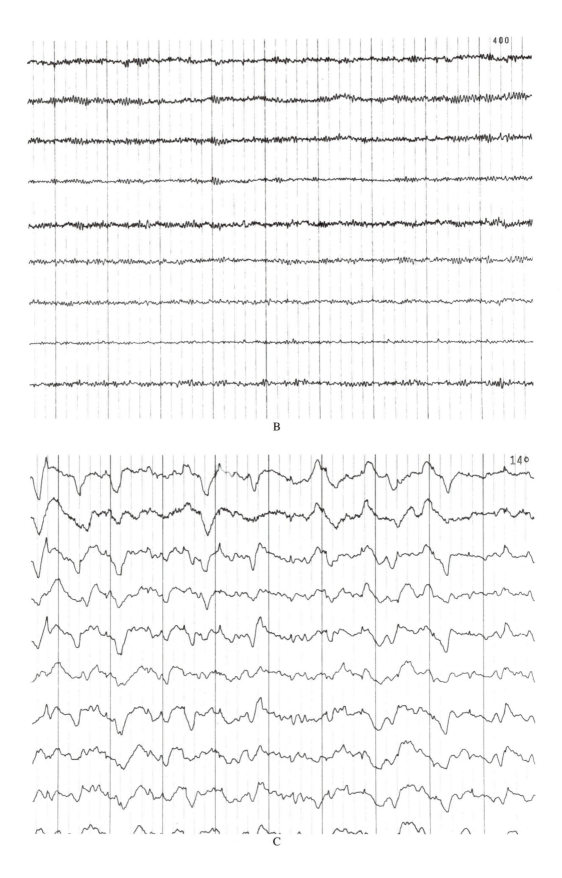

B

C

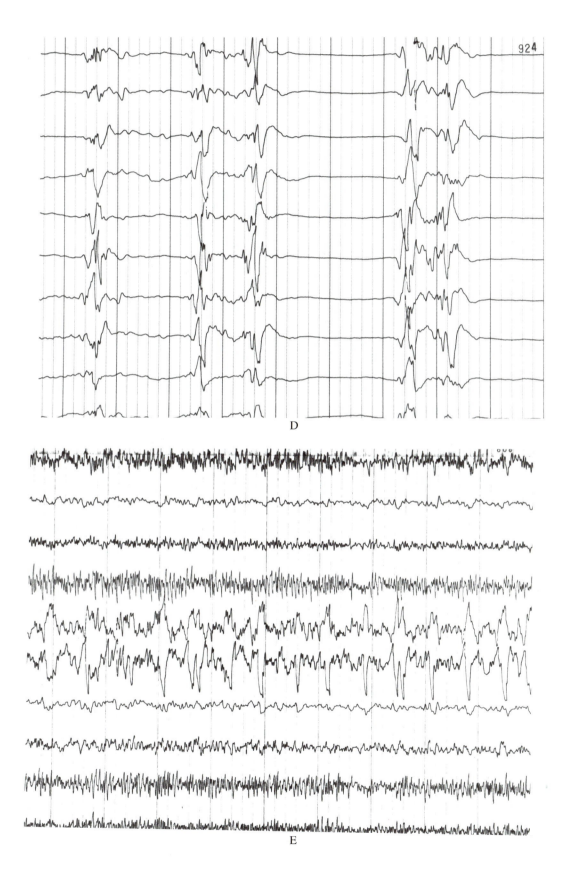

D

E

Items 419–423

The axial MRI scan below is of a 9-month-old infant at the level of the third ventricle and basal ganglia. Match the numbered structures with the appropriate letters on the scan.

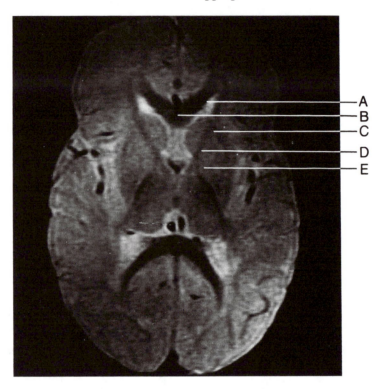

Adapted from Fischer and Ketonen, Fig. 2-71, with permission.

419. Genu of corpus callosum

420. Head of caudate nucleus

421. Anterior limb of internal capsule

422. Frontal horn of lateral ventricle

423. Globus pallidus

Items 424–427

Match the following.

    (A) Raphe nuclei
    (B) Nucleus basalis
    (C) Locus coeruleus
    (D) Red nucleus
    (E) Ventral tegmental area

424. Origin of long-tract dopaminergic projections

425. Origin of cholinergic pathways

426. Primary serotonin cell bodies

427. Numerous noradrenergic projections

BIOLOGIC DIMENSIONS OF PSYCHIATRY

ANSWERS

381. The answer is E. (Schatzberg, pp 45–50.) Brain dopamine projections are organized into four major components: the nigrostriatal, mesolimbic, tuberoinfundibular, and incerto-hypothalamic systems. The *nigrostriatal system* is one of the most extensive parts of the dopaminergic system and includes the A_8 and A_9 dopaminergic neurons (located in the mesencephalic reticular formation and substantia nigra, respectively). Projections from these sites travel via the medial forebrain bundle to terminate in the caudate, putamen, and central amygdaloid nucleus. The *mesolimbic system* originates in the A_{10} neurons found in the ventral tegmental area, which have widespread connections with limbic and paralimbic structures, including the nucleus accumbens, olfactory tubercle, stria terminalis, lateral septum, cingulate cortex, and entorhinal cortex. The tuberoinfundibular system arises in the A_{12} region of the caudal hypothalamus and projects to the hypothalamic-hypophyseal portal vessels. The incertohypothalamic system arises from dopaminergic neurons in regions A_{11}, A_{13}, A_{14}, and A_{15} of the diencephalon and project to the hypothalamus, where they modulate many aspects of hypothalamic function. Five subtypes of dopamine receptor have been identified.

382. The answer is B. (Cooper, 7/e, pp 363–383.) Serotoninergic neurons are restricted to cell clusters found in the midline of the pons and brainstem. They exhibit rhythmic pacemaker activity and are capable of autoregulation via feedback from presynaptic autoreceptors (5-HT1a). Activity within serotoninergic neurons is highest during periods of activity or arousal. The diffuse projections of these serotoninergic receptors suggest that they play an important role in modulating neural excitability at diverse sites within the CNS. Dysfunction within serotoninergic projections is postulated to play an important role in clinical disorders of arousal (e.g., posttraumatic stress disorder).

383. The answer is B. (Kaplan, 6/e, pp 907–909.) Studies that take gender differences in age of onset into consideration have demonstrated no difference in the prevalence of schizophrenia between males and females. Females tend to experience the onset of the disease between 25 and 34 years, whereas males tend to present earlier between 15 and 24 years. Males tend to display more profound negative symptoms with a more chronic debilitating course. Schizophrenics are more likely than the general population to have been born during the winter months. This correspondence has been used to support a viral etiology of the illness. Replicated retrospective studies have found a high incidence of perinatal birth injuries among schizophrenics and suggest that this is associated with more negative symptomatology and a poorer prognosis. The concordance rate for schizophrenia among monozygotic twins is 33 to 78 percent and in dizygotic twins is 8 to 28 percent.

384. The answer is E. (Schatzberg, pp 17–18.) Second messenger systems, including G proteins, allow the integration and amplification of neurotransmitter signals at the cell membrane. The G proteins are a family of enzymes that contain GTPase activity (hence the term *G proteins*).

385. The answer is C. (Schatzberg, pp 47–50.) Five different subtypes of dopamine receptor are currently identified (D_1–D_5). Each of these receptor subtypes has a distinct anatomic distribution and exhibits specific affinities for various psychotropic agents. These specific characteristics suggest that each dopamine receptor has a different function. D_1 receptors are located in the caudate-putamen, olfactory tubercle, nucleus accumbens, amygdala, and cortex. D_2 receptors are found in highest concentration in the caudate-putamen and nucleus accumbens and also in the substantia nigra ventral tegmentum and olfactory tubercle; they exhibit a high affinity for typical antipsychotic drugs, including haloperidol. Dopamine receptors appear to have both pre- and postsynaptic functions. The presynaptic receptor is often referred to as an *autoreceptor* because it regulates the release of dopamine into the synapse.

386. The answer is A. (Schatzberg, pp 129–130.) The cytochrome P-450 enzymes (CYP) are involved in the metabolism and detoxification of many different drugs. A number of isoenzymes (believed to have evolved from a common ancestral gene) are coded by separate loci. There at least 12 isoenzymes, including CYP-2D6, CYP-3A4, CYP-2C19, CYP-1A2, CYP-2A6, and CYP-2E1. People may be classified as fast or slow metabolizers based on their ability to metabolize a reference compound such as dextromethorphan. The efficiency of the CYP system is adversely influenced by inhibitors such as paroxetine, fluoxetine (and its metabolite norfluoxetine), and to a lesser extent other SSRIs, including sertraline and fluvoxamine. The drug substrates of the various clinically important CYP-450 isoenzymes are as follows:

CYP-2D6 (potent inhibition by paroxetine, (nor)fluoxetine; modest inhibition by sertraline; weak inhibition by fluvoxamine)
  - Tricyclics: desipramine, nortriptyline
  - Antiarrhythmics: encainide, flecainide, mexiletine, propafenone
  - Neuroleptics: haloperidol, thioridazine, perphenazine
  - Beta blockers: metoprolol, propranolol, bufarolol
  - Codeine
  - Dextromethorphan
  - Indoramin
  - Phenformin

CYP-2C19 (modest inhibition by fluoxetine and fluvoxamine)
  - Tricyclics: imipramine, clomipramine
  - Diazepam
  - Hexobarbital
  - Mephenytoin

CYP-3A4 (modest inhibition by all SSRIs but probably only significant with [nor]fluoxetine)
  - Tricyclics: imipramine, amitriptyline
  - Antiarrhythmics: quinidine
  - Calcium channel blockers: diltiazem, nifedipine, felodipine, verapamil
  - Cyclosporine A
  - Tamoxifen
  - Lovastatin
  - Terfenadine
  - Astemizole

CYP-1A2 (potent inhibition by fluvoxamine)
  - Xanthines: theophylline
  - Tricyclics: imipramine, clomipramine, amitriptyline
  - Clozapine
  - Warfarin
  - Propranolol

387. The answer is C. (Schatzberg, pp 129–131.) The combined use of drugs that inhibit CYP-3A4 is probably contraindicated in patients receiving terfenadine or astemizole because of the risk of fatal cardiac arrhythmias.

388. The answer is C. (Strub, pp 18–31.) The limbic system derives its name from the Greek word *limbus*, which means *rim*. The system has a vital role in determining the emotional valency of and appropriate behavioral response to environmental stimuli. Despite its pervasive and critical role in behavior, the neuroanatomic boundaries of the system are poorly defined. The system contains the hypothalamus, thalamic nuclei, limbic components of the cortex (i.e., orbitofrontal and mediotemporal structures), and the limbic striatum (i.e., nucleus accumbens, olfactory tubercle, and ventral tegmentum). The circuit of Papez forms an integral pathway linking the components of the limbic system and includes the hippocampus, fornix, anterior thalamus, hypothalamus, and cingulate gyrus.

389. The answer is C. (Schatzberg, pp 215–230.) Benzodiazepines are well absorbed from the gastrointestinal tract and metabolized primarily through the liver via phase I metabolism. Their mechanism of action is proposed to be via their binding to $GABA_A$ receptor sites. The principal action of GABA is to increase the frequency of the opening of chloride channels, which in turn decreases neuronal excitability. Three subtypes of benzodiazepine receptor have been identified. Type 1 receptors are found in high concentrations in the cerebellum and low concentrations in the hippocampus. Type 2 receptors are found in high concentrations in the hippocampus, striatum, and spinal cord. Type 3 receptors are found primarily in the cerebellum and are relatively insensitive to benzodiazepines.

390. The answer is D. (Strub, p 291.) Bilateral destruction of the anterior temporal lobes produces a distinct neurobehavioral disorder—the Klüver-Bucy syndrome. This disorder was first described in monkeys who had undergone surgical ablation of both anterior temporal lobes but is now well recognized in humans. The most common causes are limbic encephalitis, head trauma, Alzheimer's disease, and anoxia. Clinical features consist of placidity, hypersexuality with indiscriminate sexual interest in both animate and inanimate objects, amnesia, hyperorality, and visual agnosia.

391. The answer is B. (Adams RD, 5/e, pp 16–17.) Although MRI represents the most sensitive neuroimaging tool available, it is essentially "blind" to calcified structures. The technology offers particular advantages for the visualization of lesions of matter, brainstem, posterior fossa, and the anterior temporal region. The ability of MRI to produce multiplanar images provides more potential information than standard CT procedures. The adjunctive use of paramagnetic contrast materials further improves resolution and increases the sensitivity of the procedure.

392. The answer is C. (Kaplan, 6/e, pp 75–77.) In simple terms, evoked potentials are the electrical response produced by specific sensory stimuli and represent the neural conduction of modality-specific (e.g., vision, hearing) information. They have been recorded from cortical areas, brainstem, spinal cord, and peripheral nerves. The primary clinical use of evoked potentials is to determine the integrity of the visual, auditory, and somatosensory systems. The presence of normal evoked response patterns is helpful in confirming the diagnosis of conversion disorder. Although the use of evoked potentials in psychiatric disorders remains unclear, several studies have suggested that a reduced P300 amplitude is found in schizophrenia. The P300 late evoked potential is becoming of increasing interest to psychiatrists and may represent the motivational valence attributed by the subject to a particular environmental stimulus.

393. The answer is C. (Schatzberg, pp 84–101.) A number of animal models have provided valid models for investigating the pathophysiology and treatment of depression. These experimental models have included reserpine-induced reduction in motor activity, swim test immobility, clonidine withdrawal, tail suspension, lesioning of the dorsomedial amygdala, isolation/separation-induced depression, exhaustion stress, chronic mild stress, and learned helplessness. The learned helplessness model has proved a particularly powerful model in which an animal is exposed to multiple electrical shocks that it is unable to control. Symptoms induced by learned-helplessness include decreased appetite, loss of body weight, loss of competitiveness, loss of grooming activity, and an inability to initiate normal activities. These symptoms are reversed by the administration of antidepressant medications but not by antipsychotic medications. Conditioned avoidance response (in which neuroleptics are observed to produce a deficit in avoidance behavior) is the most widely used animal model of schizophrenia.

394. The answer is E. (Adams RD, 5/e, pp 22–29.) When the subject is at rest with the eyes closed, the normal EEG pattern consists of a background alpha frequency within the range of 8 to 13 Hz. This pattern is replaced by a faster, lower-voltage beta activity when the subject is anxious, concentrating, or using minor tranquilizers. Stroboscopic visual stimulation will produce an evoked response (photic driving) in the occipital lobes if the subject can perceive light. Normal sleep produces a decrease in the background frequency through stages 1 through 4 with the appearance of 1 to 3 Hz activity during the deep sleep of stages 3 and 4. Rapid eye movement (REM) sleep is associated with asynchronous, low-voltage fast activity.

395. The answer is A (1, 2, 3). (Kaplan, 6/e, p 30.) The activation of adenylate cyclase is mediated via guanosine triphosphates (GTP), which act as coupling proteins. The presence of different mediating (G) proteins, which may be either facilitory or inhibitory, allows several different neurotransmitters to activate the adenylate cyclase cascade. Adenylate cyclase can therefore be activated by dopamine, norepinephrine, serotonin, and histamine. This type of second messenger transmission is slower than simple "lock and key" allosteric transmission. The second messenger system is also capable of amplifying the initial signal because of the initiation of a cascade response. The opening of a chloride channel is produced by the binding of γ-aminobutyric acid (GABA) at its particular receptor site and is an example of allosteric binding.

396. The answer is C (2, 4). (Kaplan, 6/e, pp 29–30.) Autoreceptors are situated on the presynaptic membrane and respond to increased levels of a particular neurotransmitter (e.g., dopamine) by activating an inhibitory feedback on the synthesis and release of that neurotransmitter. Blocking the dopamine postsynaptic receptor will therefore result in increased dopamine synthesis and release. Some degree of tolerance, however, eventually develops. Autoreceptors are therefore responsible for autoregulation at the synapse.

397. The answer is B (1, 3). (Kaplan, 6/e, p 25.) Catecholamines are inactivated at the synapse either by active reuptake at the nerve terminal or by enzymatic catabolism. The two enzymes involved in this breakdown are monoamine oxidase and catechol-*O*-methyltransferase (COMT). Monoamine oxidase is situated on the external mitochondrial membrane and is available to catabolize free catecholamines within the cell cytosol. COMT is situated on the outer cell membrane and involved with the degradation of catecholamines in the synaptic cleft. These catabolic enzymes are found not only in the central nervous system but also in the intestine and liver. Tyrosine hydroxylase and dopamine decarboxylase are involved in the synthesis of the catecholamines. Tyrosine hydroxylase is the rate-limiting enzyme in this pathway.

398. **The answer is C (2, 4).** (Kaplan, 6/e, pp 37–39, 69–70.) GABA and glycine are both inhibitory neurotransmitters. Both of these neurotransmitters act rapidly via allosteric (i.e., "lock and key") binding at their receptor sites and induce a rapid hyperpolarization by increasing the chloride permeability of the neuronal cell membrane. GABA receptor activity is gaining increasing interest and importance in psychopharmacology. In particular, benzodiazepines have been found to bind at GABA receptors and act as agonists by increasing the affinity of these receptors for GABA. The development of a benzodiazepine antagonist offers the potential for the rapid, controlled reversal of benzodiazepine activity. This may offer important clinical uses in anesthesia and benzodiazepine overdose. GABA agonists are also under development and may have therapeutic uses in seizure disorders and behavioral disorders. Glycine is an inhibitory neurotransmitter confined to the brainstem and spinal cord. Both aspartate and glutamate are excitatory amino acids.

399. **The answer is C (2, 4).** (Kaplan, 6/e, pp 893–894.) Prolactin is secreted in the anterior pituitary. Its secretion is directly inhibited by dopamine released into the tuberoinfundibular system. Secretion is further modulated by negative feedback. Thyrotropin-releasing hormone (TRH), endogenous opiates, and L-tryptophan stimulate prolactin secretion. Somatostatin inhibits response. Patients with hyperprolactinemia report dysphoria, reduced tolerance to stress, oligomenorrhea, and galactorrhea. There is a sharp rise in plasma prolactin following generalized seizure activity.

400. **The answer is E (all).** (Kaplan, 6/e, pp 34–35.) *N*-methyl-D-aspartate (NMDA) is one of several agonists for the excitatory receptors. Through its actions at ion channels, it produces depolarization and therefore excitation. Intracerebral injection of NMDA results in tonic clonic convulsions and neuronal degeneration at the site of injection. This phenomenon has been now termed "excitotoxicity." Antagonists to these excitatory neurotransmitters offer promise as anticonvulsants and as a means of reducing neuronal injury following seizures, anoxia, hypoglycemia, or cerebrovascular accidents. Other potentially neurotoxic excitatory amino acids include quisqualate and kainate. Each excitatory amino acid appears to have a distinct receptor distribution in the brain.

401. **The answer is C (2, 4).** (Kaplan, 6/e, pp 31–32.) The 5-HT2 serotonin receptors are found primarily in the cortex. They are the primary site of action of fluoxetine as well as LSD and other hallucinogens and have therefore been implicated in the production of psychotic states. Buspirone is thought to act as a 5-HT1a receptor agonist. An increasing number of heterogeneous serotonin receptors with diverse activities are being discovered.

402. The answer is E (all). (Kaplan, 6/e, p 938.) Raised serum levels of the endorphins have been found in each of the situations described. The pattern of endorphins in psychiatric disorders is less clear. The endorphins increase appetite and have been shown to rise significantly with exercise. Endorphins are a heterogeneous group of peptides derived from one of three precursor proteins: proenkephalin, prodynorphin, and pro-opiomalanocortin (POMC). Unlike monoamines, which are metabolized in the nerve terminal from dietary sources, neuropeptides are synthesized in the ribosomes and require mRNA. Neuropeptides appear to exert a neuromodulating effect upon monoaminergic neurotransmission. Other neuropeptides include substance P, cholecystokinin, vasoactive intestinal polypeptide, somatostatin, bombesin, and neurotensin.

403. The answer is C (2, 4). (Davis, p 73.) Neurotransmitters are released into the synaptic cleft from the presynaptic terminal when depolarization occurs. A number of criteria for neurotransmitters have been outlined. These include the following: (1) they should be present in highest concentration in the presynaptic terminal; (2) they should be released with depolarization; (3) they should produce a similar response to electrical stimulation at the receptor; (4) there must be a method of rapid inactivation; (5) they should bind to the receptor in a selective manner; and (6) presynaptic electrical stimulation and neurotransmitter application should be similarly altered by drug actions.

404. The answer is E (all). (Kaplan, 6/e, pp 130–131.) Melatonin is an indoleamine produced in the pineal gland. The synthesis of melatonin requires tryptophan as a precursor. The uptake of tryptophan into the pineal is increased by noradrenaline. The production of melatonin is highest at nighttime with a peak at about 0300 hours and is suppressed by light stimulation. Melatonin synthesis follows a circadian 24-h cycle, which is entrained via environmental light and the suprachiasmatic nucleus. Its production appears to be unaffected by other circadian components such as the sleep/wake cycle or temperature. Melatonin is under increasing scrutiny as a potential marker for several psychiatric disorders.

405. The answer is B (1, 3). (Kaplan, 6/e, pp 2038–2054.) There are two types of monoamine oxidase (MAO): MAO-A and MAO-B. MAO-A selectively inhibits serotonin and noradrenaline, whereas MAO-B deaminates phenylethylamine, tyramine, tryptamine, and phenylethanolamine. MAO-A is selectively inhibited by clorgiline, whereas pargyline selectively inhibits MAO-B activity. Currently used MAO inhibitors such as phenelzine, tranylcypromine, and isocarboxazid are nonselective and influence both enzymes. Most MAO inhibitors irreversibly inhibit the activity of the enzyme, and although they have a short half-life will result in a depletion of enzyme activity that lasts several weeks after discontinuation of the drug.

406. The answer is B (1, 3). (Kaplan, 6/e, pp 55–58.) Second messengers are intracellular mediators for other neurotransmitters. Most monoamine neurotransmitters operate via a second messenger. These second messengers may amplify an initial response and therefore serve a modulatory function. Three broad groups of second messengers are currently recognized: cyclic nucleotides (cAMP, cGMP), calcium ions, and phospholipid metabolites (ITP, arachidonic acid). A single neurotransmitter can activate several second-messenger systems.

407. The answer is D (4). (Kaplan, 6/e, pp 30–31.) There are at least two different subtypes of dopamine postsynaptic receptors: D_1 and D_2 receptors. The D_1 receptor has been identified in the parathyroid gland (and influences parathormone secretion) and in the retina. The D_2 receptor is more widely distributed in the dopaminergic system and is found in mesostriatal, mesolimbic, mesocortical, and tuberoinfundibular distributions. Most currently available neuroleptics are nonselective and produce blockade at both receptor subtypes. Flupenthixol appears to have the highest affinity for D_2 receptors, while domperidone and sulpiride exhibit a high affinity for D_2 receptors.

408. The answer is C (2, 4). (Schatzberg, pp 204–205.) Venlafaxine is a novel bicyclic compound that is chemically unrelated to any other antidepressants. It actively inhibits the neuronal reuptake of serotonin, norepinephrine, and (to a lesser extent) dopamine. The drug undergoes extensive first-pass metabolism in the liver to its metabolite, desmethylvenlafaxine (ODV). The protein binding of venlafaxine is 27 percent and that of ODV is 30 percent. It has very little affinity for muscarinic, histaminic, or α_1-adrenergic receptors.

409. The answer is E (all). (Kaplan, 6/e, pp 1391–1395.) Characteristic changes are found in major depressive disorder. These changes include decreased REM latency, prolonged first REM period, decreased slow-wave sleep, more frequent awakenings, and early morning awakening. These changes mean that sleep is likely to be less refreshing, and excessive daytime drowsiness is often reported.

410. The answer is D (4). (Kaplan, 6/e, p 2576.) There are significant alterations in sleep architecture with aging. Total sleep, slow-wave sleep, and REM sleep all attain peak duration during childhood, stabilize after puberty, and then go into a steady decline with advancing age. These are normal physiologic changes and are not indicative of pathology. Although there may be variation among different persons, the sleep pattern of an individual is relatively stable. As a result of these changes, elderly people may complain of sleeping problems and therefore receive more sedatives. Older patients may also take more daytime naps to compensate for these changes.

411. The answer is B (1, 3). (Kaplan, 6/e, pp 1392–1393.) Chronic alcohol abuse leads to a significant disruption of sleep architecture. Changes include fragmented and decreased REM duration, decreased sleep time, and increased awakenings. Alcohol withdrawal produces decreased slow-wave sleep, difficulty initiating sleep, and usually REM rebound. In severe alcoholics REM may remain depressed.

412. The answer is B (1, 3). (Kaplan, 6/e, p 1376.) Narcolepsy is characterized by the classic tetrad of sleep attacks, cataplexy, sleep paralysis, and hypnopompic/hypnogogic hallucinations. In reality all four of these symptoms are seldom present and the sleep attacks usually precede the other symptoms. The disease usually has its onset in the second decade. There is a strong familial trend with equal frequency in both sexes. An association of HLA-B7 and HLA-DR2 with narcolepsy has been postulated. Diagnosis is made by demonstrating a shortened REM latency on polysomnography. Psychostimulants are the treatment of choice.

413. The answer is B (1, 3). (Cooper, 7/e, pp 493–495.) The dopamine hypothesis states that schizophrenia is the consequence of a relative excess of central dopaminergic neuronal activity and is founded primarily on the clinical efficacy of D_2 receptor antagonists (i.e., typical antipsychotics) and on the induction of psychosis by the chronic administration of amphetamine. However, no direct evidence of increased dopamine turnover has been obtained. D_4 receptors in the schizophrenic brain have been shown to have an increased affinity for atypical antipsychotic drugs (e.g., clozapine). The density of D_2 receptors is increased in the schizophrenic brain. However, whether or not this reflects a consequence of neuroleptic treatment is uncertain. The negative symptoms of schizophrenia are correlated with decreased prefrontal lobe activity that may reflect an adaptive down-regulation of dopaminergic activity in this region.

414. The answer is E (all). (Kaplan, 6/e, p 1377.) The disorders of excessive somnolence (DOES) have been classified by the Association of Sleep Disorders Centers (ASDC) under a number of different subheadings: (1) psychophysiologic (causes under this heading include acute or chronic stress situations); (2) associated with psychiatric disorders (e.g., mood disorders); (3) associated with drug use; (4) sleep apnea; (5) narcolepsy; (6) "restless legs" syndromes; (7) environmental; and (8) Kleine-Levin syndrome. The appropriate treatment will of course depend on the etiology.

415–418. The answers are 415-B, 416-D, 417-A, 418-C. (Adams RD, 5/e, pp 22–29. Kaplan, 6/e, pp 74–77.) EEG tracing B demonstrates the expected findings in a subject who is using minor tranquilizers. These findings are typically low-voltage, symmetric, fast-frequency wave forms found particularly over the frontal areas. The encephalopathy produced by lithium is characterized by diffuse slowing of the background rhythm. The EEG may provide valuable clues when investigating any alteration in attention, particularly when a drug overdose is suspected.

Tracing D demonstrates spike discharges localized to the left hemisphere. These changes are consistent with partial focal epilepsy of the right hemisphere. Although this is a classic ictal pattern, it is important to remember that 40 percent of patients with generalized epilepsy will have a normal EEG on single random recording. A single normal EEG tracing does not rule out epilepsy and the procedure should be repeated if necessary. All electrophysiologic data should only be interpreted in the context of the clinical findings.

Tracing A demonstrates the typical features of a hepatic encephalopathy. These changes include background slowing and bilateral synchronous "triphasic waves." The EEG abnormality closely correlates with the clinical stage of coma and may be helpful in following the patient's clinical course.

Tracing C demonstrates the "sleep spindles," K complexes, and background theta waves normally found in stage 2 sleep. Stage 1 sleep consists of an increasing percentage of theta-wave activity (4 to 7 Hz) with low-voltage, fast-background activity and vertex sharp waves. Stages 3 and 4 sleep are characterized by delta-wave predominance (1.5 to 3 Hz). The EEG of REM sleep closely approximates the waking state with the occurrence of hypotonia and REMs.

419–423. The answers are 419-B, 420-C, 421-D, 422-A, 423-E. (Fischer, p 125.) The structures shown on the axial MRI scan in the question are identified in the figure below.

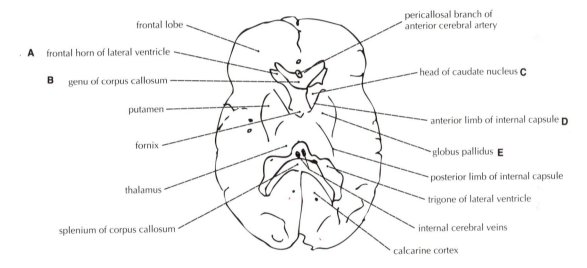

Adapted from Fischer and Ketonen, Fig. 2-71, with permission.

424–427. The answers are 424-E, 425-B, 426-A, 427-C. (Davis, pp 74–81.) There is a clear neuroanatomic distribution of the major biogenic amines and their projections. Five distinct dopaminergic tracts exist: (1) nigrostriatal, (2) mesolimbic, (3) mesocortical, (4) tuberoinfundibular, and (5) retinal. Long tracts arise from areas A9 (substantia nigra) and A10 (ventral tegmental area), while medium tracts arise from the hypothalamus. The nigrostriatal tract regulates motor activity and innervates the striatum. The mesocortical tracts and mesolimbic tracts are involved in the motor expression and the subjective experience of emotional states. The tuberoinfundibular system influences the activity of the anterior pituitary gland.

The cell bodies of the noradrenergic system lie in the hindbrain; the major collection is found in the locus coeruleus. The diffuse projections from these sites to virtually all areas of the neuraxis suggest primarily a neuromodulatory function.

The raphe nuclei are the major sites for serotoninergic projections to diffuse areas of the brain including the cortex, limbic structures, spinal cord, and lateral geniculate nucleus. The system appears to have inhibitory effects on behavioral response to environmental cues, including the suppression of aggression, sexual interest, and arousal. This neuro-modulating activity is supported by the tonic firing of the raphe nuclei, which appears to act as a behavioral "pacemaker."

Cholinergic projections arise from cell bodies situated around the medial septal area: the nucleus basalis, preoptic nucleus, and diagonal band of Broca. Destruction of the nucleus basalis, which has dense projections to the hippocampus, has been postulated to be partly responsible for the memory disturbances found in Alzheimer's disease. Diffuse cholinergic projections are to (1) ventral horn cells to all muscles, (2) striatal interneurons, (3) cortex, and (4) hippocampus.

PSYCHOSOCIAL ISSUES AND PHENOMENOLOGY

Directions: Each item below contains five suggested responses. Select the **one best** response to each item.

428. Each of the following is considered a mature ego defense mechanism EXCEPT

(A) sublimation
(B) humor
(C) repression
(D) suppression
(E) altruism

429. According to classical psychoanalytic theory, the functions of the ego include each of the following EXCEPT

(A) the control of instinctual drives
(B) development of moral codes of behavior
(C) maintenance of an appropriate relationship to reality
(D) reality testing
(E) development of satisfying object relationships

430. According to Margaret Mahler's object relations theory, the period of consolidation and object constancy is characterized by each of the following EXCEPT

(A) the child becomes comfortable during periods of mother's absence
(B) the child internalizes an image of the mother as stable and reliable
(C) the child is able to accept substitutes for the mother
(D) the child develops a social smile
(E) this stage of development is usually reached by age 3

431. The ego defense mechanism of splitting

(A) is a neurotic level defense mechanism
(B) transforms one unacceptable impulse into its opposite
(C) results in the suppression of conflict-ridden impulses
(D) produces oscillating interpersonal relationships
(E) isolates ego dystonic affect

432. Each of the following statements about Erik Erikson's theory of personality development is true EXCEPT

(A) integrity versus despair represents the final stage of personality development
(B) personality development follows a predictable sequence of critical stages
(C) trust versus mistrust represents the first developmental stage
(D) a person must accomplish each developmental task before progressing to the next stage
(E) personality development is completed by early adulthood

433. True statements regarding the pleasure principle include

(A) it is a learned function
(B) it is modulated by the reality principle
(C) it is directed toward increasing tension
(D) it attempts to create disequilibrium within the organism
(E) it persists only until late adolesence

434. Formal operational thinking is characterized by which of the following?

(A) It is usually achieved by the end of the latency period
(B) It is necessary for the development of social skills
(C) It is necessary for abstraction
(D) It heralds the acquisition of speech
(E) It is achieved by the majority of adults

435. The ego defense mechanism of projective identification

(A) is the product of a rigid superego
(B) is the prominent defense of the compulsive personality
(C) is a manifestation of the ego-ideal
(D) often makes the therapist uncomfortable
(E) produces a sudden change in the subject's character

436. The psychiatrist's obligation to maintain confidentiality may be waived in all the following circumstances EXCEPT

(A) involuntary committal
(B) child abuse
(C) medical emergency
(D) venereal disease in a sexually active patient
(E) a request for information by the patient's lawyer

437. The competency of a patient is

(A) task-specific
(B) determined by the psychiatrist
(C) necessary for involuntary commitment
(D) necessary for confidentiality
(E) necessary if informed consent is to be obtained

438. The principle of *respondeat superior*

(A) determines the patient's moral sanity

(B) describes the patient's right to dictate treatment decisions

(C) demands the confidentiality of medical records

(D) involves the vicarious responsibility an attending physician has for the treatment decisions of his resident

(E) dictates the moral imperative

439. The elements of medical malpractice include each of the following EXCEPT

(A) the presence of a doctor-patient relationship

(B) the dereliction of duty by the physician

(C) a direct causation between the physician's behavior and the damage experienced by the patient

(D) injury as a direct result of the physician's negligence

(E) the competency of the patient

440. The American Law Institute rule

(A) provides the basis of the insanity law

(B) dictates the requirements for any malpractice suit

(C) states the requirements for the right to refuse treatment

(D) outlines the requirements of seclusion and restraint

(E) provides guidelines for involuntary commitment

441. Which of the following statements regarding the Tarasoff II decision is true?

(A) It determines the requirements for involuntary hospitalization

(B) It does not influence confidentiality

(C) It dictates the clinician's responsibility to inform any person who might be harmed by the patient

(D) It is binding on all psychiatrists in the U.S.

(E) It does not apply to patients who are psychotic

442. The patient's right to bar from judicial hearings the information shared within the professional relationship is referred to as

(A) confidentiality

(B) privilege

(C) *parens patriae*

(D) *respondeat superior*

(E) obstruction

443. The structural model of family therapy considers family dysfunction to be a result of

(A) communication deficits

(B) deficient reward systems within the family

(C) poor problem-solving within the family

(D) malfunctioning boundaries within the family

(E) triangulation within the family

444. An accurate characterization of cognitive behavioral therapy is that it

(A) relies heavily on negative reinforcers

(B) is contraindicated in patients with borderline personality disorder

(C) requires multiple and prolonged sessions if it is to be effective

(D) employs flooding as a means of altering behavior

(E) requires the patient to practice techniques outside the sessions

445. Each of the following is a true statement about incest EXCEPT

(A) the majority of cases involve father-daughter relationships

(B) mothers are very rarely aware of the incest

(C) alcoholism in the family is a risk factor

(D) the mother in the family is often physically abused

(E) the victim is usually a prepubertal child

446. The number of cases of an illness at a particular time is known as the

(A) incidence

(B) point prevalence

(C) frequency

(D) risk factor

(E) cohort

447. The results of an experimental drug trial demonstrate that a drug definitely known to be effective is ineffective. This is an example of a

(A) negative skew

(B) between-sample variance

(C) standard error

(D) type I error

(E) type II error

448. A 70-year-old woman who is experiencing a normal grief reaction

(A) may experience a disrupted sleep pattern

(B) may, at times, experience the presence of the deceased person

(C) is likely to experience suicidal ideation

(D) typically experiences symptoms of grief for several years

(E) usually benefits from antidepressant medication

449. According to classical psychoanalytic theory, conversion disorder

(A) represents fixation at the oral phase of ego development

(B) is the consequence of a rigid superego

(C) indicates an unresolved oedipal conflict

(D) is an extension of female penis envy

(E) suggests inappropriate toilet training

450. Which of the following clinical features would mitigate against a diagnosis of conversion disorder?

(A) A dermatome distribution of sensory loss

(B) Convulsive movements

(C) Astasia-abasia

(D) Coordination disturbance

(E) Rhythmic tremors

451. Each of the following is a true statement about the prognosis of conversion disorder EXCEPT

(A) the majority of conversion symptoms rapidly resolve

(B) at least 25 percent of patients will develop another conversion disorder

(C) recurrent conversion symptoms are not always the same

(D) the presence of another psychiatric disorder is a poor prognostic indicator

(E) the presence of a severe psychosocial precipitant is a poor prognostic indicator

452. Monosymptomatic delusional hypochondriasis is correctly characterized by which statement?

(A) It is most effectively treated with a high-potency neuroleptic

(B) It frequently remits with hypnosis

(C) It is more common in males

(D) It usually has its onset in adolescence

(E) It seldom interrupts the affected person's life-style

453. Following a cerebrovascular accident, an elderly man claims that he can no longer recognize friends or relatives. This is most likely to be

(A) a conversion disorder

(B) Balint's syndrome

(C) prosopagnosia

(D) confabulation

(E) Capgras syndrome

454. Catatonia is characterized by each of the following features EXCEPT

(A) negativism

(B) echopraxia

(C) stereotypy

(D) mutism

(E) perseveration

455. Acute confusional states are characterized by each of the following EXCEPT

(A) complex motor tics

(B) perseveration

(C) lack of persistence

(D) distractibility

(E) fluctuating consciousness

456. The ego defenses of isolation of affect, reaction formation, and undoing are employed by which of the following personalities?

(A) Histrionic

(B) Sociopathic

(C) Compulsive

(D) Borderline

(E) Self-defeating

457. The primary ego defense mechanism employed in the development of a specific phobia is

(A) acting out

(B) isolation of affect

(C) somatization

(D) displacement

(E) suppression

458. A young woman meets a man only once. Following this encounter, she "falls madly in love" with him and writes about their love affair in her secret diary each day for the next year. This is best described as

(A) acting out
(B) an erotic transference
(C) anticipation
(D) a schizophreniform psychosis
(E) schizoid fantasy

459. At the end of the oedipal stage a boy becomes allied with his father. This is the classic example of

(A) acting out
(B) identification with the aggressor
(C) sublimation
(D) idealization
(E) reaction formation

460. A patient with borderline personality disorder would be expected to employ each of the following ego defenses EXCEPT

(A) reaction formation
(B) projective identification
(C) regression
(D) splitting
(E) somatization

Directions: Each item below contains four suggested responses of which **one or more** is correct. Select:

A	if	**1, 2, and 3**	are correct
B	if	**1 and 3**	are correct
C	if	**2 and 4**	are correct
D	if	**4**	is correct
E	if	**1, 2, 3, and 4**	are correct

461. Alexithymia is characterized by

(1) an inability to appreciate the feelings of others
(2) an association with chronic pain syndromes
(3) prolonged periods of depression
(4) a subjective unawareness of one's emotions

462. Secondary process thinking may be described as

(1) a consequence of thought derailing
(2) a phenomenon found in schizophreniform psychosis
(3) a manifestation of a core delusional experience
(4) a logical process

463. The positive symptoms of schizophrenia

(1) tend to be resistant to neuroleptic medication
(2) imply a poor prognosis
(3) are more common in male schizophrenics
(4) include paranoid delusions

464. Schneiderian first-rank symptoms include

(1) thought withdrawal
(2) auditory hallucinations
(3) thought broadcasting
(4) thought hearing

465. The classic interictal personality disorder is characterized by

(1) hypergraphia
(2) hyperviscosity
(3) hypermoralism
(4) hyposexuality

466. Characteristics of hypnopompic hallucinations include that they

(1) occur at sleep onset
(2) are associated with narcolepsy
(3) usually indicate psychosis
(4) often occur in normal persons

467. Typical features of a fugue state include

(1) the assumption of a new identity
(2) repetitive stereotypic movements
(3) amnesia for previous life experiences
(4) bizarre somatosensory experiences

468. An uncomplicated grief reaction may include which of the following?

(1) Somatic symptoms such as insomnia, weight loss, and loss of appetite
(2) Social withdrawal
(3) Emotional numbing
(4) Marked functional impairment and psychomotor retardation

SUMMARY OF DIRECTIONS

A	B	C	D	E
1,2,3	1,3	2,4	4	All are
only	only	only	only	correct

469. The speech of a schizophrenic patient may be characterized by

(1) neologisms
(2) mutism
(3) verbigeration
(4) dysprosody

470. Obsessive ruminations may be found as a manifestation of

(1) major depressive disorder
(2) schizophrenia
(3) Tourette's disorder
(4) conversion disorder

471. Trichotillomania may be characterized as

(1) a mood-congruent psychotic disorder
(2) a disorder usually associated with advanced dementia
(3) an example of a factitious disorder
(4) an irresistible urge to pull out one's hair

472. Symptoms typical of posttraumatic stress disorder include

(1) emotional numbing
(2) increased distractibility
(3) amnesia for the traumatic event
(4) social avoidance

473. Alcoholic hallucinosis may be described by which of the following?

(1) It is associated with an acute confusional state
(2) It may persist for several weeks
(3) It only involves visual hallucinations
(4) It usually occurs within 48 h of cessation of alcohol use

Directions: Each group of questions below consists of lettered options followed by a set of numbered items. For each numbered item, select the **one** lettered option with which it is **most** closely associated. Each lettered option may be used **once, more than once, or not at all.**

Items 474–477

For each definition appearing below, choose the statistical term that is most appropriate.

(A) Mean
(B) Median
(C) Standard deviation
(D) *t*-Distribution
(E) Normal distribution

474. A bell-shaped frequency distribution curve such as would be generated by plotting the height of a large number of people

475. The arithmetic sum of the observations divided by the number of observations

476. A bell-shaped curve with the tails containing more area than a *z*-distribution

477. The square root of the variance

Items 478–481

For each definition appearing below, choose the type of validity that it most accurately describes.

(A) Construct validity
(B) Predictive validity
(C) Correlative validity
(D) Concurrent validity
(E) Content validity

478. Extent to which the items in a rating scale sample the universe of behaviors to the observer, e.g., in a rating scale for depression, how well the items of the rating scale reflect the behaviors actually found in depression

479. Relation between test results and another criterion evaluated at about the same time, e.g., a comparison of self-rating depression scale results with ratings made on the basis of clinical judgment

480. Ability of a measuring instrument to forecast another measurement by a different criterion at a different time, e.g., comparison of results of a self-rating depression scale

481. Demonstration that certain explanatory constructs—e.g., depression or anxiety—account for some portion of variability of the ratings

Items 482–485

For each set of primary goals of psychotherapy listed below, select the originator with whom it is most closely identified.

   (A) Alfred Adler
   (B) Harry Stack Sullivan
   (C) Karen Horney
   (D) Jules Masserman
   (E) Eric Berne

482. To relieve immediate distress and guide the patient by any ethical means to more satisfying ways of living and a new life philosophy

483. To increase the patient's social interest so that the patient can feel an equal among peers and abandon unrealistic views of life

484. To free the patient from compulsions and resistance to change so that creative forces can be expressed

485. To develop and maintain a patient's self-esteem and interpersonal security

Items 486–490

Match the following.

   (A) *Mens rea*
   (B) *Lex talionis*
   (C) *Non compos mentis*
   (D) *Habeas corpus*
   (E) *Parens patriae*

486. The right to challenge the lawfulness of detention

487. Lack of capacity to exercise sound judgment

488. The guilty mind

489. Retributive justice

490. The right of the state to hold a dangerous person in custody

Items 491–496

For each clinical vignette, choose the defense mechanism of which it is illustrative.

(A) Fixation
(B) Resistance
(C) Dissociation
(D) Displacement
(E) Restitution

491. An epileptic adult, with no cognitive deficits, continually forgets to buy his medication, loses it when he buys it, and forgets to take it when his wife brings it home for him

492. A juvenile male enters therapy because of an inordinate feeling of anger toward and hatred of policemen. He fears that he will attack or assault a policeman because he becomes enraged by the sight of any male wearing a uniform. The patient comes from a broken home with a harsh, punitive father whom he, nevertheless, claims to love

493. An adult in psychoanalytic therapy is making satisfactory progress but then begins to arrive late at therapy sessions and seems disgruntled with the therapist

494. A 20-year-old woman who had recently become engaged experienced three episodes in which she wandered aimlessly on the streets; she did not harm herself or others during these episodes. She describes complete amnesia for these episodes. Neurologic examination and EEG results were normal

495. An 18-year-old woman enters therapy after having a child out of wedlock. The conception occurred several months after her younger sister died from rheumatic heart disease. The patient expresses strong feelings of guilt and responsibility for her sibling's death and the grief it has caused in her parents

496. A 9-year-old boy is presented for therapy because of his mother's complaints of his excessive mouthing of objects, excessive appetite, and thumb sucking. These have been lifelong behaviors. The child is dressed like—and acts like—a much younger child

Items 497–501

For each clinical sketch below, choose the type of resistance to which it most closely corresponds.

(A) Secondary gain resistance
(B) Superego resistance
(C) Id resistance
(D) Transference resistance
(E) Conscious resistance

497. During a session of free association, a patient thinks about describing having masturbated the night before but does not tell the analyst because of feelings of shame and embarrassment

498. During a therapy hour, a patient begins by freely discussing his feelings about his father, using veiled criticism with no display of affect. The therapist listens quietly. The patient becomes silent for a period, then somewhat angrily says, "Why don't you say something? You are just sitting there"

499. In discussing her repetitious hand-washing, a patient is unable to connect the act with the early desire she had to handle her brother's genitals. On many occasions, the therapist had, by gentle interpretation, suggested to the patient the possibility of a connection when the hand-washing and early fantasy had been repeatedly linked by the patient while free associating

500. A patient struggling with an offer of a job far better than any held by his siblings or father is unable to make a decision to accept it. The analysis discloses strong feelings that the patient wants to be the most loved and successful member of the family, and this is attended by much guilt

501. With many years of indulgence on the part of her husband for her headaches and infirmities, a patient has improved in her ability to work and complete household chores like grocery shopping. She cannot induce herself to learn to drive, however, and insists that her husband drive her wherever she goes

PSYCHOSOCIAL ISSUES AND PHENOMENOLOGY

428. The answer is C. (Kaplan, 6/e, pp 451–452.) Repression is considered a neurotic ego defense. It describes the process of expelling a thought or feeling from consciousness without being aware that one is doing it. The ego defense of suppression describes the process whereby one consciously and deliberately avoids paying attention to a thought or feeling. A hierarchy of ego defense mechanisms has been described by Dr. George Vaillant: psychotic (narcissistic), immature, neurotic, and mature ego defenses. Other mature ego defenses are anticipation and asceticism.

429. The answer is B. (Kaplan, 6/e, pp 451–452.) The ego essentially functions as a mediator between a person's instinctual libidinous drives and instincts and the reality of the outside world. Each of its functions is therefore directed toward this goal. According to classical psychoanalytic theory, the ego is responsible for the following functions: (1) control and regulation of instinctual drives; (2) development of an appropriate relationship to reality; (3) the capacity to develop and sustain appropriate object relationships; and (4) primary autonomous functions such as speaking, thinking, learning, intelligence, perception, and intuition. The ability to "self-evaluate" one's behavior is a function of the superego, which emerges with resolution of the Oedipus complex. It represents the incorporation and integration of parental standards and the development of an "ego-ideal."

430. The answer is D. (Kaplan, 6/e, pp 458–459.) Margaret Mahler described three developmental phases based on the theory of object relations. In the normal autistic phase (birth to 4 weeks), the major task is to achieve homeostatic equilibrium with the environment. In the normal symbiotic phase (4 weeks to 4 months), the child behaves as if he or she and the caretaker were undifferentiated. The child also develops a social smile at this age. The third phase is separation/individuation (5 to 36 months). This phase is further divided into four subphases: differentiation, practicing, rapprochement, and consolidation and object constancy. During the subphase of differentiation (5 to 10 months), the child is emerging from his or her cocoon and exploring the outside world. The sensorium therefore develops and the child exhibits stranger anxiety. Practicing (10 to 16 months) is typified by further exploration and walking. The child will also develop separation anxiety during this period. During the rapprochement subphase (16 to 24 months), the child is ambivalent about separation from the mother and may both seek and reject nurturance by her. The final subphase of separation-individuation (24 to 36 months), which is consolidation and object constancy, is characterized by the child's development of a stable internal image of the mother. The child is able to tolerate periods of separation and accept brief maternal substitutes and also develops a better sense of time and improved verbal skills during this period.

431. The answer is D. (Kaplan, ed 6, pp 493–495.) Splitting is a narcissistic (or psychotic) level ego defense mechanism in which all objects are experienced by a person as either "good" or "bad." These subjective categorizations are unstable and may oscillate rapidly between the two extremes. This process, by necessity, dictates that objects (including the self) must either be idealized or devalued. This defense mechanism therefore results in unstable relationships and extremes in the subject's mood. Splitting is considered to be the primary defense used by the borderline personality structure.

432. The answer is E. (Kaplan, 6/e, pp 404–408.) Erik Erikson postulated eight stages of personality development extending from infancy into old age. Each stage of development is critical and each developmental task must be accomplished before progressing to the next stage. Erikson described a tripartite model for understanding personality development. This model includes the somatic, ego, and cultural-historical aspects of the person's experience, and the resolution of each developmental "crisis" is influenced by each of these factors. Erikson's eight stages of personality development are trust vs. mistrust, autonomy vs. shame and doubt, initiative vs. guilt, industry vs. inferiority, identity vs. role confusion, intimacy vs. isolation, generativity vs. stagnation, and finally integrity vs. despair.

433. The answer is B. (Kaplan, 6/e, p 441.) The pleasure principle was conceptualized by Sigmund Freud. It refers to the inborn tendency of the organism to seek equilibrium by the discharge of tension. This is achieved by seeking pleasure rather than pain. The pleasure principle is modulated by the reality principle, which develops with maturation of the ego. The delay of immediate gratification by the reality principle was postulated to result eventually in greater pleasure. Freud postulated that a disequilibrium between these two systems results in psychopathology.

434. The answer is C. (Kaplan, 6/e, pp 292–296.) Formal operational thinking is the final stage of Piagetan cognitive development and begins in early adolescence. The acquisition of this degree of cognitive sophistication is not universal, however, and it is estimated that approximately 25 percent of adults are capable of formal operational thinking. It is characterized by the ability to abstract and manipulate theoretical concepts. Entry into this stage invites an increasing interest in politics, religion, and philosophy. The four stages of Piagetan cognitive development are sensorimotor (birth to 2 years), preoperational thought (2 to 7 years), concrete operations (7 to 11 years), and formal operational thinking (11 years to adulthood).

435. The answer is D. (Kaplan, 6/e, pp 458–459.) Projective identification is a narcissistic level ego defense mechanism. Through this mechanism subjects deposit uncomfortable aspects of themselves on the observer and thereby distance themselves from these experiences. These experiences are modified by the recipient. This defense is commonly employed by persons with borderline personality disorder and often makes the therapist uncomfortable.

436. The answer is E. (Kaplan, 6/e, pp 2760–2761.) Confidentiality is defined as the responsibility of the physician not to disclose to any third party information shared by the patient. Breach of confidentiality is grounds for, and is a common cause of, litigation by patients against their physicians. The exceptions to the confidentiality rule are (1) emergency situations (since there is no clear definition of what constitutes an emergency, the physician must use sound clinical judgment as to what constitutes an emergency); (2) patient incompetence—in this situation the patient's guardian or the court should be asked permission to release information; (3) information necessary to commit a patient; (4) reportable conditions—the abuse of minors or the presence of communicable diseases requires reporting to the appropriate agency; (5) the legal right of third-party payers to some aspects of the patient's record.

437. The answer is A. (Kaplan, 6/e, pp 2754–2755.) *Competence* is a task-specific term that refers to a person's ability to perform certain tasks through a capacity to use information and make a decision based on the person's own value system. The concept of global competency is therefore invalid and each determination of competency should be made with only the particular task in mind; for example, a patient may be competent to make decisions regarding treatment choices but incompetent to handle finances. Informed consent is obtained through the patient's guardian. Although the psychiatrist may be asked to make a professional assessment of a person's competence, the court ultimately makes the ruling. A patient's competency does not influence confidentiality.

438. The answer is D. (Simon, pp 386–388.) The term *respondeat superior* (literal translation from the Latin: "Let the master respond") refers to the vicarious responsibility that attending physicians have for the negligence of those they directly supervise (e.g., resident staff or paramedical therapists). This legal concept has important implications for physicians working in multidisciplinary settings such as community mental health centers. In any situation where the physician is responsible for signing insurance forms to enable nonmedical therapists to receive payment, that physician is considered ethically, morally, and medically responsible for the treatment that those personnel provide.

439. The answer is E. (Kaplan, 6/e, pp 2748–2753.) The elements of malpractice incorporate four factors often referred to as the "4 D's": (1) *dereliction* or negligence by the physician, (2) a breach of the physician's *duty* to his patient, (3) *damages* (injury) experienced by the patient, and (4) a *direct* causation between the physician's negligence and the damage. All these factors must be present for a claim of medical malpractice to be successful.

440. The answer is A. (Kaplan, 6/e, p 2764.) The American Law Institute rule has become an integral part of American insanity law. It states that a person is not responsible for an alleged crime if that person (1) lacks the ability to appreciate that the alleged act was wrong or (2) is incapable of behaving in accordance with the law. This law provides the judge and jury with considerable flexibility in reaching their determination about a particular defendant's sanity.

441. The answer is C. (Kaplan, 6/e, p 2761.) The Tarasoff II decision held that therapists have a duty to take all reasonable steps to protect a third party from physical assault by their clients. This represents an extension of the Tarasoff I decision, which stated that the therapist simply had a responsibility to warn any potential victim. According to this ruling, the therapist therefore has a responsibility to both the patient and third parties. It determines that the therapist should predict the likelihood of potential violence and overrides the confidentiality of the patient-doctor relationship. The specific Tarasoff II ruling applies only to therapists in California; each state has its own precedents.

442. The answer is B. (Kaplan, 6/e, pp 2761–2762.) Privilege is the right of the patient to bar from the court (or any judicial hearing) any information disclosed within the doctor-patient relationship. Exceptions to the rule of privilege are (1) patient litigation, (2) the patient's making his or her mental state part of the legal argument, (3) child custody, and (4) duty to protect third parties. Confidentiality is the obligation of the therapist not to disclose any information about the patient without the patient's permission.

443. The answer is D. (Kaplan, 6/e, pp 1838–1847.) The structural model of family therapy is based on the concept that families require clearly defined boundaries with a strong parental hierarchy. The system must, however, be adaptive to environmental change and allow for the growth of individual family members. Family malfunction stems from deficits in defined but malleable boundaries. The goal of therapy is to disrupt the family's current dysfunctional system and establish these clear boundaries and parental hierarchy.

444. The answer is E. (Gelder, 3/e, pp 629–630.) Cognitive therapy has proven to be an effective treatment for many psychiatric disorders. The first step in attempting to change the patient's disordered patterns of thinking is to help the patient to become aware of these disordered, or maladaptive thinking patterns. Next an attempt is made to change or suppress these ideas through verbal and/or behavioral measures. Cognitive strategies may include thought stopping, distraction and identifying logical errors in thinking patterns. Patients are encouraged to be aware of their thought patterns and practice techniques for altering these.

445. The answer is B. (Gelder, 3/e, pp 765–766.) Although it is difficult to estimate the true incidence of incest, most recent statistics suggest that approximately 15 percent of women and 6 percent of men have been sexually abused and that about half of these cases involve incest. Father-daughter incest accounts for 75 percent of incest and often involves more than one daughter. Most cases involve the eldest daughter around the age of 10. Risk factors include fathers with a history of alcoholism, poor impulse control, psychosis, depression, or chronic illness. A higher incidence of incest has been reported in lower socioeconomic groups and in families where a parent has been married before. Several characteristic patterns of family dynamics have been described. One typical pattern is a father characterized by alcohol abuse and a mother who is habitually physically assaulted and sanctions the incest.

446. The answer is B. (Kaplan, 6/e, pp 383–384.) *Point prevalence* refers to the number of cases of a disorder at a specific point in time. *Period prevalence* is the number of cases present within a certain period. The *incidence* is the number of new cases of a disorder that have their onset within a specific time period. A *cohort* is a sample of a well-specified population. The *relative risk* is the incidence in the group with the risk factor divided by the incidence in the group without the risk factor.

447. The answer is E. (Kaplan, 6/e, p 428.) The null hypothesis states that differences between samples are secondary to chance alone, i.e., that the effect being investigated does not exist. A type I error occurs when the null hypothesis is rejected when it should have been retained. A type II error occurs when the null hypothesis is retained when it should have been rejected.

448. The answer is B. (Gelder, 3/e, pp 151–154.) The normal grief reaction is a continuous process that resolves in less than 6 months. The first stage typically lasts from hours to a few days and is characterized by emotional numbing, denial, and a feeling of unreality. The second stage usually lasts a few weeks to 6 months and includes sadness, weeping, poor sleep, diminished appetite, guilt or blame, social withdrawal, and restlessness. Grieving persons may at times have a sense that the deceased is present. In the final stage, symptoms resolve and the person resumes social activities, although symptoms may recur at anniversaries.

449. The answer is C. (Kaplan, 6/e, pp 1252–1253.) Conversion disorder describes the subjective alteration of a particular bodily function in the absence of any identifiable physical pathology. The incidence of the condition appears to be decreasing and is more common among females, lower socioeconomic groups, and rural and poorly educated persons. The presence of other psychiatric disease also predisposes to the condition. It usually occurs in persons with histrionic, passive-aggressive, and dependent personalities. Conversion disorders were the breeding ground for early psychodynamic theory and inspired Freud's attempts to outline psychoanalytic principles. These earliest psychodynamic constructs considered conversion disorders to be a failure to resolve incestuous oedipal conflicts. They have been expanded to include the presence of any unconscious intrapsychic conflict and the presence of any primary or secondary gain. Neurobehavioral theory suggests that the conversion disorder is secondary to alterations in cortical arousal served primarily by the right hemisphere. This theory would explain why the majority of conversion symptoms are left-sided.

450. **The answer is A.** (Kaplan, 6/e, pp 1254–1256.) Conversion disorders may present with motor or sensory symptoms or both. The most common are hemianesthesia, gait disturbance (astasia-abasia), glove-and-stocking anesthesia, tunnel blindness, pseudoseizures, and tremors. Symptoms that correlate with neuroanatomic boundaries (e.g., dermatome sensory loss) suggest physical pathology. *La belle indifference* describes the patient's apparent lack of concern for his or her predicament, and although this symptom was once considered pathognomonic of conversion, it is now considered an unreliable sign.

451. **The answer is E.** (Kaplan, 6/e, pp 1257–1258.) Although the initial conversion symptom remits rapidly in 90 percent of patients, at least 25 percent have a recurrence within 6 years. It has been estimated that as many as 60 percent of patients initially diagnosed as suffering from a conversion disorder will eventually be found to have an organic etiology for their symptoms. After excluding any physical basis for the symptom, treatment focuses on reassuring the patient and identifying psychosocial precipitants. Hypnosis and amobarbital (Amytal) may be helpful in identifying occult factors. Once these precipitants have been identified, individual, family, and behavioral therapy may all be effective in developing more productive coping skills in the patient and family.

452. **The answer is A.** (Kaplan, 6/e, pp 1025–1027.) Monosymptomatic delusional hypochondriasis refers to the delusion that one is suffering from a single, specific physical affliction. The most common example is delusional parasitosis (i.e., the belief that one is infested by a parasite). The disorder is more common in females with an average age of onset of 55. The disease may profoundly negatively influence the life-style of the person and may occasionally result in suicide. High-potency neuroleptics (pimozide has been most extensively studied) are effective in alleviating the delusion.

453. **The answer is C.** (Strub, pp 277–278.) The term *agnosia* describes a deficit in cognition. In particular, *prosopagnosia* describes an inability to recognize familiar faces. A person with prosopagnosia may be able to recognize the voices of family members without recognizing their facial features. The condition is caused by bilateral lesions in the visual association cortices. Many other modality-specific agnosias have been described; these include tactile, auditory, and visual agnosias.

454. **The answer is E.** (Kaplan, 6/e, p 1132.) Catatonia is currently divided into two broad subtypes: stuporous and excited catatonia. Stuporous catatonia is characterized by stereotypy, bizarre postures, mutism, waxy flexibility, negativism, echolalia, and echopraxia. *Excited catatonia* appears to be a misnomer and is now seldom used. The excited catatonic is described as agitated, talkative, and driven by delusions. It is most likely that these patients are in fact suffering from manic psychosis. Perseveration describes a person's inability to change set and is normally associated with prefrontal lesions.

455. **The answer is A.** (Adams RD, 5/e, pp 729–732.) The acute confusional state (delirium) is a rapidly developing alteration in the level of arousal and attention. The disorder is a nonspecific symptom of an encephalopathy of any etiology. The clinical features of an acute confusional state include perseveration, distractibility, lack of persistence, alteration in consciousness, and hallucinations. Since attention is the "bedrock" of cognitive functioning, it is misleading to interpret higher cognitive functioning in the context of an acute confusional state. The presence of an encephalopathy is confirmed by diffuse background slowing on electroencephalography.

456. The answer is C. (Kaplan, 6/e, pp 1220–1221.) The obsessive-compulsive personality uses the ego defenses of isolation of affect and reaction formation as a means of controlling uncomfortable, ego-dystonic affect. This need for control results in perfectionism and undoing, which paralyzes the person's attempts at decision-making. A genetic predisposition to obsessive-compulsive personality has been documented. Freud conceptualized these persons as fixated at the anal stage of psychosexual development and bound in a conflict between libidinous drives and parental expectations. Erikson postulated that this arrest at the anal stage leads to a dilemma between the choices of autonomy and shame.

457. The answer is D. (Kaplan, 6/e, p 457.) Phobias provided Freud with material for much of his early work in psychoanalysis. In particular, his study of little Hans who suffered from a phobia of horses provided the template for the development of his theory that displacement is the mechanism necessary for the development of phobias. By this mechanism, affect can be directed from the initial object toward one less threatening and can be thus avoided. In the case of Hans, Freud postulated that the boy's repressed and hostile feelings (oedipal conflict) toward his father could be redirected toward horses. Since Hans was able to avoid horses, his anxiety could be subjectively avoided.

458. The answer is E. (Kaplan, 6/e, p 451.) Schizoid fantasy is an immature level ego defense mechanism. Through this mechanism the person retreats into an autistic environment in which conflicts can be resolved and gratification obtained without the perceived threat of intimacy. The person does not believe the content of the fantasy and does not act it out. Other immature ego defenses include acting out, blocking, hypochondriasis, introjection (e.g., identification with the aggressor), passive-aggressive behavior, projection, regression, and somatization.

459. The answer is B. (Kaplan, 6/e, p 375.) Identification with the aggressor is an example of introjection—an immature ego defense mechanism. Although the internalization of objects is a necessary part of development, the introjection of the punitive traits of the aggressor will result in self-punitive symptoms. By introjecting a feared object, one feels more control of the anxiety-provoking affect.

460. The answer is A. (Kaplan, 6/e, pp 1438–1441.) The borderline personality uses narcissistic level ego defenses. In particular, splitting and projective identification are considered to be the primary defensive strategies of the borderline personality. In splitting, external objects are viewed as either "all good" or "all bad" and the subject's perception of the object may change rapidly. This instability will result in unstable and volatile dyadic relationships.

461. The answer is C (2, 4). (Kaplan, 6/e, p 662.) Alexithymia describes the inability to experience emotions at a subjective level. The alexithymic person can be expected to respond to situations of emotional conflict and dysphoria with somatic complaints. These persons therefore have a higher incidence of chronic pain syndromes and somatization disorders. The genesis of alexithymia is unknown, but it does appear to be a disorder of temperament.

462. The answer is D (4). (Kaplan, 6/e, p 439–441.) The concept of primary and secondary process thinking was introduced by Freud. Primary process thinking uses symbols, metaphors, and images to produce an illogical cognitive style. Freud considered that this form of thinking was involved in dreaming and creative thinking. Secondary process (primarily language-based) thinking relies on sequential, rational processes in the production of a predictable, logical cognitive style. Secondary process thinking is therefore helpful in abstract thinking, planning, and problem-solving.

463. The answer is D (4). (Kaplan, 6/e, pp 774–775.) There has been a resurgence in interest in attempting to define the positive and negative subtypes of schizophrenia. Positive symptoms include hallucinations, delusions, and agitation. Negative symptoms include apathy, social withdrawal, poverty of affect of speech, and cognitive deficits associated with schizophrenia. Positive symptoms are associated with an acute episode or acute exacerbation of illness and tend to respond to neuroleptics. Negative symptoms tend to be insidious and associated with poor social functioning. Females tend to exhibit more positive symptoms.

464. The answer is E (all). (Kaplan, 6/e, p 170.) Schneider attempted to delineate symptoms that could distinguish the psychosis of schizophrenia from other secondary psychoses (i.e., those secondary to an "organic" process). Although experience has demonstrated that the Schneiderian first-rank symptoms are not pathognomonic for process schizophrenia, they are still frequently referred to and have been incorporated into current nosology such as that found in the *DSM IV*. First-rank symptoms include audible thoughts, thought hearing, broadcasting and withdrawal, auditory hallucinations, experiences of influence, and alienation. Schneider also described the nonspecific second-rank symptoms of emotional impoverishment, depressed or elevated mood, and other perceptual disturbances.

465. The answer is E (all). (Strub, pp 410–411.) The features of the classic interictal personality of temporo-limbic epilepsy include (1) hyperviscosity (not being able to change the subject of conversation); (2) hypergraphia (excessive writing); (3) hypermoralism; (4) a sense of personal destiny; (5) hyposexuality; (6) circumstantiality; (7) dependence and passivity; (8) lack of humor; (9) elation or euphoria; (10) compulsive behavior; (11) hostility and aggressive behavior; (12) paranoia; (13) increased emotionality; and (14) depression. These represent stable characteristics in the temperament of some patients with temporo-limbic epilepsy and are probably not influenced by anticonvulsants.

466. The answer is C (2, 4). (Kaplan, 6/e, p 654.) Hypnopompic and hypnagogic hallucinations are predominantly visual and occur at the time of waking and falling asleep, respectively. They are frequently experienced by normal persons and are not suggestive of any underlying psychotic disorder. The hallucinations have a "dreamlike" quality and may elicit extreme anxiety in those who first experience them. They are found in as many as 50 percent of patients with narcolepsy and they have also been reported with increased frequency in patients with temporo-limbic epilepsy.

467. The answer is B (1, 3). (Kaplan, 6/e, pp 1285–1286.) Fugue states are characterized by the sudden onset of periods of altered identity often associated with travel away from the person's usual place of routine. These persons are unaware that they are in an altered state of perception and, while in the fugue, have amnesia for past life experience. Their actions appear purposeful and seldom appear unusual to those unfamiliar with the person. Once they have returned to their usual mental status, they have no recollection of their behaviors during the period of fugue.

468. The answer is A (1, 2, 3). (Kaplan, 6/e, pp 1723–1728.) As described by *DSM IV*, an uncomplicated grief reaction may last several months and include feelings of depression associated with somatic symptoms such as insomnia and loss of energy, appetite, and weight. The development of functional impairment and psychomotor slowing suggests the emergence of a complicated grief reaction. Survivors may hoard and "enshrine" the possessions of the deceased and may imagine that they see that person during the first few months after death. Complicated grief may be characterized by prolonged denial, clinical major depressive disorder, or a failure to resolve the affective distress associated with the initial stages of an uncomplicated grief.

469. The answer is E (all). (Kaplan, 6/e, pp 974–975.) The speech of the schizophrenic may exhibit each of the features listed. Verbigeration describes the repetitive use of meaningless words or phrases. The schizophrenic may invent new words (neologisms) or simply refuse (or be unable) to communicate. Apart from the semantic and lexical errors described, the schizophrenic may also exhibit abnormalities in the nonverbal aspects of communication, which results in the production of inappropriate emotional coloring to a conversation (dysprosody). The automatic repetition of what the schizophrenic hears (echolalia) and word salad have also been described.

470. The answer is A (1, 2, 3). (Kaplan, 6/e, pp 996–997.) Obsessive ruminations do not constitute an encapsulated psychiatric syndrome but a symptom with a differential diagnosis. Approximately 30 percent of patients with a major depressive disorder exhibit obsessive ruminations, which will be considerably diminished once the patient is euthymic. Transient obsessive ruminations may be found in process schizophrenia, but their incidence is probably much less than previously thought. Approximately 3 to 12 percent of patients with obsessive-compulsive disorder (OCD) will develop a schizophreniform psychosis. There is an increased incidence of OCD among patients with Tourette's disorder.

471. The answer is D (4). (Kaplan, 6/e, pp 1412–1415.) Trichotillomania describes the irresistible urge to pull one's hair. Delaying the act causes increasing tension and the pulling of hair produces immediate reduction in anxiety—in this respect the disorder resembles obsessive-compulsive disorder. The incidence of the condition is unknown but is estimated at 1 to 3 percent of the population. A higher incidence is found among the mentally retarded. Behavior modification has been the major therapeutic modality although several recent studies have demonstrated the efficacy of tricyclic antidepressants.

472. The answer is E (all). (Kaplan, 6/e, pp 1227–1236.) The symptoms of posttraumatic stress disorder may occur at any time after the initial stressor. In simple terms, these symptoms may be divided into two broad categories: intrusive and avoidant. These symptoms essentially represent the person's attempts to cope with the initial stressor and avoid further incidents. Intrusive symptoms include distractibility, decreased sleep, nightmares, increased startle response, irritability, and difficulty concentrating. The person may reexperience the traumatic event with recurrent flashbacks or subjective reenactments. Avoidant symptoms include social withdrawal, emotional numbing, attempts to avoid reminders of the event, diminished interest in activities, and psychogenic amnesia for the event.

473. The answer is C (2, 4). (Kaplan, 5/e, p 635.) Alcoholic hallucinosis describes the development of auditory and visual hallucinations that normally occur within 24 to 48 h of alcohol withdrawal in an alcohol-dependent person. The hallucinations occur in the presence of a clear sensorium and last several weeks after cessation of alcohol use. Neuroleptics are effective in reducing the hallucinosis.

474–477. The answers are 474-E, 475-A, 476-D, 477-C. (Kaplan, 6/e, pp 412–429.) No physician can read the clinical or experimental literature critically without at least a minimum knowledge of experimental design and statistics. Many statistical analyses compare the mean of some variable in an experimental group with the mean of a control group. The mean, or arithmetic average, is defined as the total value of the observations added together, divided by the number of observations. The mean is usually the most useful measure of the central tendency of the data.

Other measures of central tendency are the median and the mode. The median is the midpoint between the highest and lowest points. The mode is the most frequently occurring value.

To describe the numerical characteristics of a population requires knowledge of the variation of the data. The values used for this purpose are the range, variance, and standard deviation. The range is the difference between the highest and lowest values in the data. The variance is the average squared deviation of the individual values of the mean.

A t-distribution resembles a bell-shaped normal distribution but has more area in the two tails of the curve. The t-distribution reflects the fact that for small samples (less than 30), the standard deviation will, on average, be larger than in an infinite population. Therefore, in order to achieve statistical significance with small numbers of subjects, the difference between the control groups has to be greater than is the case with large numbers of subjects.

478–481. The answers are 478-E, 479-D, 480-B, 481-A. (Kaplan, 6/e, pp 381–383.) Behavior rating instruments are usually examined for several kinds of validity. Before the validity of any scale can be determined, its reliability must be examined. Reliability, defined as the consistency of the instrument in differentiating one subject from the other, is most efficiently determined by applying correlational measures to ratings established by different judges.

While all forms of validity are interrelated, there are differences. A rating scale may have one form of validity and not another. Before researchers decide to employ a certain scale, they must determine whether the scale has content validity, i.e., whether it measures the behavior it is meant to measure.

A second important type of validity, concurrent validity, is determined by comparing test results with some other independent criterion of measurement. For example, the scores of a self-rated depression scale could be compared with the clinical judgment of a psychiatrist following an interview.

In predictive validity, a determination is made as to how well a measurement can predict another measure by another means at a later time. The difference between concurrent and predictive validity involves differences in time periods when the criterion measures are obtained; i.e., concurrent validity measures are performed at the same time and predictive measures at different times.

Construct validity refers to the extent to which an instrument measures an explanatory construct. A researcher must make predictions that certain types of scores will be obtained if the test adequately measures the researcher's construct.

482–485. The answers are 482-D, 483-A, 484-C, 485-B. (Kaplan, 6/e, pp 492–506.) Six people are commonly thought of as belonging to the cultural and interpersonal school of psychoanalytic thought, and all are widely acclaimed as effective and innovative therapists. Alfred Adler (1870–1937) was a member of Freud's circle from 1902 to 1911. When Adler disputed Freud's theory of innate aggressive drive, he became dissociated from Freud. Best known for his theory of the "inferiority complex" and striving for superiority as motivating human behavior, Adler also introduced a number of other widely held theories regarding the basic social nature of humans and the necessity for taking responsibility for one's own behavior. In his therapeutic practice, he finally came to stress that patients must increase their social interest in order to increase their self-esteem.

Karen Horney (1885–1952) was trained in psychoanalysis by Karl Abraham and his school in Berlin and came to the United States, where her creativity was encouraged. In her famous book *The Neurotic Personality of Our Time*, she presented evidence to demonstrate that culture and environmental events are potent etiologic factors in the production of neurosis. Horney based her therapy primarily on the reduction of "blockages," or resistances, in order to free patients from a "compulsive," stereotyped approach to life.

The name Harry Stack Sullivan (1892–1949) is practically synonymous with the "interpersonal" approach to psychiatry and human behavior. Trained in the United States, he underwent classical analysis but early in his career rejected classical psychoanalysis on both theoretical and pragmatic grounds. Sullivan's guiding principle in therapy was to preserve and increase a patient's self-esteem. He also regarded each psychiatric interview, no matter how short, as an opportunity for therapy.

Sandor Rado (1890–1971) materially tried to change the field of psychoanalysis, but never broke from it. He endeavored to increase the scientific underpinning of psychoanalysis and keep it within the fold of medicine. Rado defined an emotionally healthy person as self-reliant and capable of experiencing affection, pride, friendliness, optimism, and joy. Accordingly, his therapy was aimed at enhancing these characteristics in his patients in addition to developing their independence.

Jules Masserman was trained in psychoanalysis by Franz Alexander and in psychobiology by Adolf Meyer. His research and clinical career have been devoted to an amalgamation of biologic and psychological concepts. He has used laboratory methods to investigate methods of psychotherapy and has evolved an eclectic approach that invokes all ethical procedures in helping patients find a better life-style and life-view.

Transactional analysis was developed by Eric Berne in the fifties after he decided traditional psychoanalysis took too long to effect change in patients. He was originally influenced by Paul Federn and the Vienna Psychoanalytic Society, but parted ways in a friendly spirit from classical analysis. Berne developed not only script analysis but also a total theory of personality in which he took ideas from California group therapists. Frederick Perls' gestalt techniques were particularly useful to Berne in delineating ego states and interpersonal games. In his therapy, Berne tried to demystify the complexities of human behavior by reducing problem behavior to its simplest form, thereby helping patients to see destructive forms of human interaction ("games"). The final phase of therapy was to help patients interrupt their games.

The above six pioneers, through their writings and speeches, have influenced not only several generations of psychiatric trainees but the general public as well. Adlerian groups exist throughout the world, and Berne fostered a creativity in his followers that has enabled transactional analysis to grow in the decade since his death.

486–490. The answers are 486-D, 487-C, 488-A, 489-B, 490-E. (Kaplan, 6/e, pp 2756–2764.) The traditional approach to crime and punishment holds that persons are endowed with free will and therefore are responsible for their behavior, and that the threat of punishment deters antisocial behavior. According to these concepts, a person who by free will chooses to commit antisocial acts should receive punishment as a deterrence against such acts in the future, as well as a deterrence to persons who might otherwise be tempted to commit similar acts. When an antisocial act has been judged the result of free will, the doctrine of *lex talionis* applies. This doctrine, enunciated in the code of Hammurabi, justifies the taking of "an eye for an eye or a tooth for a tooth." Offenders are punished in kind for their misdeeds. Traditional doctrine holds that the degree of punishment depends on the state of mind of the person, which supposedly can be determined by the court's evaluation of legal and psychiatric evidence. It is, of course, possible to challenge every one of these assumptions. Nevertheless, some legal machinery is required to protect society.

The doctrine of *parens patriae* holds that the state may intervene and hold in custody persons deemed dangerous to themselves or others. This doctrine leads to commitment procedures for those persons judged incompetent, insane, or dangerous to self or others.

All societies recognize that mental illness and dementia may ameliorate the doctrine of responsibility. The doctrine of *non compos mentis* recognizes that patients thus affected may lack the capacity to exercise free will and therefore are less responsible for their behavior.

The concept of *mens rea*, the guilty mind, applies to a person accused of an antisocial act who is capable of having committed the act with deliberation and malice aforethought. If the accused person is judged not to have the guilty mind, the punishment is correspondingly ameliorated. The psychiatrist's role has been to advise the court of the mental state of the accused person. The court then decides on the weight to be accorded this information in setting the sentence, either for a prison term or detention in a mental institution.

Habeas corpus refers to the right of any detained person to have a hearing to determine the legality of the detainment. At a hearing, a judge will decide on the legality of the procedures involved in confining the person. This right applies to prisoners as well as to patients in mental institutions.

491–496. The answers are 491-B, 492-D, 493-B, 494-C, 495-E, 496-A. (Kaplan, 6/e, pp 451–452.) Ego defense mechanisms attempt to counter the anxiety generated by unresolved drives. Although these defenses diminish anxiety, if they become rigid and inflexible they may produce psychopathology.

Fixation describes the persistence of an immature mode of coping. It is postulated to occur as a result of stress during critical periods of ego development. The described patient's mouthing, sucking, and oral manipulation represent fixation at the oral stage.

Resistance describes opposition to the therapeutic process. In its simplest form, it describes a patient who "forgets" or refuses to comply with the terms of the therapeutic relationship. To the described patient, his medication symbolized his illness and he therefore believed that by not taking his medication he could deny the existence of his illness. This represents a prelogical or magical form of thinking. Resistance in the psychotherapeutic relationship provides productive material for the therapist to work with.

In displacement, the person transfers affect from one object to another more acceptable object. Through this mechanism the person may be able to tolerate the expression of an uncomfortable affect toward a less anxiety-provoking object. In the patient described, the link between his father and other authority figures is not difficult to extrapolate; the connection to the displacement object, however, is not always so clear.

In restitution, the subject relieves guilt by committing an act or adopting a life-style that is intended to atone for a perceived transgression. This should not be confused with reaction formation in which subjects do the opposite of their ego-dystonic drives.

497–501. The answers are 497-E, 498-D, 499-C, 500-B, 501-A. (Kaplan, 6/e, pp 1767–1788.) A keystone of psychoanalysis is the recognition and management of resistances. Resistances arise when some distressing material in a person's unconscious threatens to become conscious.

Conscious resistance takes the form of deliberate censorship of material during free association, material that patients feel will cause the analyst to think poorly of them, or that will engender within themselves feelings of shame, guilt, or embarrassment.

The ego may expend much energy in repression resistances, which keep instinctual impulses from reaching conscious recognition. Repression resistance describes the efforts of the ego to prevent disclosures during the analytic process. If analysts can help their patients overcome the repression resistances, the ego will finally accept or reject the repressed instinctual material, thereby disposing of a permanent threat and the need to expend energy previously required to maintain the repression.

Patients with transference resistance transfer to the therapist significant feelings generated by some previously encountered person for whom the therapist acts as a symbol. Transference resistance has the particular quality of both reflecting and expressing the patient's struggle with early experience and feeling. Although the transference can be positive, it frequently takes a negative form that may be evidenced by silence, sarcasm, or by a veiled or overtly hostile question or remark. Therapists must recognize these kinds of responses as clinical transference phenomena and not respond in kind. The patient described in the question may have been struggling to cope with feelings about his father, but he was unable to connect his veiled criticisms of his father with their instinctual origins—an example of repression resistance. He then transferred the resistance to recognizing his feelings about his father to the analyst, whom he criticized for being silent. Such resistances appearing as transference can be dealt with very effectively by the analyst. A transference resistance can become a transference attachment. Alternatively, the negative aspects of the transference resistance may dominate and seriously impede the therapeutic relationship.

Id resistance refers to the inability to change some ingrained behavioral pattern, often in the form of a compulsion, which derives from a particular instinctual drive that is very powerful. The washing of hands as a manifestation of unacceptable sexual impulses is an example. The resistance is to unlearning the ingrained, maladaptive pattern of behavior that serves to mask, as it were, unacceptable impulses from which the behavior originates.

In superego resistance, patients on the verge of achieving some seemingly cherished goal find themselves too guilt-ridden about the achievement to accept it. Such promptings of the conscience prevent these patients from making their desired changes.

Patients with secondary gain resistance cling to the advantages that stem from their sick role, such as attention, comfort, and avoidance of responsibility. This is often seen in cases where financial compensation is involved.

ANXIETY DISORDERS

Directions: Each item below contains five suggested responses. Select the **one best** response to each item.

502. Panic disorder may be characterized as

(A) usually having its onset in middle age
(B) being a self-limiting disorder
(C) occurring in approximately 10 percent of the population
(D) having equal sex distribution
(E) tending to run in families

503. A 65-year-old man with severe chronic obstructive airways disease complains of severe generalized anxiety. The most appropriate psychotropic would be

(A) alprazolam
(B) carbamazepine
(C) fluvoxamine
(D) buspirone
(E) clonazepam

504. According to classical psychoanalytic theory, anxiety represents

(A) unresolved separation from the mother
(B) an undifferentiated id
(C) the cause of repression
(D) fixation at the oral stage of ego development
(E) anger directed against the self

505. Each of the following is a true statement about posttraumatic stress disorder (PTSD) EXCEPT

(A) the majority of a population experiencing a natural disaster will exhibit PTSD

(B) the onset of the disorder may be delayed weeks or years after the stressor

(C) PTSD is more common in children than in adults following a stressor

(D) symptoms usually resolve within 1 week

(E) PTSD is a frequent consequence of rape

506. The symptoms of generalized anxiety disorder

(A) tend to worsen with age

(B) are precipitated by intravenous lactate infusion

(C) demonstrate diurnal variation

(D) include difficulty initiating and maintaining sleep

(E) have a 1-year prevalence of 1 percent in the general population

507. All the following statements regarding buspirone are correct EXCEPT

(A) it has significant effects on the gamma-aminobutyric acid (GABA) receptor system

(B) it is capable of reversing "learned helplessness" in animal models of anxiety

(C) it exhibits no clinically significant drug interactions

(D) it exerts its antianxiety effect by blocking serotonin (5-HT$_{1A}$) receptors

(E) it has a half-life of 1 to 10 h in healthy subjects

508. The compulsions found in a patient with obsessive-compulsive disorder

(A) are usually ego-syntonic

(B) are usually an attempt to modify or control a primary obsession or compulsion

(C) are nonpurposeful

(D) are usually considered reasonable by the patient

(E) are usually a direct acting out of the patient's obsessive thoughts

509. Flooding therapy for agoraphobia

(A) is effective in reducing symptoms in at least 60 percent of patients

(B) causes the majority of patients to drop out of therapy

(C) requires several weeks of treatment

(D) is less effective than cognitive therapy

(E) has limited efficacy because of the emergence of extinction

510. The differential diagnosis of a patient exhibiting obsessive-compulsive behavior includes each of the following EXCEPT

(A) schizophrenia

(B) panic disorder

(C) phobic disorder

(D) Tourette's disorder

(E) major depression

Directions: Each item below contains four suggested responses of which **one or more** is correct. Select:

A	if	**1, 2, and 3**	are correct
B	if	**1 and 3**	are correct
C	if	**2 and 4**	are correct
D	if	**4**	is correct
E	if	**1, 2, 3, and 4**	are correct

511. Which of the following medical conditions may mimic panic disorder?

(1) Pheochromocytoma
(2) Complex partial seizures
(3) Caffeine intoxication
(4) Hypoglycemia

512. True statements regarding buspirone include that it

(1) has a potent sedative effect
(2) has significant potential for abuse
(3) decreases psychomotor performance
(4) has dopaminergic activity

513. Agents that have demonstrated efficacy in panic disorder include

(1) clonazepam
(2) propranolol
(3) desipramine
(4) buspirone

514. Symptoms of withdrawal from diazepam

(1) usually subside within 10 days of discontinuing the drug
(2) may include generalized convulsions
(3) are unlikely if the drug was used at therapeutic dosage
(4) may include paranoid delusions

515. Sleep terrors in children

(1) occur during rapid eye movement (REM) sleep
(2) are heralded by a scream
(3) are usually indicative of psychopathology
(4) normally occur during the first half of the night

516. Which of the following medications should alleviate the symptoms of alprazolam withdrawal?

(1) Carbamazepine
(2) Clonazepam
(3) Propranolol
(4) Buspirone

517. Patients with somatoform pain disorder are often

(1) alexithymic
(2) workaholics
(3) suffering from a major depressive disorder
(4) counterdependent

SUMMARY OF DIRECTIONS

A	B	C	D	E
1,2,3	1,3	2,4	4	All are
only	only	only	only	correct

518. A 30-year-old woman is referred to a psychiatrist by her family doctor. Despite the fact that she is extremely attractive, she ruminates constantly over her perception that her nose is huge, bulbous, and deformed. Her distress

(1) is likely to resolve spontaneously
(2) will be alleviated by plastic surgery
(3) should resolve with cognitive psychotherapy
(4) may necessitate neuroleptic medication

519. The symptoms of posttraumatic stress disorder

(1) may be aggravated by unrelated life stressors
(2) include cognitive difficulties
(3) may include psychogenic amnesia
(4) usually disappear with time

520. Premature ejaculation is accurately described by which of the following statements?

(1) It is more common among college-educated males
(2) It is frequently associated with an anxiety disorder
(3) It may be caused by urethritis
(4) It occurs in approximately 30 percent of males

521. Appropriate initial treatment interventions for premature ejaculation include

(1) hypnosis
(2) anxiolytics
(3) topical lidocaine jelly
(4) the "squeeze technique"

522. True statements regarding sexual aversion disorder include that it

(1) is almost completely confined to females
(2) usually necessitates psychopharmacologic intervention
(3) carries a poor prognosis despite treatment
(4) is often found in association with panic disorder

523. The person who engages in "cross-dressing"

(1) is almost always male
(2) is usually homosexual
(3) has frequently been engaged in other paraphiliac behavior
(4) has a female sexual identity

524. When prescribing a benzodiazepine to an 80-year-old woman, the physician should expect

(1) an increased half-life of the drug
(2) increased absorption
(3) decreased hepatic metabolism
(4) decreased CNS sensitivity to the drug

ANXIETY DISORDERS

A N S W E R S

502. The answer is E. (Kaplan, 6/e, pp 1191–1204.) Panic disorder is a common condition with an estimated 6-month prevalence of 0.6 to 1.0 percent. The prevalence of agoraphobia may be as high as 6 percent. Anxiety disorders are more common among females and usually have their onset in adolescence or young adulthood. Although genetic factors have been demonstrated in both generalized anxiety and panic disorders, the evidence suggests that there is a stronger genetic loading in panic disorder. The long-term course of panic disorder remains uncertain; it is clear, however, that most patients continue to experience recurrent episodes. The prognosis of generalized anxiety tends to be more favorable than that of panic disorder.

503. The answer is D. (Kaplan, 6/e, pp 1957–1961.) The treatment of anxiety disorders in patients with compromised respiratory function often presents a therapeutic dilemma. Conventional anxiolytics (i.e., sedative hypnotics) may depress respiratory drive and further aggravate the patient's condition. Since it produces no such respiratory depression, the novel anxiolytic buspirone offers significant advantages in treating this group of patients. Buspirone produces no more sedation than a placebo. Indeed, several studies have suggested that the drug may improve psychomotor performance.

504. The answer is C. (Kaplan, 6/e, pp 464-465.) Freud's earliest theory postulated that anxiety was the result of a failure to discharge libidinous energy. Later, he developed a more complex theoretical framework that included the concept of repression. According to this scheme, conscious ideas, emotions, and impulses that are unacceptable to the ego are forced into the unconscious by repression. Freud postulated that anxiety is secondary to that repression. Finally, as part of his structural model of the psyche, Freud postulated that anxiety is an expression of the ego's response to instinctual forces arising from the id. According to this theory, anxiety is considered to arise from the ego and is a primary psychological force.

505. The answer is D. (Kaplan, 6/e, pp 1227–1236.) As many as 80 percent of people who experience a catastrophic stressor will develop posttraumatic stress disorder (PTSD). Although symptoms may occur almost immediately following the stressor, they are more usually delayed weeks or years. PTSD may occur in any age group but is most common in children. Rather than resolve, the symptoms of PTSD may grow worse. A 20-year follow-up study of World War II veterans demonstrated an increase in symptoms with time. Although longitudinal studies are limited, it appears that PTSD is a cyclical disorder with periods of exacerbation precipitated by life stressors.

506. The answer is D. (Kaplan, 6/e, pp 1236–1244.) Generalized anxiety disorder usually has its onset in late adolescence or young adulthood and is more common in women. The onset of the disorder after age 40 should raise the suspicion of an underlying medical precipitant. Physical symptoms reflect autonomic arousal. Although the condition tends to be chronic, the symptoms do subside with age. The 1-year prevalence in the general population is estimated at 6.4 percent.

507. The answer is A. (Schatzberg, pp 234–241.) Buspirone is a member of a group of compounds known as the azapirones. Its clinical action as an antianxiety medication is mediated via its action at 5-HT_{1A} presynaptic and postsynaptic receptors. It has no effect on the GABAergic systems in the brain. Buspirone has a short half-life (1 to 10 h) in healthy subjects. In addition, buspirone prevents neuroleptic-induced catalepsy in rodents and binds to dopamine receptors throughout the brain. Azapirones have exhibited efficacy in reversing "learned helplessness" in animal models of anxiety. Buspirone lacks any abuse potential and does not adversely influence psychomotor functions. It appears to be an ideal anxiolytic in patients with chronic obstructive airways disease and has been demonstrated to improve respiratory function in these patients. Buspirone has exhibited no significant drug interactions.

508. The answer is B. (Kaplan, 6/e, pp 994–995.) The compulsive act is normally an attempt to control a primary obsession or compulsion. The compulsive ritual is seldom a direct acting out of the primary impulse and is therefore unlikely to dissipate the anxiety provoked by the primary obsession. The compulsions are usually ego-dystonic and are recognized by the subject as being irrational.

509. The answer is A. (Kaplan, 6/e, p 1794.) The behavioral technique of flooding is an effective treatment for agoraphobia and has proved superior to all other treatment modalities. This technique exposes the patient to the feared stimulus for brief but intense periods. Flooding is rapidly effective in reducing symptoms, but for the most sustained results the exposure should be spaced and regularly repeated. The goal of flooding is extinction—the elimination of the dysfunctional response to the feared stimulus. Ideally this technique should be used in conjunction with psychopharmacologic interventions.

510. The answer is B. (Kaplan, 6/e, pp 1222–1224.) Attempting to separate the syndrome of obsessive-compulsive disorder from other psychiatric disorders may be difficult. Patients with a number of psychiatric conditions may exhibit obsessive-compulsive behavior as part of their condition. Differentiating the obsessive-compulsive syndrome from other conditions is important if appropriate treatment modalities are to be selected. Approximately 30 percent of patients with depressive disorder exhibit obsessive-compulsive symptoms and a similar fraction of patients with obsessive-compulsive disorder will develop a major depressive disorder. Patients with process schizophrenia often exhibit obsessive-compulsive behavior. It may also be difficult at times to distinguish the bizarre magical thinking of obsessive-compulsive disorder from schizophreniform delusions.

511. The answer is E (all). (Kaplan, 6/e, pp 477–478.) Prior to commencing treatment, the physician should consider and exclude medical conditions that mimic panic disorder. A number of conditions may produce similar symptoms. These symptoms essentially represent marked autonomic sympathetic overflow and may be caused by acute myocardial infarction, pheochromocytoma, hypoglycemia, caffeine or cocaine intoxication, and complex partial seizures. The relationship between mitral valve prolapse and panic disorder remains unclear, and although the two conditions may be found together, no direct causal relationship has been established. An electroencephalogram with anterior temporal or nasopharyngeal leads should be obtained for all patients to explore the possibility of a complex partial seizure disorder.

512. The answer is D (4). (Kaplan, 6/e, pp 1957–1961.) Buspirone is a novel anxiolytic with demonstrated efficacy and a benign side effect profile. The drug is thought to act at the 5-HT$_{1A}$ autoreceptor with additional dopaminergic activity at higher doses. The drug produces no sedation and has been shown to improve psychomotor testing in the laboratory. Apart from mild dizziness, no significant side effects have been reported and the drug is safe far in excess of the therapeutic dosage.

513. The answer is B (1, 3). (Kaplan, 6/e, pp 1201–1207.) A number of psychotropic drugs have proven efficacy in panic disorder. Tricyclic antidepressants and SSRIs take several weeks to produce maximum benefit and should be used in doses equivalent to those required for antidepressant effect. Monoamine oxidase inhibitors are effective in as many as 90 percent of patients but have a limited clinical role because of their potentially hazardous side effects. High-potency benzodiazepines (e.g., clonazepam, alprazolam) are rapidly effective and are useful adjuncts to antidepressants, particularly during the initial phase of treatment. Although beta blockers are probably effective in generalized anxiety disorder, they are not effective in panic disorder.

514. The answer is C (2, 4). (APA Task Force Report, pp 15–21.) Physical dependence on benzodiazepines may occur at therapeutic dosage after just a few weeks' use. The temporal pattern of symptoms of discontinuance is largely dependent on the pharmacokinetic characteristics of the particular benzodiazepine. There may be an initial rebound of anxiety symptoms within a few days of stopping the drug. With a benzodiazepine of long half-life, such as diazepam or clonazepam, this period is followed in the first 10 days by a confusional state with tachycardia, hallucinations, and autonomic overflow. Paranoid delusions or frank psychosis may persist for as long as several months. Withdrawal seizures normally occur within a few days and are more common with high-potency benzodiazepines.

515. The answer is C (2, 4). (Kaplan, 6/e, pp 1386–1387.) Sleep terrors usually have their onset before age 12 but may occasionally occur as late as the third decade. Their occurrence does not usually indicate underlying psychopathology in young children, but adults with the condition have a high incidence of anxiety disorders. Each episode is usually heralded by a scream and occurs during the first half of the evening during stages 3 and 4, that is, during non-rapid eye movement (NREM) sleep. Subjects are unable to remember the content of their "terror," and this distinguishes the disorder from nightmares.

516. The answer is A (1, 2, 3). (APA Task Force Report, pp 35–38.) Patients are more likely to experience symptoms following the withdrawal of short half-life, high-potency benzodiazepines (e.g., alprazolam, triazolam). The recent increase in the therapeutic use of these agents has increased the frequency of withdrawal symptoms. Tapering doses of long half-life benzodiazepines (e.g., clonazepam) usually provides an effective means of reducing withdrawal. Early data suggest that carbamazepine is effective in preventing withdrawal symptoms, although the drug's mode of action in this situation remains a matter of debate. Beta blockers and clonidine are helpful in reducing the autonomic overflow usually associated with withdrawal from benzodiazepines. Finally, phenobarbital substitution and tapering has also demonstrated efficacy in this situation.

517. The answer is E (all). (Kaplan, 6/e, pp 1251–1270.) Somatoform pain disorder is a common and disabling condition in which the patient experiences severe disabling pain with no identifiable etiology. The symptoms must be present for at least 6 months to meet criteria for a diagnosis of this condition. It has been estimated that as many as half of these patients are suffering from a major depressive disorder and the remainder usually meet criteria for a dysthymic disorder. Several personality styles have been associated with the condition. These include the "pain-prone" patient who is pessimistic and self-punitive, the alexithymic patient who is unable to generate affective experience at a conscious level, and the counterdependent workaholic who finds nurturance unacceptable and therefore develops somatic complaints to validate dependent needs.

518. The answer is D (4). (Kaplan, 6/e, pp 1268–1269.) Body dysmorphic disorder (which is also referred to as *monosymptomatic delusional hypochondriasis*) describes an irrational preoccupation with a symptom or perceived body deformity. Common examples include delusional parasitosis and a preoccupation with one's body odor or physical imperfections. The disorder may occur in isolation or in association with other psychiatric disorders such as major depression or schizophrenia or following neurologic injury. The illness tends to run a chronic, relapsing course. Treatment is primarily pharmacologic. The high-potency neuroleptic pimozide has documented efficacy. In addition, there have been isolated reports of a positive response to other neuroleptics, tricyclics, and monoamine oxidase inhibitors.

519. The answer is A (1, 2, 3). (Kaplan, 6/e, pp 1227–1236.) Symptoms of posttraumatic stress disorder may occur immediately following the stressor or more typically may be delayed months or years. Symptoms may be divided into the three broad categories of intrusion, hyperarousal, and avoidance. Patients frequently exhibit deficits in attention with subsequent difficulties in short memory. The majority of patients experience chronic symptoms with periods of acute exacerbation.

520. The answer is E (all). (Kaplan, 6/e, pp 1309–1310.) There is no single definition of premature ejaculation. Masters and Johnson define it as an inability of the male to satisfy his female partner 50 percent of the time. This definition of course implies that the female partner is capable of achieving orgasm normally. Premature ejaculation implies ejaculation within ten thrusts or within 2 min of penetration. The condition occurs in 30 percent of males and is often associated with sexual naivete, anxiety disorders, and the male's pre-occupation with satisfying his partner. The condition may be caused by abdominal and pelvic surgery, lower spinal cord lesions, prostatitis, and urethritis. The higher incidence of premature ejaculation among men with college education probably reflects their increased concern for their partner's satisfaction.

521. The answer is D (4). (Kaplan, 6/e, pp 1309–1310.) Treatment of premature ejaculation consists primarily of the squeeze technique in which the female partner squeezes the coronal ridge of the penis just prior to ejaculation. In most circumstances this will eventually result in more sustained periods of penile erection and decreased performance anxiety on the part of the male. Although patients are frequently anxious, psychotropic medications are seldom indicated. Psychodynamic psychotherapy may be helpful in some cases in which the patient appears to harbor deep hostility toward women.

522. The answer is C (2, 4). (Kaplan, 6/e, p 1050.) Sexual aversion disorder describes a persistent avoidance of almost all sexual contact. Patients will describe their repulsion for the sexual act. The disorder often has its genesis in previous episodes of abuse or assault or in dyspareunia. Patients usually require multimodal treatment and assessment.

523. The answer is B (1, 3). (Kaplan, 6/e, pp 1075–1076.) Transvestite fetishism usually occurs in males and has its onset in adolescence. The transvestite is usually heterosexual and has a male sexual identity. These persons have frequently been involved in other paraphilias, such as exhibitionism, frottage, or voyeurism.

524. The answer is B (1, 3). (Jenike, pp 254–256.) Significant alterations in drug metabolism occur with aging. Decreased splanchnic blood flow and an increased gastric pH result in decreased absorption from the gut. The higher percentage of body fat in the elderly prolongs the half-life of lipid-soluble drugs, while the decreased relative water content increases the effective concentration of water-soluble drugs. Decreased serum albumin increases the percentage of unbound, i.e. "active," drug. Decreased cytochrome P-450 activity and renal clearance prolong excretion. The elderly brain tends to be more sensitive to the effects of psychotropics.

CHILDHOOD DISORDERS

Directions: Each item below contains five suggested responses. Select the **one best** response to each item.

525. Each of the following is a characteristic of the fragile X syndrome EXCEPT

- (A) macro-orchidism
- (B) large ears
- (C) occurrence limited to males
- (D) mental retardation
- (E) short stature

526. The mother of a 4-year-old girl complains that the child wets her bed three times a week. She should be told that

- (A) bed-wetting is the result of premature toilet training
- (B) the family should come in for evaluation
- (C) the child requires imipramine
- (D) the child requires a physical examination and urinalysis
- (E) the child should receive psychotherapy

527. A child suffering from reactive attachment disorder

- (A) usually has delayed developmental milestones
- (B) is frequently mentally retarded
- (C) seldom responds to treatment
- (D) often has motor abnormalities
- (E) is usually male

528. A child with an IQ of 60

- (A) is usually diagnosed before attending school
- (B) usually requires institutional care
- (C) may be able to live independently as an adult
- (D) seldom learns vocational skills
- (E) is unlikely to develop stable relationships

529. Compared with the pervasive developmental disorders, schizophrenia with childhood onset

(A) usually has a later age of onset
(B) has a higher incidence of perinatal complications
(C) has a worse prognosis
(D) is more likely to be found in association with mental retardation
(E) is seldom associated with a family history of schizophrenia

530. A 14-year-old child who commits suicide

(A) is unlikely to have suffered from a major depressive disorder
(B) is unlikely to have exhibited prior signs of psychopathology
(C) is more likely to be female
(D) is more likely to be black
(E) often has a family member who had attempted or completed suicide

531. All the following neuroendocrine findings are associated with anorexia nervosa EXCEPT

(A) increased 24-h plasma cortisol levels
(B) dexamethasone nonsuppression
(C) normal thyroid-stimulating hormone
(D) increased follicle-stimulating hormone
(E) blunted adrenocorticotropic response to corticotropin-releasing hormone

532. A person with trisomy 21 has a higher incidence of

(A) hyperthyroidism
(B) hyperparathyroidism
(C) hypertonia
(D) hearing impairment
(E) diabetes mellitus

Items 533–534

A 10-year-old boy is referred to you for evaluation of his behavior. His parents describe 2 years of rudeness, disobedience, and cheekiness. The boy refuses to participate in family activities and "throws a tantrum" when he is confronted about his behavior. The child has broken furniture, smashed ornaments, and kicked his mother. His schoolteacher has made no derogatory comments about his behavior and his grades have been satisfactory.

533. The most appropriate initial diagnostic step would be

(A) electroencephalography
(B) projective psychological testing
(C) formal school reports
(D) family interview
(E) methylphenidate treatment trial

534. The child's most likely diagnosis is

(A) conduct disorder—aggressive type
(B) attention-deficit hyperactivity disorder
(C) oppositional defiant disorder
(D) identity disorder of childhood
(E) inhalant substance abuse

Directions: Each item below contains four suggested responses of which **one or more** is correct. Select:

A	if	**1, 2, and 3**	are correct
B	if	**1 and 3**	are correct
C	if	**2 and 4**	are correct
D	if	**4**	is correct
E	if	**1, 2, 3, and 4**	are correct

535. Enuresis in a 7-year-old child

  (1) is likely to be a manifestation of underlying psychological problems

  (2) is likely to resolve spontaneously

  (3) requires a prompt behavioral intervention

  (4) occurs more frequently in boys

536. The core symptom complexes of infantile autism include

  (1) deficits in reciprocal social interaction

  (2) restricted repertoire of activities

  (3) impaired verbal communication

  (4) absence of imaginative behavior

537. True statements regarding normal adolescence include

  (1) gender identity disturbances are usual

  (2) emotional turmoil is an expected part of this developmental period

  (3) acting out is an appropriate ego defense during this stage of development

  (4) rebellious behavior is normal

538. Medications with proven efficacy in attention-deficit hyperactivity disorder include

  (1) pemoline

  (2) clorgyline

  (3) desipramine

  (4) tranylcypromine

539. A 30-year-old man has a history of attention-deficit hyperactivity disorder. He is more likely than the general population to suffer from

  (1) Briquet's syndrome

  (2) obsessive-compulsive disorder

  (3) dysthymia

  (4) schizotypal personality disorder

540. Asperger's syndrome may be accurately characterized by which of the following statements?

  (1) It is more common in males

  (2) It includes deficits in social communication

  (3) It persists into adulthood

  (4) It is associated with normal language skills

541. You examine a child in the emergency room who you believe has been the victim of child abuse. As the treating physician

  (1) you must report the case to the police immediately

  (2) you should consult a social worker immediately

  (3) you must obtain a sworn statement from the child's parents

  (4) you should perform all necessary diagnostic procedures even without the parent's consent

SUMMARY OF DIRECTIONS

A	B	C	D	E
1,2,3	1,3	2,4	4	All are
only	only	only	only	correct

542. A child receiving psychotropic medications

    (1) will exhibit greater tolerance to the drug than will an adult

    (2) will require higher dosages compared with an adult

    (3) requires therapeutic plasma levels similar to those of an adult

    (4) will frequently exhibit a paradoxical response

543. Medical complications of bulimia nervosa include

    (1) metabolic alkalosis

    (2) hypercarotenemia

    (3) parotid enlargement

    (4) thrombocytopenia

544. Characteristics of complex motor tics include that they

    (1) are stable over time

    (2) are purposeless

    (3) cannot be suppressed by the patient

    (4) are nonrhythmic

545. In the first week of life, the behavior of a normal neonate includes

    (1) orienting the head toward a human voice

    (2) a long latency between a painful stimulus and crying

    (3) a tendency to fix the eyes on a human face

    (4) absence of a grasp reflex

546. True statements concerning the pharmacologic treatment of attention-deficit hyperactivity (ADHD) disorder include

    (1) bupropion is an effective treatment

    (2) monoamine oxidase inhibitors have demonstrated efficacy

    (3) the cardiac status of children receiving a tricyclic antidepressant should be followed closely

    (4) tricyclic antidepressants are the first-line treatment option

Directions: Each group of questions below consists of lettered options followed by a set of numbered items. For each numbered item, select the **one** lettered option with which it is **most** closely associated. Each lettered option may be used **once, more than once, or not at all.**

Items 547–550

Match the descriptions below with the appropriate test.

- (A) Peabody
- (B) Rorschach
- (C) Halstead-Reitan
- (D) Bender
- (E) Wechsler

547. A test originally designed to disclose the structure, dynamics, and boundaries of personality and which may also produce inferences about intelligence

548. A test originally designed to test visuomotor abilities in children but which may also serve as a memory and projective test

549. A test battery originally designed to disclose the effects of brain lesions on mental, motor, and sensory performance

550. A test battery originally designed to evaluate cognitive, verbal, and performance abilities; it can also disclose patterns of organic deficit and be used projectively

Items 551–554

For each of the following sets of essential clinical information, select the *DSM IV* diagnosis with which it is most closely associated.

   (A) Oppositional disorder
   (B) Avoidant disorder
   (C) Overanxious disorder
   (D) Separation anxiety disorder
   (E) Generalized anxiety disorder

551. Great distress when either parent or child leaves the home; persistent fears of danger to self or close relatives; phobias about monsters, death, or being kidnapped; sleep disturbances and nightmares

552. A failure to involve self with unfamiliar peers, embarrassment, timidity, and lack of social contact even though it is desired; lack of motor activity and initiative; poor articulation despite good language skills

553. Excessive worry and fear unrelated to stress or specifics of the environment; excessive worry about possible injury, school tests, or friendships; excessive self-doubt; sleep difficulties and psychophysiologic symptoms

554. Resistance to authority and to demands; unresponsiveness to persuasion; provocativeness, stubbornness, and procrastination

CHILDHOOD DISORDERS

A N S W E R S

525. The answer is C. (Kaplan, 6/e, pp 2216–2217.) The fragile X syndrome is the second most common cause of mental retardation (behind Down's syndrome). Females are the carriers of the gene. Although it was thought that the clinical syndrome was limited to males, it is now recognized that it may also be expressed in females. In fact, only one-third of female carriers are normal; the remainder are either learning disabled or mentally retarded. Phenotypically normal males with the fragile X have also been reported. Physical characteristics are short stature, long face, large ears, pectus excavatum, and macroorchidism. Cognitive deficits typically involve functions of the right hemisphere.

526. The answer is D. (Kaplan, 6/e, pp 2337–2340.) Over 80 percent of 2 year olds, 50 percent of 3 year olds, 25 percent of 4 year olds, and 7 percent of 5 year olds are enuretic. There is often a family history of enuresis. The condition is more common in lower socioeconomic groups and broken homes and in neglected and abused children. It is crucial to evaluate children for a medical cause of their enuresis (e.g., infection, posterior urethral valves, meatal stenosis, spina bifida occulta, or diabetes). A physical etiology will be found in 5 percent of enuretics. Psychotropics should be reserved for children who have failed to respond to more conservative treatment (i.e., behavioral methods).

527. The answer is A. (Kaplan, 6/e, pp 2354–2359.) The reactive attachment disorder of infancy or early childhood is a result of social deprivation. Although the child may exhibit delays in developmental milestones, these are a result of an impoverished psychosocial experience rather than indicative of neurodevelopmental deficits. The child usually has the capacity for normal social interaction and development. The majority of children have the capacity to benefit considerably from treatment interventions provided the period of deprivation has not been too prolonged. It is important, therefore, to evaluate a child's psychosocial experience before concluding that he or she is mentally retarded.

528. The answer is C. (Kaplan, 6/e, pp 2209–2210.) The IQ range of 50 to 70 is defined as mild retardation and accounts for 85 percent of all retarded persons. Most persons with mild retardation are capable of learning prevocational skills and eventually living independently. They are also capable of developing long-term, stable interpersonal relationships. These children are seldom recognized prior to attending school and even then the diagnosis may be significantly delayed. It is important to realize that the IQ score is not necessarily an accurate indication of the person's functional capacity.

529. The answer is A. (Kaplan, 6/e, pp 2393–2398.) The onset of schizophrenia before age 12 is rare, particularly in girls. The genetic basis for the childhood onset form of the illness appears to be similar to that for the adult onset form of schizophrenia. A high incidence of abnormalities on electroencephalography has been demonstrated; however, the incidence of perinatal complications is lower than that found in patients with pervasive developmental disability. The majority of children with childhood onset schizophrenia have IQ scores within the normal range, while 75 percent of autistic children are retarded. The long-term prognosis for childhood-onset schizophrenia is unknown.

530. The answer is E. (Kaplan, 6/e, pp 2431.) Adolescent suicide is a common and increasing problem with no predilection for any particular social class or racial group. Although the incidence of suicide attempts is higher in adolescent females than in adolescent males, the incidence of completed suicide is higher in males. The majority of adolescents who attempt suicide are suffering from a major depressive disorder or substance abuse or have been the victims of abuse. The majority will also have communicated their suicidal ideation prior to their suicidal act.

531. The answer is D. (Kaplan, 6/e, p 1365.) The neuroendocrine changes found in anorexia nervosa are a reflection of both weight loss and the mood disorder that accompanies the disorder. The amenorrhea that accompanies the profound weight loss is reflected in decreased FSH and LH levels. Approximately 90 percent of patients will have nonsuppression on dexamethasone challenge and will have consistently raised plasma cortisol levels. Thyroid function is usually normal or marginally diminished. Bulimia nervosa is not normally associated with dexamethasone nonsuppression or alterations in gonadotropic hormones.

532. The answer is D. (Kaplan, 6/e, pp 718–719.) Down's syndrome is the most common cause of mental retardation in the developed world. The condition is associated with a high incidence of a number of physical abnormalities including duodenal atresia, hypotonia, seizures, endocardial cushion defects, hypothyroidism, and hearing loss. Neuropathologic changes similar to those of Alzheimer's disease are commonly seen in Down's syndrome. These persons do not often demonstrate the typical dementia associated with the neurofibrillary plaques and tangles.

533–534. The answers are 533-D, 534-C. (Kaplan, 6/e, pp 2317–2319.) Children with oppositional defiant disorder are often simply described as "difficult kids." The majority of their behavioral problems occur in the context of their relationship with parents or other emotionally concerned adults. The clinical features essentially reflect the normal behavioral problems seen in the "terrible 2's." These children are described as rude, resentful, touchy, hostile, impertinent, and often precocious. They typically confront their parents' authority, although their behavior with teachers and other authority figures is usually less trouble-some. Their behavior does not include the antisocial problems demonstrated by children with conduct disorders. Family dysfunction is often a precipitant for this behavior and the children may be performing their roles as scapegoats within this family system. Family therapy with particular emphasis on behavioral control by the parents is the mainstay of treatment. The concurrence of an attention-deficit disorder should be evaluated by a thor-ough examination of the child and his or her social system.

535. The answer is C (2, 4). (Kaplan, 6/e, pp 2237–2240.) Enuresis is defined as a frequency of urinary incontinence of at least twice per week for a period of at least 3 consecutive months or the presence of significant distress or impairment in social or academic settings due to incontinence. The prevalence of enuresis is relatively high from ages 5 to 7 (approx-imately 15 percent), but the vast majority of cases remit spontaneously so that the preva-lence in 14-year-old boys is approximately 1 percent. The decision as to whether to treat enuresis in a particular child is largely determined by the disability incurred and whether the disorder occurs at an age when spontaneous remission is likely (i.e., 5 to 7 years). In most cases, treatment should begin with conservative methods such as a bell and pad. Unfortunately, most children treated by a physician immediately receive pharmacologic, rather than behavioral, interventions.

536. The answer is E (all). (Kaplan, 6/e, p 2277–2288.) Numerous items are listed in the cri-teria of infantile autism. They may be divided into three broad groups: (1) Impairment in reciprocal social interaction. This includes behaviors such as an indifference to other people's feelings, an inability to make friends, impaired imitation, and lack of social play. (2) Qualitative impairment in verbal and nonverbal (prosodic) communication and ima-gination. This includes absent or abnormal communication such as grunting or echolalia and an inability to maintain gaze or use body language appropriately. (3) Restricted reper-toire of motor behaviors. This describes stereotypic movements, compulsive rituals, and a preoccupation with maintaining routine.

537. The answer is D (4). (Kaplan, 6/e, pp 2185–2188.) Contrary to public opinion, emo-tional turmoil is not an expected part of adolescent development. Although teen-agers may experience transient periods of dysphoria and anxiety, these reach significant pro-portions in only approximately 7 percent of subjects. Rebelliousness toward authority fig-ures represents a normal part of the emancipation process. Despite this rebellion, the majority of teen-agers continue to share their parents' belief and value systems. When adolescents do suffer from significant psychological difficulties, there is no reason to believe that they will necessarily outgrow these difficulties. The limited repertoire of symptoms exhibited by these teen-agers often makes it difficult to precisely categorize their psychiatric disorder.

538. The answer is E (all). (Kaplan, 6/e, p 2304–2308.) There is no doubt that methylphenidate is an effective treatment for attention-deficit hyperactivity disorder (ADHD). But the drug's short half-life and side effect profile (insomnia, growth retardation, motor tics, and appetite suppression) and the development of tolerance to the drug have prompted alternative treatment strategies. Both the monoamine oxidase inhibitors and tricyclic antidepressants have proven efficacy in reducing the child's hyperactivity and improving attention.

539. The answer is B (1, 3). (Kaplan, 6/e, p 2152.) Approximately one-third of adults with a history of ADHD in childhood will eventually develop a psychiatric disorder in adulthood. The most common disorders in this group are antisocial personality disorder, alcoholism, ADHD (residual type), and Briquet's syndrome (somatization disorder). Many will also complain of chronic dysphoria, low self-esteem, and poor career achievements. The dysphoric symptoms usually respond to psychotropic treatment of the ADHD.

540. The answer is E (all). (Kaplan, 6/e, pp 2291–2293.) Asperger's syndrome describes a disorder characterized by restricted social skills; restricted, repetitive, stereotypic movements; and difficulty with complex motor tasks. Children with the syndrome do not exhibit any delay in language functions. The condition occurs more frequently in males (9:1). The long-term prognosis of the disorder is unknown, but the deficits appear to persist into adulthood.

541. The answer is C (2, 4). (Kaplan, 6/e, pp 2455–2469.) It is the responsibility of the physician to report suspected child abuse to the appropriate agency immediately. All states have an identified agency responsible for the investigation of all such cases. This agency is required to make a determination about the most suitable placement for the child. Many hospitals have an identified department or person who can facilitate these referrals. The physician's duty to protect the child against further injury overrides any consideration of confidentiality. The physician may pursue any investigations or treatment considered necessary for the child's care.

542. The answer is A (1, 2, 3). (Kaplan, 6/e, pp 2196–2198.) The increased metabolism and renal clearance of medications in children necessitates the use of higher oral dosages. It is important to monitor serum levels in children rather than rely on oral dosage. Children usually tolerate psychotropics well and should not exhibit paradoxical responses.

543. The answer is E (all). (Kaplan, 6/e, pp 1367–1368.) The medical complications of the eating disorders may be life-threatening. Recognized sequelae to anorexia nervosa include osteoporosis, hypothermia, bradycardia, arrhythmias, hypotension, edema, reduced renal clearance, renal calculi, and pancytopenia. The repeated vomiting of bulimia nervosa results in a metabolic alkalosis, parotid enlargement, dental caries, and traumatic injury to the upper gastrointestinal tract. The chronic abuse of ipecac by bulimic patients is reported to produce a myopathy that may include a cardiomyopathy.

544. The answer is C (2, 4). (Kaplan, 6/e, pp 2325–2326.) Tics may be motor, vocal, or sensory. They are rapid, brief, nonrhythmic, and purposeless. Although they are involuntary, they can usually be suppressed by the sufferer for short periods. Tics have a variable response to stress and may be aggravated, unchanged, or improved. The nature and pattern of the tic may change over time and may include other modalities. Motor tics are the most common type and account for three-quarters of initial presentations with the facial muscles the area most frequently involved.

545. The answer is B (1, 3). (Kaplan, 6/e, p 2202.) Neonates exhibit a number of innate responses that appear to promote infant-maternal interaction. A neonate will orient its head to a human voice and learn to respond preferentially to its own mother's voice. It will fix its eyes on the human face. The grasp reflex allows the infant to grasp its mother, just as an arboreal primate would. The normal infant cries immediately following a painful stimulus.

546. The answer is A (1, 2, 3). (Kaplan, 6/e, pp 2304–2310.) Numerous psychotropics have been reported to have therapeutic utility in ADHD. The antidepressants are recognized as effective second-line treatments (behind psychostimulants) and appear to be particularly effective in reducing motor hyperactivity. In addition to tricyclics, monoamine oxidase inhibitors, bupropion, and selective serotonin reuptake inhibitors have also been reported to be effective in ADHD. Several sudden deaths in children receiving tricyclics have been attributed to conduction abnormalities and highlight the importance of cardiac monitoring in children receiving these agents.

547–550. The answers are 547-B, 548-D, 549-C, 550-E. (Strub, pp 76–89.) Among the widely used psychological tests with clinical application are those devised by Rorschach, Wechsler, Bender, and Halstead and Reitan. As originally designed, each test was meant to serve some specific purpose, such as intelligence testing, assessment of personality structure, or evaluation of sensory perception. Some of the tests also assess motor function. Although designed to serve a specific goal, each test allows the interpreter to draw certain conclusions about a patient's mental capacity, psychodynamics, and the organic integrity of the patient's brain. Clinicians must have knowledge of the validity and sensitivity of the tests for each of these various aspects of brain function.

Wechsler tests are available in two forms, one for adults and another for children. Results of these tests are widely used by clinicians to derive IQ scores and to make inferences about the organic integrity of the brain, although in this regard the tests' limitations need fuller appreciation. While some examiners use the Wechsler test results projectively to assess personality structure, either the Rorschach or Bender tests or the Minnesota Multiphasic Personality Index is much more commonly used for this purpose. The IQ score is derived as a full-scale score, a verbal score, and a performance score. Certain brain lesions will be reflected in the test scores, but a normal Wechsler score does not exclude organic disorders of the brain. In general, patients with lesions of the right hemisphere score poorly on the performance scales, and those with lesions of the left hemisphere score poorly on the verbal scales. As arbitrarily incorporated in the scaling, the verbal and performance IQs in normal subjects should be about the same. Any large discrepancy suggests an organic disorder, but Wechsler test results alone can neither establish nor exclude an organic lesion. The results have to be integrated with the information from a patient's history, physical examination, neuroradiologic studies, EEG, or autopsy findings before a diagnosis can be made.

Lauretta Bender adopted the Gestalt figures of Wertheimer to test the visuomotor skills of children as a function of their maturation and to study the effects of brain lesions and retardation. The patient copies nine designs, which are then scored for accuracy, rotation, relation to each other, excesses or deletions, size, and pressure of lines. Generally, children younger than age 3 cannot perform the test, whereas most normal 12-year-old children can. Because the examiner gives few instructions, patients are compelled to call upon their own resources. While some overlap exists between subjects who are normal and those who have brain damage, brain-damaged subjects in general perform less well than normal subjects. Usually, patients with lesions of the right parietal lobe perform most poorly, whereas patients with lesions in other locations may produce essentially normal results. By asking a subject to produce the designs without looking at the originals, the examiner can test the patient's memory. By interpreting the distortions in the patient's drawings, the examiner may make inferences about the personality dynamics of the patient.

The Rorschach test requires the subject to respond to ten cards with inkblot figures, some of which are multicolored. What patients perceive in the relatively formless figures expresses their personality. A major criticism of the test is that the personality of the interpreter cannot always be separated from that of the patient. The examiner scores a patient's responses according to location, determinants, and content. The location refers to the areas of the figure to which the patient responds, as well as to whether the response involves the figure partially or as a whole. A large number of responses to the figure as a whole is associated with high intelligence and organizational ability. The content score indicates the breadth and range of the patient's interests and includes whether the patient responds in human, animal, sexual, or natural terms. The determinants of each response indicate the factors that made the patient produce the particular response, such as the form, shading, color, and sense of apparent movement. For example, an overemphasis on form would suggest an inhibited, rigid personality; a lack of perception of form might suggest inadequate control, inability to comply, or poor organizational ability. (The Murray Thematic Apperception Test has applications similar to the Rorschach. The Sentence Completion Test also has similar projective uses, but is thought to tap data at a more conscious level than the other projective tests like the Rorschach and the Murray.)

The Halstead-Reitan battery was devised because the psychological instruments available in the 1940s—such as the Wechsler, Rorschach, and Bender tests—too often failed to disclose abnormalities in patients with confirmed brain lesions. Halstead at the University of Chicago and Reitan at Indiana University School of Medicine worked with patients from neurologic and neurosurgical services who had confirmed brain lesions. They devised new tests and new interpretations of old tests based on empirical correlations of test results with clinical, neuroradiologic, and postmortem findings. The resultant battery includes the new versions of the Wechsler, the Halstead category tests, and a variety of motor and sensory tests. Originally designed to evaluate adults, a battery is now available for children as young as 5 years. The battery requires several hours to administer but includes the widest variety of tests and yields the most complete assessment of brain function of any neuropsychological instrument now available. The work has put to final rest a holy grail of psychologists, which was to develop a single test for evaluating brain damage. The complexity and range of brain functions cannot be tested on one dimension. Clinical conclusions based on converging lines of evidence from many sources are far more secure than conclusions relying on a single pathognomonic finding, which, when present, relieves the clinician of having to struggle with the diagnosis. The Halstead-Reitan battery, with its many cognitive, performance, and sensory tasks—some taken from the standard neurologic examination—recognizes this principle.

551–554. The answers are 551-D, 552-B, 553-C, 554-A. (Kaplan, 6/e, p 2345.) Anxiety disorders make up a considerable part of the practice of child psychiatry. Anxiety-ridden children struggle with the burden of terror-filled ideas that disaster awaits them or those they love. When the child is unable to displace anxiety onto a symbolic object or situation, the anxiety becomes free-floating rather than phobic. This free-floating anxiety may manifest as separation anxiety, avoidant disorder, or overanxious disorder. These conditions are manifestations of the child's fear of separation, contact, or both. Although a certain amount of oppositional behavior is normal to the development of a clear ego identity, when it becomes prolonged and intense and interferes with social functioning, it is regarded as an oppositional disorder. This disorder is more common in males, while anxiety disorders are more common in females. In separation disorder the family tends to be enmeshed. Avoidant children usually have at least one parent who is avoidant. The parents of a child with oppositional disorder are often preoccupied with issues of control.

MOOD DISORDERS

Directions: Each item below contains five suggested responses. Select the **one best** response to each item.

555. The term *double depression* describes

    (A) a particularly severe episode

    (B) melancholic depression

    (C) coincident mood disorder and substance abuse

    (D) iatrogenic exacerbation of depressed mood

    (E) major depression coincident with a dysthymic disorder

556. Patients with bipolar II disorder exhibit

    (A) only episodes of hypomania

    (B) prolonged periods of mania and depression

    (C) mania induced only by antidepressants

    (D) brief periods of hypomania followed by a major depressive disorder

    (E) consecutive manic episodes

557. The period between cycles of depression

    (A) remains stable

    (B) rarely exceeds 5 years

    (C) decreases with age

    (D) exhibits no clear pattern

    (E) averages 1 year in bipolar mood disorder

558. Adjustment disorders are accurately described by the statement that they

    (A) are most common in adult males

    (B) are most commonly associated with an anxious mood

    (C) are usually present for more than 6 months

    (D) seldom interfere with occupational functioning

    (E) carry a worse prognosis in adolescents than in adults

559. Atypical depression is characterized by

(A) a rapid response to electroconvulsive therapy
(B) early morning awakening
(C) poor response to all anti-depressants
(D) melancholia
(E) mood reactivity

560. All the following medications exhibit an adverse drug interaction with lithium EXCEPT

(A) terfenadine
(B) hydrochlorothiazide
(C) naproxen
(D) haloperidol
(E) ibuprofen

561. Following a serious suicide attempt, a 72-year-old man presents with the clinical features of a major depressive disorder with mood-congruent psychotic features. On examination, the patient exhibits moderate Parkinsonism and mild congestive heart failure. An electrocardiogram demonstrates a left bundle branch block and frequent ventricular extrasystoles. The most appropriate treatment at this time would be

(A) supportive psychotherapy
(B) electroconvulsive therapy (ECT)
(C) nortriptyline and haloperidol
(D) deprenyl
(E) thioridazine

562. Each of the following is a true statement about suicide EXCEPT

(A) females complete suicide more frequently than males
(B) most suicide victims have identifiable axis 1 disorders
(C) suicide ranks among the top 10 causes of death in the United States
(D) suicide tends to run in families
(E) the majority of suicide victims have communicated their intent prior to the act

563. The natural course of unipolar depression is characterized by which of the following statements?

(A) The first episode is by age 20 in the majority of patients
(B) The untreated episode lasts an average of 3 months
(C) The mean is six episodes per lifetime
(D) Twenty percent of patients will have more than one episode
(E) Sixty percent of patients will become chronically disabled

564. Major depressive disorder in childhood

(A) carries a good long-term prognosis
(B) is estimated to occur in 15 percent of 10-year-old children
(C) fails to respond to antidepressants
(D) seldom has somatic symptoms
(E) is frequently associated with mood-congruent psychotic features

565. Each of the following statements about the postpartum blues is true EXCEPT

(A) it normally occurs shortly after delivery
(B) it is self-limiting
(C) there is a significant risk of suicide
(D) it occurs in up to 50 percent of women
(E) it lasts less than 30 days

566. Which of the following statements about lithium maintenance therapy is true?

(A) It is effective prophylaxis in 50 percent of patients with bipolar illness
(B) It is indicated in all patients with bipolar illness
(C) It may cause sustained leukopenia
(D) It invariably impairs thyroid function
(E) It should maintain blood levels between 0.8 and 1.2 meq/L

567. The presence of melancholia with a major depressive disorder is associated with each of the following EXCEPT

(A) diurnal variation in symptoms
(B) anorexia
(C) good response to ECT
(D) anhedonia
(E) premorbid personality disorder

568. According to Sigmund Freud, melancholia develops as a consequence of

(A) a self-defeating cognitive stance
(B) anal-sadistic impulses
(C) the internalization of a "bad object" during infancy
(D) harsh criticism by the superego
(E) a diminished sense of self

569. Each of the following is a true statement about late luteal phase dysphoric disorder EXCEPT

(A) the onset of the disorder tends to be after age 30
(B) oral contraceptives are effective in reducing symptoms
(C) symptoms worsen with age
(D) symptoms remit a few days after onset of the follicular phase
(E) the disorder causes disruption in work and social activity

570. Diagnostic criteria for anorexia nervosa include each of the following EXCEPT

(A) in females, the absence of at least three consecutive menstrual cycles
(B) an intense fear of gaining weight
(C) weight loss of at least 15 percent
(D) distorted body image
(E) delusions about food

571. Sodium valproate is characterized by which of the following?

(A) It may decrease the blood levels of carbamazepine with co-administration
(B) It has a half-life of approximately 24 h
(C) It has teratogenic effects
(D) It exhibits low protein binding
(E) It has dopamine agonist effects

572. Which of the following is an absolute contraindication to electroconvulsive therapy (ECT)?

(A) Intracranial tumor
(B) Hypertension
(C) Myocardial infarction within 6 weeks
(D) Seizure disorder
(E) None of the above

Directions: Each item below contains four suggested responses of which **one or more** is correct. Select:

A	if	**1, 2, and 3**	are correct
B	if	**1 and 3**	are correct
C	if	**2 and 4**	are correct
D	if	**4**	is correct
E	if	**1, 2, 3, and 4**	are correct

573. Which of the following psychotropics should be avoided in a breast-feeding patient?

(1) Diazepam
(2) Lithium
(3) Phenothiazines
(4) Barbiturates

574. For augmenting tricyclic antidepressants in a treatment-resistant major depressive disorder, agents with demonstrated efficacy include

(1) cyproheptadine
(2) triiodothyronine (T_3)
(3) nifedipine
(4) lithium

575. Rapid-cycling bipolar mood disorder

(1) describes four or more episodes of mood disorder per year
(2) occurs in 25 percent of bipolar patients
(3) is more common in females
(4) may indicate occult hyperthyroidism

576. The patient with chronic intractable pain

(1) most often has a family history of mood disorder
(2) is most likely a blue-collar worker
(3) is often alexithymic
(4) is most often male

577. According to Beck's cognitive theory, elements essential to the development of depression include

(1) logical errors
(2) the cognitive triad
(3) silent assumptions
(4) parataxic distortion

578. Dysthymic disorder is correctly characterized by which of the following statements?

(1) It seldom improves with antidepressants
(2) It is often accompanied by mood-congruent psychotic features
(3) It usually responds to long-term psychotherapy
(4) It is often complicated by a superimposed major depressive disorder

579. Suicide in the elderly

(1) is more common than in other age groups
(2) is highest in men age 80 to 89
(3) is usually associated with a major depressive disorder
(4) is increasing

580. True statements regarding fluoxetine include that

(1) it is primarily metabolized by the liver
(2) it is extensively bound to serum proteins
(3) it takes more than 1 month to achieve steady state
(4) its absorption is not influenced by food intake

581. Dexamethasone nonsuppression is accurately described by which of the following?

(1) It persists well beyond treatment response
(2) It is found most commonly among patients with a major depression with psychotic features
(3) It predicts a rapid response to antidepressants
(4) It is found in anorexia nervosa

582. In the treatment of a major depressive disorder,

(1) cognitive psychotherapy has been shown to be effective
(2) antidepressants are most effective in alleviating vegetative symptoms
(3) combined psychotherapy and pharmacotherapy is most effective
(4) placebo is as effective as psychotherapy

583. Characteristics of phototherapy include that it

(1) may be used to augment antidepressants
(2) may cause hypomania
(3) is more effective if administered in the morning
(4) is most effective at 400 lux

584. An appropriate candidate for short-term dynamic psychotherapy must

(1) be motivated
(2) not be suffering from a mood disorder
(3) possess at least average intelligence
(4) be capable of tolerating inter-personal conflict

585. According to Bowlby's theory of separation, the infant demonstrates which of the following stages?

(1) Denial
(2) Protest
(3) Distortion
(4) Detachment

586. The serum lithium level will be raised by which of the following?

(1) Furosemide (Lasix)
(2) Naproxen
(3) Aspirin
(4) Low-salt diet

587. Which of the following investigations would be necessary prior to starting lithium therapy in a healthy 25-year-old man?

(1) CBC
(2) BUN and creatinine
(3) T4 and TSH
(4) Creatinine clearance test

588. Risk factors for completed suicide in a patient with a major depressive disorder include

(1) female sex
(2) low social class
(3) age of less than 30 years
(4) psychotic features

SUMMARY OF DIRECTIONS

A	B	C	D	E
1,2,3	1,3	2,4	4	All are
only	only	only	only	correct

589. According to Elisabeth Kübler-Ross, the stages of dying

(1) are successfully negotiated by most people
(2) follow a predictable sequence
(3) are shaped by cultural attitudes and beliefs
(4) usually include a period of panic

590. ECT that uses a brief-pulse waveform current pattern as opposed to a sine-wave current pattern

(1) produces a longer seizure
(2) produces less confusion in the subject
(3) is less effective in treating depression
(4) requires less energy

591. Depression following a left frontal cerebrovascular accident

(1) is usually resistant to antidepressants
(2) is seldom incapacitating
(3) is a manifestation of pseudobulbar affect
(4) is more likely with opercular lesions

592. Carbamazepine can accurately be described by which of the following?

(1) It is as effective as lithium in preventing relapse in bipolar affective disorder
(2) It is effective in preventing only the depressive phase of bipolar illness
(3) It is an effective antimanic agent
(4) It is ineffective in patients with rapid-cycling bipolar mood disorder

593. Acute severe lithium toxicity

(1) is usually secondary to deliberate overdose
(2) may require emergency hemodialysis
(3) is likely to produce a fulminant hepatitis
(4) may produce cardiac arrhythmias

594. Mood disorders in the mentally retarded are

(1) not usually accompanied by somatic symptoms
(2) usually resistant to psychotropics
(3) usually short-lived
(4) often accompanied by aggressive behavior

595. Side effects of monoamine oxidase (MAO) inhibitors include

(1) significant weight gain
(2) suppression of rapid eye movement (REM) sleep
(3) peripheral neuropathy
(4) generalized edema

596. Cardiovascular effects of tricyclic antidepressants include

(1) quinidine-like actions
(2) decreased sensitivity to circulating catecholamines
(3) prolonged QT interval
(4) prominent P waves

597. Which of the following are considered valid animal models of depression in humans?

(1) Maternal separation
(2) Learned helplessness
(3) Reserpine administration
(4) Chronic stress

MOOD DISORDERS

ANSWERS

555. The answer is E. (Kaplan, 6/e, p 1166.) *Double depression* describes patients who develop a major depression in addition to a concurrent dysthymic disorder. These patients are at higher risk for recurrence of their major depression and are less responsive to medication.

556. The answer is D. (Kaplan, 6/e, p 1143.) Bipolar II disorder is characterized by brief periods of hypomania followed by a major depressive disorder. According to *DSM IV* this would be classified as "bipolar disorder not otherwise specified." Although the characteristics of patients with this type of mood disorder have not been fully elaborated, certain features have been reported. These patients appear to have a higher incidence of other psychopathology, including alcoholism, drug abuse, obsessive-compulsive disorder, and antisocial personality. They also appear to have an earlier age of onset and higher risk of suicide than patients with bipolar I or unipolar depression.

557. The answer is C. (Kaplan, 6/e, p 1167.) The duration of the period between successive episodes of mood disorder in unipolar and bipolar patients decreases with increasing age. This decrease with each successive cycle is approximately 20 percent in unipolars and 10 percent in bipolars. The average cycle length in bipolar mood disorder is 33 months and in unipolar mood disorder 45 months.

558. The answer is E. (Kaplan, 6/e, pp 1418–1424.) An adjustment disorder is a reaction, within 3 months, to an identifiable psychosocial stressor. The maladaptive reaction includes occupational impairment or symptoms that are in excess of the expected norm or both. The adjustment disorder does not, by definition, persist beyond 6 months. Adjustment disorders carry a poor prognosis in adolescents and 56 percent will have evidence of a psychiatric disorder 5 years after the initial adjustment disorder. There are nine subtypes of adjustment disorder; depression is by far the most common.

559. The answer is E. (Schatzberg, p 583.) Patients suffering from an atypical depression meet *DSM-IV* criteria for major depression but still exhibit significant mood reactivity (i.e., their moods may improve briefly in response to environmental factors). Patients with atypical depression are usually rejection sensitive, xenophobic, and hypersomnolent. The disorder exhibits a differential treatment response to MAO inhibitors and possibly electroconvulsive therapy.

560. The answer is A. (Schatzberg, pp 327–329.) Lithium exhibits several significant, sometimes life-threatening drug interactions. Although all diuretics may produce increases in serum lithium levels, the thiazide diuretics are most likely to raise lithium levels significantly. Via their inhibition of renal tubular prostaglandin, nonsteroidal anti-inflammatory agents increase serum lithium levels. Lithium may worsen the extrapyramidal symptoms of neuroleptics. In addition, the combination of high-potency neuroleptics with lithium has been reported to result in a toxic encephalopathy. Lithium may decrease conduction in the sinus node and potentiate antiarrhythmic drugs (e.g.,quinidine, digoxin). Patients on this combination should be followed closely and undergo regular electrocardiograms.

561. The answer is B. (Kaplan, 6/e, pp 2129–2140.) The main indications for ECT in patients with a major depressive disorder are (1) failure to respond to psychotropics, (2) mood-congruent delusions or hallucinations, (3) high suicide risk, (4) life-threatening psychomotor retardation, (5) previous response to ECT, and (6) medical contraindications to the use of standard psychotropics. The patient described clearly meets these criteria. ECT provides a safe, rapid, and effective treatment of major depression in the elderly.

562. The answer is A. (Kaplan, 6/e, pp 1739–1752.) Suicide is the fifth most common cause of death in the Western world. It has been estimated that approximately 90 percent of patients who commit suicide are suffering from a psychiatric illness. There is a strong familial and genetic determinant to suicide. The vast majority of persons who attempt or complete suicide will have informed someone of their intention prior to the act. Although the incidence of suicide attempts is higher among females, males complete suicide more frequently. Males tend to employ more violent means of self-destruction (e.g., guns, hanging).

563. The answer is C. (Kaplan, 6/e, pp 2380–2381.) The majority of patients with unipolar depression will have their first episode by age 40. As many as 50 to 85 percent of patients will have at least two episodes. The mean number of episodes per lifetime is six. The average duration of an untreated unipolar depression is 6 to 13 months, while treated depressions last approximately 3 months. An attempt to withdraw antidepressants in less than 3 months will almost always result in immediate recurrence of symptoms. Approximately 20 percent of patients with unipolar mood disorder will exhibit a significant chronic impairment in functioning. Men carry a poorer long-term prognosis.

564. The answer is E. (Kaplan, 6/e, p 2367.) It is estimated that the incidence of major depressive disorders in 10 year olds is 1.7 percent. The illness is more likely to be found in the children of parents with mood disorders; the incidence is doubled with one afflicted parent and quadrupled with both parents afflicted. Children may frequently develop somatic complaints, agitation, and mood-congruent psychotic features. The onset of a major depressive disorder suggests a poor long-term prognosis. Children will respond to antidepressants in a similar fashion to adults. There is a much higher incidence of oppositional behavior, learning problems, and substance abuse among children with major depression.

565. The answer is C. (Kaplan, 6/e, pp 1062–1063.) The postpartum blues is considered to fall under the category of an adjustment disorder with depressed mood. Postpartum dysphoria, headaches, tearfulness, and irritability occur in 50 percent of women. This disorder is most common in primiparae and symptoms usually peak within 10 days and resolve within 30 days of delivery. No formal psychiatric intervention is normally required, although a small percentage of these patients may go on to develop a major depressive disorder. The etiology is unknown but presumed to be secondary to rapid alterations in estrogen, progesterone, and prolactin.

566. The answer is D. (Kaplan, 6/e, pp 2022–2031.) Lithium maintenance therapy is effective in preventing relapse in 70 to 80 percent of patients with bipolar illness. There are no well-defined criteria for implementing long-term lithium therapy. Most clinicians would agree that two or three episodes within a few years or devastating episodes are an indication for maintenance therapy. Ultimately the decision should be made only after discussion with the patient. Long-term side effects include a uniform suppression of thyroid function, tremor, weight gain, and diarrhea. High peak levels have been associated with encephalopathy and nephrotoxicity. In order to minimize these possible side effects, the recommended maintenance blood level is 0.5 to 0.8 meq/L. Lithium may produce a leukocytosis rather than leukopenia.

567. The answer is E. (APA, DSM IV, p 224.) According to *DSM IV,* a major depressive disorder with melancholia is associated with at least five of the following: (1) loss of interest or pleasure in all, or almost all, activities, (2) lack of reactivity to usually pleasurable stimuli, (3) depression worse in the morning, (4) early morning awakening, (5) psychomotor retardation or agitation, (6) anorexia or weight loss, (7) no significant premorbid personality disorder, (8) one or more previous major depressive episodes followed by recovery, (9) previous good response to somatic therapies.

568. The answer is D. (Kaplan, 6/e, pp 1068–1069.) Freud outlined his early theory about melancholy in the 1915 treatise "Mourning and Melancholia." He postulated that in mourning the psychic pain is the consequence of the loss of an external object, whereas in melancholia this pain may be precipitated by an actual or perceived loss. The self-reproach and self-punitive attitude of the melancholic is the consequence of a harsh superego activated by the aggressive impulses generated by the ego's sense of abandonment. The melancholic directs this hostility inward rather than against the lost object.

569. The answer is B. (Kaplan, 6/e, p 1124.) Late luteal phase dysphoric disorder has been included in the appendix of the *DSM IV* but remains a controversial diagnostic entity since 90 percent of women experience some symptoms during the premenstrual period. The varied symptoms of the disorder have their onset during the late luteal phase (i.e., the week before menses) and remit a few days after the onset of the follicular phase (i.e., a few days after the menses). The disorder usually starts after age 30 and the symptoms often increase with age. Typical symptoms include affective lability, irritability, decreased interest, difficulty concentrating, hypersomnia/insomnia, and numerous physical symptoms. Oral contraceptives are ineffective in reducing symptoms. Recent studies suggest that fluoxetine may be helpful in reducing affective symptoms and bromocriptine is effective in reducing breast swelling.

570. The answer is E. (Kaplan, 6/e, p 1364.) The presence of delusional thought content is not necessary to make a diagnosis of anorexia nervosa, though patients do exhibit a distorted body image that is not malleable to outside suggestion. The illness may, however, coexist with schizophrenia, obsessive-compulsive disorder, or anxiety disorders.

571. The answer is C. (Schatzberg, pp 360–366.) Valproic acid is a unique, branched-chain carboxylic acid that increases GABA levels and responsivity in the central nervous system. The drug is well absorbed from the gastrointestinal tract and is extensively metabolized in the liver with a half-life of 6 to 16 h. The drug is extensively protein-bound and its competitive displacement by agents such as aspirin may significantly increase the free fraction of the drug. Valproate tends to inhibit hepatic metabolism and may, therefore, raise serum concentrations of other anticonvulsants (e.g., carbamazepine, phenobarbital) and psychotropic medications. Serum concentraions may be elevated by inhibitors of the CYP450 enzyme system. The incidence of neural tube defects in children born to mothers receiving valproate has been reported at 1 to 1.5 percent.

572. The answer is E. (APA, Treatments, pp 1805–1806.) According to the recent report of the APA Task Force, there are no absolute contraindications to performing electroconvulsive therapy; however, a number of medical conditions place the patient at higher risk. The most important physiologic stress is increased cardiac output and also possibly an immediate 5- to 10-s period of bradycardia or asystole immediately following the electrical stimulus. Patients with a history of hypertension, recent myocardial infarction, or compromised cardiac function are at increased risk for complications. Digoxin therapy may in particular predispose to prolonged bradycardia. Modern cardiac pacemakers are electrically shielded and therefore relatively immune to any interference. The degree of raised intracranial pressure that occurs during the ECT-induced seizure does not represent an absolute contraindication to ECT in patients with intracranial tumors and arteriovenous malformations. ECT may be safely administered at any stage of pregnancy.

573. The answer is E (all). (Kaplan, 6/e, pp 1700–1701.) As a rule of thumb, all psychotropics should be avoided if a mother is breast feeding. Benzodiazepines and barbiturates in the mother's milk will produce drowsiness in the child. Lithium concentrations in breast milk may approach those of maternal serum and present a potent potential hazard to the child (e.g., encephalopathy). Although the concentrations of tricyclic antidepressants and fluoxetine are generally lower in breast milk than in the maternal circulation, their use in the lactating woman should be undertaken with caution.

574. The answer is C (2, 4). (APA, Treatments, pp 1792–1802.) There is no universal definition of the treatment-resistant major depressive disorder. However, it is generally agreed that a failure to respond to an adequate dose (i.e., >150 mg daily) of imipramine after 4 to 6 weeks of treatment is resistance to treatment. The most common causes of treatment resistance are inadequate dosage or duration of treatment and noncompliance. The possibility of drug interactions or occult medical illness may also hamper treatment response. Recognized pharmacologic treatment augmenters for treatment-resistant cases include lithium, T_3, stimulants, neuroleptics, and L-tryptophan. The combination of antidepressants may also prove effective and recent research suggests that the combination of a tricyclic with fluoxetine may produce rapid response. Nonpharmacologic interventions include sleep deprivation, sleep phase advancement, and high-intensity light. Finally, ECT is often effective in those cases that fail to respond to the above interventions.

575. The answer is B (1, 3). (APA, Treatments, pp 1934–1936.) Rapid-cycling bipolar affective disorder may be defined as four or more episodes of mood disorder per year. The condition is postulated to occur in as many as 10 percent of patients with bipolar disorder. It is more common among females and in patients who have received tricyclic antidepressants for prolonged periods. A significant percentage of patients will be found to have subclinical hypothyroidism in association with long-term lithium use. Although there are no rigorous guidelines for the treatment of "rapid cyclers," a number of agents have demonstrated efficacy in this group. These include carbamazepine, valproic acid, clonazepam, propranolol, and verapamil. An attempt should be made to avoid tricyclic antidepressants.

576. The answer is A (1, 2, 3). (APA, Treatments, pp 1901–1904.) The *DSM IV* diagnosis of somatoform pain disorder describes severe, prolonged pain in the absence of plausible physical pathology. The condition is most common in females and blue-collar workers. Their family history is often positive for alcohol abuse and major depressive disorder. A significant percentage of patients will have psychophysiologic markers for depression (i.e., DST nonsuppression and shortened REM latency). Patients benefit from antidepressants and psychosocial and educational intervention. Since these patients express their affective discomfort through physical symptoms, it is not surprising that there is an increased incidence of alexithymia.

577. The answer is A (1, 2, 3). (APA, Treatments, pp 1834–1835.) The cognitive theory of depression suggests that automatic, negatively biased thinking is responsible for precipitating and perpetuating depressive episodes. The cognitive triad describes the negative view that depressives hold about themselves, their world, and their future. Silent assumptions are psychological constructs that make the person vulnerable to a helpless and hopeless depressive position. Logical errors produce a distortion that also predisposes to a depressed position. Cognitive therapy attempts to identify these self-defeating cognitive patterns and replace them with more productive patterns.

578. The answer is D (4). (Kaplan, 6/e, pp 2367–2368.) Dysthymic disorder describes a syndrome of chronic dysphoria persisting for more than 2 years (1 year in children and adolescents). There are none of the somatic symptoms usually associated with a major affective disorder. The condition may occur concurrently with other psychopathology, most commonly a major affective disorder (producing the so-called double depression). Recent research suggests that a significant percentage of dysthymic patients (50 percent) will benefit from tricyclic antidepressants. A family history of affective disorder suggests a good response to antidepressants. No psychotherapeutic techniques have demonstrated efficacy for this group of patients.

579. The answer is E (all). (Kaplan, 6/e, p 2517.) The elderly are at highest risk for suicide with a 50 percent higher rate than young adults. The incidence of suicide among the elderly is increasing, with men between 80 and 89 and women between 50 and 65 years of age at highest risk. Compared with young people, the elderly are less likely to communicate their suicidal ideation or make "manipulative" gestures and tend to employ more lethal methods. Approximately 75 percent of these elderly suicide attempters will be found to have a major depressive disorder. The presence of mood-congruent psychotic features increases the possibility of suicide.

580. The answer is E (all). (PDR, 1996, p 902.) Fluoxetine absorption is not influenced by food. The drug is metabolized by the liver to an active metabolite, norfluoxetine. The half-life of fluoxetine is 2 to 3 days and that of its metabolite is 7 to 9 days. This means that more than 30 days are required to reach steady state levels. Serum protein binds 94.5 percent of serum fluoxetine. Other protein-bound drugs, such as digoxin or warfarin, may be displaced and therefore become more bioavailable. The serum concentration of tricyclic antidepressants may be increased several fold by the concomitant use of fluoxetine.

581. The answer is C (2, 4). (Kaplan, 6/e, pp 1095–1096.) The dexamethasone suppression test is a nonspecific test for psychiatric disorders. Although a number of contradictory studies have been published, some clear patterns have emerged. The highest incidence of nonsuppression is found in patients with a psychotic depression. Patients with a family history are more likely to be nonsuppressors. The return of suppression indicates treatment response, and patients tend to "run true" with each episode of mood disorder. Any significant medical illness or weight loss can cause nonsuppression. Dementia may also produce nonsuppression.

582. The answer is A (1, 2, 3). (APA, Treatments, pp 1817–1823.) The major studies have all been consistent in demonstrating that combined psychotherapy and pharmacotherapy is most effective for treating a major depressive disorder. Psychotherapy has demonstrated the most efficacy in the areas of problem-solving and psychosocial dysfunction. Pharmacotherapy is most effective for treating vegetative symptoms and preventing relapse. Patients with an identified psychosocial precipitant responded best to psychotherapy. Combined treatment appears to produce better long-term outcome.

583. The answer is A (1, 2, 3). (Kaplan, 6/e, pp 2144–2145.) The intensity of the light source used for phototherapy should be above 2500 lux. Phototherapy is most effective if administered in the early morning for at least 30 min; it appears that 2 h is necessary for adequate clinical response, and a typical dose response curve has been demonstrated. Several cases of hypomania following light treatment have been reported.

584. The answer is E (all). (APA, Treatments, p 1876.) Appropriate patient selection is probably the most important factor in achieving a positive outcome from short-term dynamic psychotherapy. Despite the well-defined selection criteria for suitable patients, a broad range of patients will benefit from the technique. Selection criteria include (1) motivation for change, (2) ego strength, (3) psychological mindedness, (4) the ability to tolerate "focal" interpersonal conflict, and (5) the ability to develop affective involvement. Patients with narcissistic and immature level ego defense structures are unlikely to benefit from short-term psychotherapy.

585. The answer is C (2, 4). (APA, Treatments, p 1952.) Bowlby described three stages of infant response to separation from the mother. These stages are protest, despair, and detachment. Bowlby considers the mother-infant attachment bond to be a paradigm for depression. According to this theory, if the infant is separated from the mother for prolonged periods of time, a hopeless depression may persist throughout life.

586. The answer is C (2, 4). (Kaplan, 6/e, pp 2022–2031.) The excretion of lithium is almost entirely renal. Any drug that reduces the renal clearance of lithium will therefore raise serum levels. Increased levels occur with thiazide diuretics, nonsteroidal anti-inflammatory drugs, low sodium intake, and dehydration. Loop diuretics (furosemide, ethacrynic acid) increase renal clearance and may therefore reduce serum levels. Although the combination of lithium and haloperidol has been implicated in causing an encephalopathy, this association has not been confirmed. Verapamil may lower serum lithium levels. A prolonged response to neuromuscular blocking agents has been reported when they are used in conjunction with lithium.

587. The answer is A (1, 2, 3). (APA, Treatments, pp 1926–1927.) The appropriate use and efficacy of lithium therapy is dependent on a thorough evaluation, appropriate dosage, and close monitoring. Initial evaluation is necessary to ensure appropriate patient selection and objective parameters for follow-up. In addition to a thorough history and physical examination, a young (<40 years), healthy subject requires the following: weight measurement, CBC, T_4/TSH, fasting blood sugar and electrolytes, urinalysis, and BUN and creatinine. Older patients require additional evaluation, including ECG, EEG, thyrotropin-releasing hormone test, 24-h urine volume, and creatinine clearance and concentration test. In patients on a maintenance schedule, with no clinical evidence for side effects, follow-up requires annual thyroid function tests and quarterly serum creatinine and lithium levels.

588. The answer is C (2, 4). (Kaplan, 6/e, pp 1739–1740.) Although females have a higher rate of suicide attempts, males are more likely to complete a suicide. Risk factors for suicide include (1) male sex, (2) divorce or widowhood and living alone, (3) age over 45, (4) unemployment, (5) chaotic family background, (6) alcohol or drug abuse, (7) psychosis, (8) chronic illness, and (9) poor insight. Recent work suggests that there are subgroups of high-risk subjects in different age groups, each with its own demographic features; for example, the group over age 55 tends to contain less alcoholism and fewer personality disorders but more widowhood and chronic illness than the group under age 35. The demographic profile of the geriatric population at risk has yet to be established.

589. The answer is B (1, 3). (Kaplan, 6/e, pp 1718–1719.) Despite the intensity of emotional distress that the dying process involves, most people are able to cope with this period effectively. The ability to navigate this traumatic period is determined by a number of factors, including past experiences and familiarity with death, sociocultural norms, religious beliefs, cognitive development, and personality structure. Kübler-Ross has defined a number of stages in the dying process. Although they have become embedded in current medical and social thinking, these stages do not always follow a predictable sequence. The five stages are (1) shock and denial, (2) anger, (3) bargaining, (4) depression, and (5) acceptance.

590. The answer is C (2, 4). (Kaplan, 6/e, pp 2129–2140.) The goal of modern ECT equipment is to induce seizure activity with the fewest possible side effects. This is accomplished by delivering the minimum amount of current for the shortest possible duration. Traditional equipment has used the sine-wave type of electrical current available through domestic circuits. The development of brief-pulse waveforms allows the administration of the current only during a small peak period of the cycle. This produces an equivalent clinical response for only one-third of the energy expenditure and therefore reduces cognitive side effects such as postictal confusion and memory loss. The brief-pulse waveform has demonstrated efficacy equal to that of the sine-wave method.

591. The answer is D (4). (Kaplan, 6/e, pp 191–192.) Affective disorders are common following cerebrovascular accidents. The likelihood of a major depressive disorder appears to be directly proportional to the proximity of the lesion to the left frontal pole. Mania appears to be more likely with right frontopolar lesions. The development of a mood disorder during the period of rehabilitation can profoundly impede progress and diminish the possibility of functional recovery. It is therefore extremely important that the mood disorders are recognized early and treated aggressively. Nortriptyline has proved effective for the treatment of "poststroke depression."

592. The answer is B (1, 3). (Kaplan, 6/e, pp 1964–1972.) Carbamazepine has proven efficacy as prophylaxis in bipolar affective disorder and as an antimanic agent. Although the drug should theoretically possess antidepressant properties, this has yet to be confirmed clinically. The drug has been proved equivalent to lithium in preventing relapse of both the manic and depressive phases of the illness. The serum level necessary to obtain the acute and chronic effects has not been fully elaborated, but it would appear that it correlates with anticonvulsant levels. One major study suggested the following predictors of a good anti-manic response to carbamazepine: (1) greater severity of symptoms, (2) anxiety and dys-phoria, (3) rapid cycling, and (4) negative family history of mood disorder.

593. The answer is C (2, 4). (Kaplan, 6/e, pp 2022–2031.) The majority of lithium intoxica-tions occur accidentally during treatment, i.e., through the presence of dehydration or salt depletion or the addition of drugs that raise serum lithium levels (thiazides, nonsteroidal anti-inflammatory drugs). The severity of clinical symptoms does not always follow the serum lithium level. During the early stages the serum level may be highest and antecede the development of florid clinical signs. Early signs of intoxication include diarrhea, vom-iting, tremor, and lethargy. These will be followed by evidence of encephalopathy, includ-ing myoclonus, increased muscle tone, extensor plantar responses, seizures, and decreasing consciousness. Cardiac arrhythmias and respiratory arrest may be terminal events. Treat-ment of lithium intoxication includes saline alkaline diuresis with adjunctive theophylline or loop diuretics, hemodialysis, and cardiorespiratory support. Bronchial toilet is particu-larly important since viscous bronchial secretions are likely to develop. With the onset of coma, the mortality of lithium toxicity approaches 50 percent.

594. The answer is D (4). (Kaplan, 6/e, pp 2223–2232.) Mood disorders are common among the mentally retarded and are frequently unrecognized. They may exhibit both unipolar and bipolar disease. The mentally retarded will use primitive ego defenses in coping with their illness and are more likely to become aggressive or show somatization. The usual somatic symptoms found in a mood disorder will be present but sometimes difficult to recognize. These patients will respond to conventional psychotropics, but they may be more sensitive to side effects.

595. The answer is E (all). (Kaplan, 6/e, pp 2038–2054.) The primary advantage of monoamine oxidase inhibitors in the elderly is their relative lack of anticholinergic side effects. The side effects that are most common are hypotension and insomnia. The develop-ment of orthostatic hypotension is particularly hazardous in the elderly. A peripheral neuropathy can be prevented by the adjunctive use of vitamin B_6 (pyridoxine). Generalized edema, if it occurs, usually resolves within a week of commencing treatment. Weight gain with carbohydrate craving may be marked. A reversible lupuslike reaction and hyperpro-lactinemia have been reported. Reference to a standard text should always be made prior to starting any medication concomitant with a monoamine oxidase inhibitor.

596. The answer is B (1, 3). (Kaplan, 6/e, pp 1496–1497.) The tricyclic antidepressants exhibit quinidine-like effects on the cardiovascular system. Possible dose-related cardiac side effects include prolonged QT interval; flattened or inverted T waves; prominent Q waves; pro-longed AV conduction; bradycardia or tachycardia; atrial and ventricular arrhythmias; and diminished cardiac output. Accordingly, patients with compromised cardiac functioning or conduction abnormalities should not receive tricyclic antidepressants if they can be avoided.

597. The answer is E (all). (Kaplan, 6/e, pp 1074–1075.) The learned helplessness model is produced by exposing the animal to an inescapable stress such as an electric shock. Although animals will initially protest and become agitated, they will soon assume a helpless and submissive position. This state has been correlated with decreased central noradrenergic drive, which can be restored with antidepressants or by allowing the animal to regain some control over the noxious stimulus. Maternal separation results in a predictable sequence of protest, despair, and denial in the infant. The physiologic changes associated with this state are reversed by tricyclic antidepressants. The antihypertensive provided the first physiologic model of depression and produces alterations in central biogenic amines in a manner similar to that of a major depressive disorder. Chronic stress (e.g., changing cage mates or housing conditions) produces physiologic changes similar to those of depression; these changes are reversed by tricyclics and monoamine oxidase inhibitors. Chronic stress models use repeated unpredictable stressors (e.g., tail pinching) that produce a decrease in exploratory behavior. This change is reversed by antidepressants and ECT.

PERSONALITY DISORDERS

Directions: Each item below contains five suggested responses. Select the **one best** response to each item.

598. According to Otto Kernberg's theory, the basis of the borderline personality is

(A) an inability to mobilize productive ego defenses

(B) the presence of an atypical mood disorder

(C) an inability to integrate both positive and negative self and object representations

(D) an inability to differentiate the self from the maternal and paternal objects

(E) an inability to differentiate between fantasy and reality

599. The person with a schizoid personality disorder

(A) feels abandoned and alone

(B) uses fantasy as a major ego defense

(C) frequently distorts reality

(D) is seldom capable of abstract thinking

(E) is not an appropriate candidate for group therapy

600. According to Kohut's theory, narcissistic personality disorder

(A) is a consequence of unfulfilled oral needs

(B) is a consequence of the individual's inability to internalize a stable object during early childhood

(C) is caused by excessive aggressive drives

(D) is a result of parental abuse

(E) is a consequence of the parents' failure to respond to the child's need for idealization

601. Each of the following disorders has an increased incidence among the family of origin of a person with antisocial personality disorder EXCEPT

(A) substance abuse

(B) histrionic personality disorder

(C) schizophrenia

(D) somatization disorder

(E) antisocial personality disorder

602. When attempting psychotherapy with a patient suffering from a paranoid personality disorder, the therapist

(A) should avoid zealous interpretations

(B) must assume a passive position

(C) must be unusually warm and ingratiating toward the patient

(D) should assume a stance of technical neutrality

(E) almost always requires the use of adjunctive neuroleptic medication

Directions: Each item below contains four suggested responses of which **one or more** is correct. Select:

A	if	**1, 2, and 3**	are correct
B	if	**1 and 3**	are correct
C	if	**2 and 4**	are correct
D	if	**4**	is correct
E	if	**1, 2, 3, and 4**	are correct

603. According to the *DSM IV,* diagnostic criteria for borderline personality disorder include

(1) chronic feelings of loneliness and emptiness
(2) affective instability
(3) recurrent suicidal threats or gestures
(4) episodes of micropsychosis

604. Characteristics of all persons with a personality disorder include

(1) interpersonal conflict
(2) suppression
(3) inflexible responses to stress
(4) mood lability

605. The person with a passive-aggressive personality disorder

(1) is difficult to engage in psychotherapy
(2) usually had punitive, insensitive parents
(3) has learned to retroflex aggressive feelings
(4) often exhibits ideas of reference

606. A patient experiencing a dissociative fugue

(1) assumes a new personal identity
(2) is likely to be confused
(3) usually travels away from his or her usual residence
(4) is likely to exhibit an anterograde amnesia

607. Client-centered psychotherapy recognizes which of the following principles?

(1) Clients are admonished to suppress feelings about the therapist
(2) Therapists cultivate a caring, unconditional regard for the client
(3) Clients are encouraged to change their life-style
(4) Therapists express their own affecive responses generated by their relationship with the patient

Directions: Each group of questions below consists of lettered options followed by a set of numbered items. For each numbered item select the **one** lettered option with which it is **most** closely associated. Each lettered option may be used **once, more than once, or not at all.**

Items 608–611

For each of the case histories below, choose the disorder (according to *DSM IV* criteria) with which it most closely corresponds.

  (A) Schizotypal personality disorder
  (B) Schizoid personality disorder
  (C) Self-defeating personality disorder
  (D) Paranoid personality disorder
  (E) Avoidant personality disorder

608. A 39-year-old man reluctantly submits to a psychiatric examination at the urging of his siblings, whom he accuses of treachery in the family business and plotting against him. Unable to relax, he is guarded and totally humorless. He does not love his female companion but is jealous of anyone who makes amorous advances toward her. He attends the psychiatric interview only to appease his family, and he is concerned that they are attempting to institutionalize him.

609. A 24-year-old college graduate submits to a psychiatric examination more in deference to her parents than from self-concern. The patient has a degree in education but is content with a job filing books in the library. She has no friends and spends her time collecting recipes and cooking for herself. She seems indifferent to criticism and has never had a romantic relationship

610. A 46-year-old woman is referred to a psychiatrist by her 25-year-old daughter, who complains that her mother is hostile toward everyone. The daughter describes her mother as always being eccentric and superstitious. Her mother has joined a cult that believes in communicating with the dead and household pets. She believes she has telekinesis and clairvoyance and is the reincarnation of an Egyptian queen

611. A 29-year-old man comes to a psychiatrist complaining that he cannot find friends who will accept him "for who he is." In the interview, the patient appears tense and anxious. The psychiatrist encourages the patient to meet persons of both sexes, but the patient ruminates constantly over his sense of inadequacy, fear of rejection, and anxiety in social situations

PERSONALITY DISORDERS

A N S W E R S

598. The answer is C. (Kaplan, 6/e, p 458.) The concept of splitting forms the cornerstone of Kernberg's theory of the borderline personality structure. This primitive level defense is indicative of the dilemma that borderline personalities face in their inability to internalize both positive and negative self and object relations. The borderline personality is therefore incapable of developing a mature relationship, which will, by necessity, involve ambivalent feelings. Intolerable affects generated within a relationship are therefore split off and attached to another object (i.e., person). The genesis of the borderline personality's inability to integrate mixed affect is considered to be secondary to either excessive ego-dystonic aggression or an environment that has not allowed the child to integrate the polarized feelings.

599. The answer is B. (Kaplan, 6/e, pp 1444–1446.) The person with a schizoid personality disorder is incapable of generating and nurturing social relationships and leads a quiet, retiring life with virtually no intimacy with others. Rather than feeling alone and abandoned, this person uses schizoid fantasy as the major ego defense mechanism. Complex and satisfying desires are fulfilled through these fantasies, thereby limiting the need for interpersonal contact and heightening the person's social isolation. The schizoid personality is often intelligent and involved in creative, but solitary professional pursuits. Provided the therapist is patient, the schizoid person can benefit greatly from individual and group therapy.

600. The answer is E. (Kaplan, 6/e, p 467.) Kohut's "self-psychology" model of the mind focuses on the role of external experiences in creating self-cohesion and self-esteem. The theory focuses on infantile needs and how they have (or have not) been met. The goal of therapy in this approach is to build psychic structure and repair defects in the patient's sense of self. According to this theory, narcissism occurs as a consequence of the parents' failure to provide appropriate idealization of the child.

601. The answer is C. (Kaplan, 6/e, pp 1441–1444.) The transmission of antisocial personality appears to have both genetic and environmental components. Antisocial personality disorder is three times more common among males. Female siblings have a much higher incidence of histrionic personality disorder. Conversion disorder and substance abuse also cluster in these family cohorts.

602. The answer is A. (Kaplan, 6/e, pp 1434–1436.) Psychotherapy can be particularly challenging with paranoid personalities. Since these patients, by definition, have difficulty with intimacy and trust, it is difficult to establish a productive therapeutic alliance. Interpretations should be used sparingly, and it is preferable for the therapist to allow the patient to volunteer areas for discussion. The therapist should maintain a polite and professional manner and explain clearly any deviation from routine. The patient should not be made to feel humiliated at any time. The paranoid person will be frightened if the therapist is perceived as weak or disorganized. The efficacy of neuroleptics in this disorder is currently unproven.

603. The answer is A (1, 2, 3). (Kaplan, 6/e, p 1438–1441.) The diagnostic criteria for borderline personality disorder have always been an area of controversy. The most recent criteria outlined in the *DSM IV* have excluded the presence of micropsychosis. These criteria remain descriptive and have not attempted to define or identify any core pathologic process. They include intense and unstable interpersonal relationships, repetitive self-destructive behavior, chronic fear of abandonment, chronic dysphoric affect, cognitive distortions, impulsivity, and poor social adaptation.

604. The answer is B (1, 3). (Kaplan, 6/e, pp 665–666.) The basic deficit in the personality disorders is the persistent use of lower level ego defenses and an inability to be flexible in response to stress. The discomfort of the personality disordered person is played out in the context of interpersonal relationships, i.e., externalized. This defensive style makes it difficult for these persons to develop stable relationships and leaves them feeling helpless, dysphoric, and overwhelmed. It also results in a tendency to alienate and aggravate others. This maladaptive coping style therefore results in a cycle of unproductive and painful relationships that further compound the person's distress.

605. The answer is A (1, 2, 3). (Kaplan, 6/e, pp 1458–1459.) Persons with a passive-aggressive personality disorder have usually had punitive and insensitive parents. As children they have had to learn to retroflex aggressive impulses for fear of angering their parents and thereby place their relationships in jeopardy. This results in the indirect communication of negative affect, i.e., passive-aggressive behavior. They procrastinate any confrontation and become sullen and withdrawn when criticized. The passive-aggressive person is likely to experience a conflictual transference in psychotherapy and sabotage attempts to work through painful issues. This makes it difficult to sustain a productive therapeutic relationship.

606. The answer is C (2 and 4). (Kaplan, 6/e, pp 1285–1286.) Dissociative fugue is characterized by a sudden dramatic loss of autobiographical memory and personal identity.

The victims usually wander far from home and assume new identities and occupations. The disorder occurs almost exclusively in men and has its onset in the context of intense emotional distress. The disorder may be of varying duration and tends to remit spontaneously. Subjects can usually recall their previous memories while under hypnosis.

607. **The answer is C (2, 4).** (Kaplan, 6/e, pp 1446–1448.) The client-centered therapy developed by Carl Rogers demands that the therapist is genuine in response to the patient, has an unconditional regard for the patient, and is sensitive to the patient's subjective experience of the world. The method does not insist that the therapist reveal every passing thought but does require the therapist to divulge any persistent responses to the patient's behavior.

608–611. **The answers are 608-D, 609-B, 610-A, 611-E.** (Kaplan, 6/e, pp 1425–1461.) The symptoms of personality disorders usually become apparent by adolescence, are prominent features of the person's life-style, and interfere with work and relationships. The paranoid personality is characterized by extreme, unrealistic distrust and suspiciousness; exaggerated social hypersensitivity; and cold, restricted, humorless affect. The schizoid personality displays an absence of tender feelings and an indifference to the opinions or feelings of others. This person displays coldness, aloofness, and social isolation. The avoidant personality seeks intimacy but is overwhelmed by the anxiety that social contact elicits. Heightened rejection sensitivity and low self-esteem further compound the difficulty in forming relationships. The schizotypal personality exhibits odd or eccentric behavior, magical thinking, social anxiety, and few friends. Although a florid thought disorder is absent, the schizotypal personality may display ideas of reference or paranoid ideation.

SUBSTANCE ABUSE

Directions: Each item below contains five suggested responses. Select the **one best** response to each item.

612. Withdrawal symptoms from heroin

(A) occur within 4 h of the last dose
(B) reach their peak at 24 h
(C) may induce generalized convulsions
(D) may last several weeks
(E) can be alleviated by naloxone

613. The lifetime prevalence of alcoholism in the United States is approximately

(A) 2 percent
(B) 7 percent
(C) 13 percent
(D) 21 percent
(E) 32 percent

614. Alcohol-induced persistent amnestic disorder

(A) is a retrograde memory disorder
(B) is associated with folate deficiency
(C) resolves in about one-quarter of patients
(D) usually occurs following a closed head injury
(E) is more likely to occur in patients with decreased transketolase activity

615. The probability that the son of an alcoholic father will himself develop alcoholism is

(A) 5 percent
(B) 10 percent
(C) 20 percent
(D) 30 percent
(E) 50 percent

616. Alcoholics Anonymous is characterized
by each of the following statements
EXCEPT

(A) members cannot receive psycho-
active drugs
(B) the twelve-step program is an
essential component of recovery
(C) anonymity of members is preserved
(D) spirituality is a central theme in
recovery
(E) many members are from the middle and upper social classes

Directions: Each item below contains four suggested responses of which **one or more** is correct. Select:

A	if	**1, 2, and 3**	are correct
B	if	**1 and 3**	are correct
C	if	**2 and 4**	are correct
D	if	**4**	is correct
E	if	**1, 2, 3, and 4**	are correct

617. Disorders associated with an increased incidence of alcoholism include

(1) panic disorder
(2) major depressive disorder
(3) phobic disorders
(4) schizophrenia

618. True statements regarding disulfiram include that it

(1) binds irreversibly to aldehyde dehydrogenase
(2) may precipitate psychosis
(3) may be fatal in combination with alcohol
(4) may enhance the intoxication produced by alcohol

619. After prescribing disulfiram to an alcoholic man, you advise him

(1) the drug will take 2 days before it is effective
(2) reactions with alcohol may occur as long as 2 weeks after stopping the drug
(3) he may safely use rubbing alcohol topically
(4) reactions usually last a few hours

620. Clinical signs of cocaine toxicity include

(1) myocarditis
(2) formication
(3) respiratory depression
(4) visual hallucinations

621. The cocaine withdrawal syndrome is characterized by

(1) hypersexuality
(2) anorexia
(3) motor tics
(4) hypersomnia

622. Chronic cannabis abuse may result in

(1) decreased fertility in females
(2) panic attacks
(3) glaucoma
(4) bronchial carcinoma

623. Clinical features of phencyclidine (PCP) intoxication include

(1) seizures
(2) stereotypic movements
(3) muscle rigidity
(4) myoclonic jerks

624. A patient is brought to the emergency room after ingesting a large overdose of phencyclidine (PCP) 30 min earlier. Appropriate treatment interventions at this time include

(1) diazepam
(2) gastric suction
(3) isolation
(4) haloperidol

SUMMARY OF DIRECTIONS

A	B	C	D	E
1,2,3	1,3	2,4	4	All are
only	only	only	only	correct

625. Contraindications to nicotine gum include

(1) seizure disorder
(2) recent myocardial infarction
(3) peptic ulceration
(4) lactation

626. Disorders with a higher prevalence in alcoholic patients include

(1) major depression
(2) dysthymia
(3) panic disorder
(4) obsessive-compulsive disorder

627. Intrauterine cocaine exposure is associated with an increased risk of

(1) microcephaly
(2) premature birth
(3) retarded fetal growth
(4) developmental reading disability

628. True statements regarding elderly alcoholics include

(1) they often begin drinking heavily late in life
(2) they are often not recognized
(3) they are frequently suffering from a major depressive disorder
(4) they are more likely to have a family history of alcoholism than are younger alcoholics

SUBSTANCE ABUSE

A N S W E R S

612. The answer is D. (Kaplan, 6/e, p 850.) The acute phase of withdrawal from short-acting opiates usually begins 8 to 12 h after cessation of the drug and consists of craving, dysphoria, lacrimation, yawning, diaphoresis, rhinorrhea, piloerection, muscle aches, hot and cold flushes, and palpitations. This period is followed in severe cases of withdrawal by vomiting, diarrhea, low-grade fever, hypertension, and tachypnea. This initial phase of withdrawal usually lasts 7 to 10 days and is followed by a protracted period of withdrawal including insomnia, dysphoria, and generalized malaise. This final stage of withdrawal may last several weeks and contribute to relapse. The longer-acting opiates such as methadone may produce an even more prolonged period of withdrawal symptoms.

613. The answer is C. (Kaplan, 6/e, p 769.) The Epidemiological Catchment Area (ECA) study found the lifetime prevalence of alcoholism to be approximately 13 percent. The prevalence is higher in males but is rapidly increasing in females. The age of onset appears to be decreasing. The incidence is highest among 25 to 44 year olds and lowest among persons over 65.

614. The answer is C. (Kaplan, 6/e, p 785.) *Alcohol-induced persistent amnestic disorder* is the *DSM-IV* term for the amnestic disorder presumed to be associated with an acute thiamine deficiency in an alcohol-abusing patient. The acute phase of the disorder (also referred to as *Wernicke's encephalopathy*) is characterized by ataxia, ophthalmoplegia, and confusion. A dense, anterograde amnesia follows an episode of Wernicke's encephalopathy in approximately 70 percent of patients. About 25 percent of patients with a Korsakoff's amnesia will fully recover their memory, 50 percent will exhibit partial recovery, and the remaining 25 percent will exhibit a persistent, dense amnesia. Patients with a genetically determined deficiency in transketolase appear at increased risk of developing a Korsakoff's syndrome.

615. The answer is D. (Kaplan, 6/e, p 781.) The prevalence of alcoholism among the sons of alcoholic fathers is approximately 35 percent; the prevalence among grandsons of an alcoholic 12 percent. The genetic loading for alcoholism is highest in type 2 alcoholics. The concordance between monozygotic twins is estimated at 70 percent; between dizygotic twins 33 percent. The risk of recurrent alcohol abuse is 7 percent in the general population and appears to be rising.

616. The answer is A. (APA, Treatments, pp 1151–1162.) The membership of Alcoholics Anonymous is heterogeneous. Many members are middle class, employed, and married. The percentage of female members has increased to approximately 34 percent in recent years. The majority of initial contacts with AA are made during a period of crisis; these "newcomers" are allocated a more experienced member, or "sponsor," who is available to support the person's sobriety and provide advice. Although this "one to one" approach is important, the major philosophy of the AA program is a self-help process outlined by the "twelve steps." Spirituality is a cornerstone of this twelve-step recovery process, which is designed to provide the way to a "spiritual awakening."

617. The answer is A (1, 2, 3). (Kaplan, 6/e, pp 330–331.) Anxiety disorders, panic disorders, and phobias in particular are associated with alcoholism. While the lifetime prevalences of panic disorder and phobic disorders are 1 to 2 percent and 8 to 23 percent in the general population, respectively, their lifetime prevalences are more than doubled in alcoholics. Unipolar affective disorder, but not bipolar affective disorder, is also more common among alcoholics. The influence of comorbidity upon treatment outcome and sobriety has not yet been fully evaluated. The incidence of antisocial personality has been estimated as high as 79 percent in alcoholics as opposed to approximately 1 percent in the community.

618. The answer is E (all). (Kaplan, 6/e, pp 2124–2125.) Most studies have demonstrated the efficacy of disulfiram in reducing alcoholic relapse. This data is difficult to evaluate since studies have obviously been limited by their ability to select only those patients who would agree to take the drug. Disulfiram binds irreversibly to aldehyde dehydrogenase and may inhibit the activity of this enzyme for as long as 2 weeks. The drug also inhibits dopamine-dehydroxylase and may therefore precipitate a psychotic reaction in susceptible persons. Other side effects include autoimmune hepatitis, peripheral neuropathy, and cardiac conduction abnormalities. Disulfiram may enhance the intoxicating effects of small quantities of alcohol.

619. The answer is C (2, 4). (Kaplan, 6/e, p 2124.) The adverse reaction after alcohol ingestion is caused by a five- to tenfold increase in serum acetaldehyde. This produces facial flushing, headache, nausea, vomiting, palpitations, syncope, and blurred vision. Life-threatening reactions include respiratory depression, seizures, cardiac arrhythmias, and congestive heart failure. Reactions may occur as long as 2 weeks after discontinuing disulfiram and may occur following the topical application of alcohol.

620. The answer is C (2, 4). (Kaplan, 6/e, pp 821–822.) Cocaine blocks the presynaptic uptake of dopamine and norepinephrine. These changes result in euphoria and the sympathetic surge that cocaine users experience. Intoxication may produce a psychosis, cardiac arrhythmias, hypertension, hyperthermia, coronary artery spasm, seizures, and cerebrovascular accidents. Treatment of these symptoms is supportive.

621. The answer is C (2, 4). (Kaplan, 6/e, pp 822–823.) The cocaine withdrawal syndrome can be divided into three stages. Stage 1 (0 to 4 days) consists initially of agitation, depression, anorexia, and high cocaine craving. This initial period is followed by fatigue, hypersomnia or normal sleep, hyperphagia, and decreased craving. Stage 2 is initially characterized by normalized sleep, energy, and appetite but is usually followed by periods of anergy, dysphoria, and increased craving precipitated by cues associated with cocaine use. Stage 3 is a period of extended vulnerability to relapse.

622. The answer is C (2, 4). (Kaplan, 6/e, pp 815–816.) The most widely recognized consequences of cannabis abuse are euphoria, hyperphagia, altered perceptions, and apathy. In susceptible persons the drug may precipitate a panic attack, organic delusional attack, or exacerbation of comorbid schizophrenia. Chronic use in males results in smaller testicles and azoospermia. The suppression of prolactin in females actually increases fertility, although use of the drug during pregnancy inhibits fetal growth and maturation. Cannabis has powerful antiemetic effects and reduces intraocular pressure. An increased incidence of chronic obstructive airway disease and bronchial carcinoma has been reported in chronic abusers. The drug has actions on the immune system resulting in decreased humoral and cell immunity.

623. The answer is B (1, 3). (Kaplan, 6/e, pp 869–871.) Phencyclidine (PCP or "angel dust") produces alterations in neurotransmitters at multiple sites, including the hippocampus, cortex, striatum, and amygdala. Acute intoxication may present in a number of ways: catatonia, acute psychosis, or delirium. Patients will exhibit hypertension, nystagmus, seizures, diminished pain response, ataxia, and muscle rigidity. Treatment is symptomatic; benzodiazepines may reduce agitation.

624. The answer is A (1, 2, 3). (Kaplan, 6/e, pp 869–871.) Phencyclidine has been used by as many as 8 million Americans. In low doses the drug produces an intoxication similar to that of alcohol. However, in larger doses the drug has a number of potentially hazardous effects, some of which may be fatal. Clinical features include ataxia, hyperreflexia, seizures, hypertensive crisis, muscular rigidity, nystagmus, coma, and eventually death. Treatment is essentially supportive. Stimulation should be reduced as much as possible. Since the drug is extensively bound to acidic gastric contents, a gastric lavage will considerably reduce eventual absorption. Acidification of urine plus diuretics will increase urinary excretion. Diazepam is useful in reducing agitation and muscular rigidity and decreasing the chance of seizures.

625. The answer is C (2, 4). (Kaplan, 6/e, p 801.) Nicotine gum has proved to be a useful aid to smoking cessation. However, patients should have instruction in the correct method of using and chewing the gum if they are to be successful. The gum should not be used while the patient is still smoking. Contraindications to nicotine gum include recent myocardial infarction, unstable angina, severe arrhythmias, pregnancy, and lactation.

626. The answer is E (all). (Kaplan, 6/e, pp 669–670.) The ECA study (which included a survey of 20,000 community dwellers) reported that those who met criteria for alcohol abuse and dependence had a significantly higher prevalence of virtually all other psychiatric disorders. Among male alcohol abusers, the most common comorbid psychiatric disorders were antisocial personality disorder (22 percent), phobic disorders (19 percent), major depression (14 percent), and dysthymia (5.1 percent). Among female substance abusers, the most fequent comorbid disorders were phobic disorders (28 percent), major depressive disorder (28 percent), dysthymia (12 percent), and antisocial personality disorder (10 percent).

627. The answer is A (1, 2, 3). (Kaplan, 6/e, p 830.) The neonatal cocaine exposure syndrome occurs in only a minority of infants exposed to the drug in utero. Clinical features consist of poor feeding, irritability, and poor sleeping patterns. These normally occur on the second day of life and last approximately 1 week. Although further study is necessary, intrauterine cocaine exposure does not appear to be associated with long-term neurologic effects. Teratogenic effects of cocaine include microcephaly, urinary tract abnormalities, and intracerebral hemorrhage. Premature birth, placenta previa, and abruptio placentae are common among mothers who abuse cocaine.

628. The answer is A (1, 2, 3). (Kaplan, 6/e, pp 2581–2587.) Substance abuse is a common but often unrecognized problem in the elderly. As many as 60 percent of elderly patients admitted to some general hospitals may have evidence of alcoholism. Compared with younger alcoholics, older alcoholics are less likely to have a family history of alcoholism. As many as 25 percent of elderly alcoholics have a major depressive disorder and many begin drinking later in life after a significant personal loss.

THOUGHT DISORDERS

Directions: Each item below contains five suggested responses. Select the **one best** response to each item.

629. A delusional disorder with delusions of infidelity usually

(A) has its onset in early adulthood
(B) has an insidious onset
(C) resolves within 6 months
(D) is not associated with severe impairment in functioning
(E) occurs in the context of a cognitive deficit

630. All the following medications have been implicated in causing neuroleptic malignant syndrome EXCEPT

(A) clozapine
(B) amantadine
(C) L-dopa
(D) haloperidol
(E) buspirone

631. All the following factors indicate poor prognosis in schizophrenia EXCEPT

(A) poor premorbid work record
(B) low IQ
(C) early age of onset of psychosis
(D) paranoid type
(E) single marital status

632. An elderly man with no previous psychiatric history suddenly begins to ruminate continuously about his love for a woman he has never actually met. Which of the following syndromes does this describe?

(A) Capgras
(B) de Clerambeault
(C) Ganser
(D) Othello
(E) Balint

633. Risk factors for tardive dyskinesia include each of the following EXCEPT

(A) the presence of a mood disorder
(B) increasing age
(C) female sex
(D) "negative symptom" schizophrenia
(E) neuroleptic treatment of several years' duration

634. Clozapine-induced agranulocytosis is accurately described by the statement that it

(A) seldom occurs within 4 weeks of starting treatment
(B) occurs in approximately 5 percent of patients
(C) is seldom life-threatening
(D) is not an indication for discontinuing the drug
(E) is usually self-limiting

635. Which of the following descriptions of cocaine-induced psychosis is accurate?

(A) It almost always occurs in association with a delirium
(B) It is usually associated with a loss of insight
(C) It is predictably correlated with the amount of cocaine consumed
(D) It often includes delusional parasitosis
(E) It is unlikely to recur with repeated cocaine use even in susceptible individuals

636. Alcoholic hallucinosis is correctly described by which of the following statements?

(A) It occurs during alcoholic binges
(B) It may persist for several weeks
(C) It only involves visual hallucinations
(D) It occurs in the context of an attentional deficit
(E) It is more common in patients with a family history of schizophrenia

637. Which of the following statements regarding suicide in schizophrenia is true?

(A) It occurs in 10 percent of patients
(B) It is more common in females
(C) It is usually in response to command auditory hallucinations
(D) It seldom occurs in the period following discharge from the hospital
(E) It usually occurs after decades of illness

Directions: Each item below contains four suggested responses of which **one or more** is correct. Select:

A	if	**1, 2, and 3**	are correct
B	if	**1 and 3**	are correct
C	if	**2 and 4**	are correct
D	if	**4**	is correct
E	if	**1, 2, 3, and 4**	are correct

638. Prodromal symptoms of schizophrenia include

(1) decreased personal hygiene
(2) magical thinking
(3) inappropriate affect
(4) somatic delusions

639. The novel antipsychotic risperidone

(1) is a powerful serotonin antagonist
(2) has significant anticholinergic effects
(3) may produce marked orthostatic hypotension
(4) is a selective D_1 antagonist

640. A patient with catatonia may exhibit

(1) echopraxia
(2) waxy flexibility
(3) unprovoked outbursts
(4) improvement with lorazepam

641. Acute dystonic reactions are characterized by which of the following statements?

(1) They usually occur soon after starting a neuroleptic
(2) They predict the development of tardive dyskinesia
(3) They most often affect facial muscles in the elderly
(4) They rapidly respond to benzodiazepines

642. Brief psychotic disorder is correctly characterized by which of the following statements?

(1) It lasts less than 1 month
(2) It usually occurs in young adults
(3) It is likely to respond to neuroleptics
(4) It may include catatonic behavior

643. A 30-year-old woman with schizophreniform disorder

(1) is likely to respond to neuroleptics
(2) has a 50 percent probability of eventually developing schizophrenia
(3) is at increased risk for suicide
(4) is likely to return to her premorbid baseline within 4 weeks of the onset of the disorder

644. Postpartum psychosis may be characterized by which of the following descriptions?

(1) It occurs in about 0.1 percent of pregnancies
(2) It usually develops within 1 day of delivery
(3) It recurs in approximately one-third of women who have experienced an episode
(4) It usually lasts about 4 days

SUMMARY OF DIRECTIONS

A	B	C	D	E
1,2,3	1,3	2,4	4	All are
only	only	only	only	correct

645. First-rank Schneiderian symptoms of schizophrenia include

(1) thought insertion
(2) abulia
(3) auditory hallucinations
(4) ambivalence

646. The person with schizotypal personality

(1) is often paranoid
(2) more often develops schizophrenia than does the general public
(3) often uses metaphorical language
(4) usually requires maintenance neuroleptic medication

647. Ego defenses employed by the patient with an acute schizophreniform psychosis include

(1) isolation of affect
(2) denial
(3) suppression
(4) schizoid fantasy

648. The ophthalmic side effects of neuroleptics

(1) are most common with high-potency agents
(2) are promoted by exposure to sunlight
(3) include retinal degeneration
(4) are related to the total lifetime dose received

649. Compared with a male, a female suffering from schizophrenia has

(1) a later age of onset
(2) more negative symptoms
(3) more affective symptoms
(4) a poorer response to neuroleptics

650. True statements regarding delusional disorder include that it

(1) is more common in females
(2) usually has its onset in middle age
(3) is more common in lower social classes
(4) is more common among immigrants

651. A 70-year-old patient complains of the recent onset of formed visual hallucinations. This suggests

(1) the development of paraphrenia
(2) an occipital lobe cerebrovascular accident
(3) a complex partial seizure disorder
(4) probable deficits in vision

THOUGHT DISORDERS

629. The answer is D. (Kaplan, 6/e, p 1044.) The onset of delusional disorders is typically in mid to late adulthood. They do not usually result in any severe impairment in personality or functional capacity. The delusional disorders tend to be chronic and the patient is likely to develop a progressive, insidious preoccupation with the focus of the delusions. The majority of cases have an acute onset and approximately half become a chronic disorder. An acute onset of delusions is more likely to be associated with spontaneous remission. Although delusional disorders may occasionally occur in the context of a neurodegenerative disorder or stroke, they are not typically associated with any cognitive deficits. The delusional disorders are extremely difficult to treat but may respond to high-potency neuroleptics.

630. The answer is E. (Kaplan, 6/e, p 1913.) Neuroleptic malignant syndrome (NMS) has been reported with agents other than the neuroleptics. In particular, agents with dopaminergic activity (e.g., L-dopa, bromocriptine, and amantadine) have been implicated as etiologic agents. The relatively selective D_2 blocker clozapine has been associated with several cases of NMS. Characteristic features of NMS include rigidity, fever, autonomic instability, elevated creatinine phosphokinase, leukocytosis, and rhabdomyolysis.

631. The answer is D. (Kaplan, 6/e, pp 899–903.) Approximately 40 to 60 percent of patients with schizophrenia are chronically impaired by their illness. Good prognostic indicators include late age of onset, obvious precipitating factors, positive symptoms, affective symptoms, and acute onset. The absence of an appropriate social support system and the presence of predominantly negative symptoms (e.g., poverty of affect or poor motivation and organizational skills) are negative prognostic factors.

632. The answer is B. (Kaplan, 6/e, pp 169, 183.) The case describes erotomania (*psychose passionelle*, or de Clerambeault syndrome), a disorder in which the person has a delusional belief that he or she is having a love affair with someone. This may occur in the context of a delusional, mood, or organic disorder. The Othello syndrome describes a conjugal paranoia in which the subject falsely believes his or her spouse to be guilty of infidelity. Capgras syndrome (reduplicative paramnesia) describes the delusion that familiar figures are actually impostors who have assumed the identity of people known to the subject. Balint's syndrome describes a defect in visual scanning secondary to an occipital or parieto-occipital lesion.

633. The answer is D. (Kaplan, 6/e, pp 2005–2006.) Tardive dyskinesia usually develops after several years of neuroleptic treatment; however, some patients may develop the disorder in a considerably shorter period. The incidence of tardive dyskinesia is approximately 4 to 5 percent per year for the first 5 years, but this is higher in older patients. The presence of a mood disorder clearly increases the risk of developing tardive dyskinesia, and patients with schizoaffective disorders are therefore at particular risk. The symptoms of tardive dyskinesia often first appear following a reduction in neuroleptic dosage, but as many as 30 percent of patients will eventually remit off neuroleptics.

634. The answer is A. (Kaplan, 6/e, pp 996–997.) The incidence of clozapine-induced agranulocytosis is approximately 1 percent. The side effect seldom occurs during the first 4 weeks of treatment, and this allows a relatively safe window in which to determine the efficacy of the drug in a particular patient. The agranulocytosis is not self-limiting and carries a mortality of 40 percent if a superadded infection supervenes. Once clozapine is discontinued, the granulocyte count should return to normal levels in 2 to 4 weeks.

635. The answer is D. (Kaplan, 6/e, p 822.) Although many cocaine users will experience some degree of paranoia, a subgroup will also experience a more persistent psychosis characterized by suspiciousness, paranoia, visual and tactile hallucinations, and loss of insight. Patients frequently complain of parasitosis or formication. The emergence of a cocaine-induced psychosis is not necessarily directly related to the amount of cocaine consumed and some individuals may develop the disorder at relatively low doses. Cocaine-induced psychosis is likely to recur upon repeated use in susceptible individuals. It may occur with or without an alteration in attention.

636. The answer is B. (Kaplan, 6/e, p 1053.) Alcoholic hallucinosis occurs in alcohol-dependent persons within 48 h of abstinence. The hallucinations may involve any sensory modality and, unlike delirium tremens, occur in the context of a clear sensorium. The hallucinations usually remit within a few days but may persist for several months after abstinence. The patient is seldom delusional and does not meet criteria for a schizophreniform psychosis. Neuroleptics are often necessary to control symptoms.

637. The answer is A. (Kaplan, 6/e, p 984.) Suicide in the person with schizophrenia usually occurs in the context of depressive symptoms rather than as a response to command auditory hallucinations. In half the cases, the patient has been discharged from the hospital within the last few weeks and has been ill for a few years. Single males are at highest risk.

638. The answer is A (1, 2, 3). (Kaplan, 6/e, pp 899–900.) Recognized prodromal symptoms of schizophrenia include social withdrawal; impairment in social performance; blunted or inappropriate affect; vague and overelaborate speech; odd beliefs and magical thinking; unusual perceptual experiences; lack of initiative; and peculiar behavior.

639. The answer is B (1, 3). (Kaplan, 6/e, p 835.) Risperidone is a derivative of benzisoxazoles that is unlike any other antipsychotic medication. The drug is a potent 5- HT_2 and D_2 receptor antagonist but is less likely than haldol to produce catalepsy. Risperidone is also less likely to produce extrapyramidal side effects than haloperidol. The greatest improvement in positive and negative symptoms in schizophrenics is seen at doses of risperidone of 4 to 8 mg. The potent α_1 blockade accounts for the drug's association with significant orthostatic hypotension. It is only minimally sedating and has no anticholinergic side effects.

640. The answer is E (all). (Kaplan, 6/e, p 751.) The neurophysiologic and phenomenological underpinnings of catatonia remain unclear. Catatonia has classically been divided into three subgroups: stuporous, excited, and periodic. The validity of and rationale for this classification are controversial and provide no clear guidelines for etiology or treatment. Stuporous catatonia is characterized by mutism, social withdrawal, and markedly diminished motor activity. Patients demonstrate echopraxia, echolalia, and stereotypies and seldom initiate any original spontaneous motor behavior. Agitated catatonia is described as a state of extreme psychomotor agitation with increased verbal output. Whether this represents a true schizophreniform psychosis or simply mania remains unclear. Lorazepam has demonstrated efficacy in stuporous catatonia.

641. The answer is A (1, 2, 3). (Kaplan, 6/e, pp 1911–1912.) Acute dystonic reactions usually occur within a few hours of receiving the neuroleptic—50 percent of cases occur within 48 h. Episodes may last anywhere from a few minutes to several hours. Reactions usually involve the facial and neck muscles, although the extremities may occasionally be involved. Blepharospasm and an oculogyric crisis may occur. The incidence of acute dystonic reactions is uncertain and estimates range from 2 to 25 percent. Anticholinergics are the most effective treatment for acute dystonic reactions. Benzodiazepines are often helpful in akathisia.

642. The answer is E (all). (Kaplan, 6/e, pp 1028–1031.) *Brief psychotic disorder* is a new diagnostic category in *DSM IV*. It describes the acute onset of psychotic symptoms that last from 1 day to 1 month. Symptoms may include delusions, hallucinations, posturing, catatonia, disorganized speech, and affective lability. The disorder usually occurs in early adulthood and patients return to their premorbid baseline. Although a number of studies have suggested a familial vulnerability to brief psychotic disorder, its association with primary mood and thought disorders remains unclear. Short-term neuroleptics provide prompt symptomatic relief.

643. The answer is A (1, 2, 3). (Kaplan, 6/e, pp 1025–1027.) Schizophreniform disorder is essentially identical to schizophrenia with the exceptions of short duration (i.e., more than 1 but less than 6 months) and no deterioration in social functioning. Although patients who have experienced a schizophreniform psychosis do better than schizophrenics, they do not do as well as patients who suffer from a mood disorder. A significant number of patients relapse and as many as half will subsequently be reclassified as suffering from schizophrenia. Acute onset and brief duration of index episode as well as good premorbid functioning and the absence of affective blunting are considered good prognostic signs. As a group, patients with schizophreniform disorder have a higher mortality and suicide rate than the general population. Since there are no controlled studies of the treatment of schizophreniform disorder, the clinician should attempt to control symptoms with the lowest effective dose of neuroleptics and provide the patient a supportive, nonintrusive, and safe environment until the psychosis has resolved.

644. The answer is B (1, 3). (Kaplan, 6/e, pp 1062–1063.) Postpartum psychosis occurs in about 0.1 percent of mothers. Its onset is usually 3 to 14 days post partum and it typically has a duration of 2 to 3 months. The disorder recurs in about one-third of susceptible mothers and usually with increasing severity. As many as 4 percent of mothers suffering from postpartum psychosis will commit infanticide.

645. The answer is B (1, 3). (Kaplan, 6/e, p 970.) Schneider attempted to identify some symptoms that, in the absence of organic mental disease, he considered to be diagnostic of a process schizophrenia. His "first-rank" symptoms were auditory hallucinations, experiences of influence, experiences of alienation (this will include the experience that "foreign thoughts" are being inserted into one's head), and thought broadcasting. These symptoms are now recognized in association with affective disorders and are therefore no longer considered diagnostic of schizophrenia.

646. The answer is A (1, 2, 3). (Kaplan, 6/e, p 1438.) As many as 10 percent of patients with a diagnosis of schizotypal personality disorder will eventually develop schizophrenia. Overall, the long-term prognosis for the person with a schizotypal personality disorder is better than that of a schizophrenic. Brief periods of paranoid ideation are not unusual, and these personalities often employ magical thinking and consider themselves to have special powers.

647. The answer is C (2, 4). (Kaplan, 6/e, pp 451–452.) The person with a schizophreniform psychosis uses psychotic level defenses that, in simple terms, attempt to distort the external world to comply with that person's experience. Examples of these narcissistic level defenses include denial, distortion, projection, schizoid fantasy, projective identification, and splitting.

648. The answer is C (2, 4). (Kaplan, 6/e, pp 2008–2009.) Several ophthalmologic side effects have been reported with neuroleptics. Retinitis pigmentosa is associated with high maintenance doses of thioridazine and may result in blindness. Whitish-brown granular deposits have been found in the anterior chamber and lens of patients on long-term maintenance chlorpromazine; however, these do not present a hazard to eyesight. These "benign" ocular changes appear to correlate with the development of a bluish-gray skin discoloration and are accelerated by exposure to sunlight.

649. The answer is B (1, 3). (Kaplan, 6/e, p 2394.) Although the incidence of schizophrenia is similar in both sexes, there are significant differences in symptoms. Females tend to have a later age of onset with more positive symptoms and a somewhat better response to neuroleptics. The concordance rate for schizophrenia is higher between monozygotic females.

650. The answer is E (all). (Kaplan, 6/e, pp 980–981.) The delusional disorders are a heterogeneous group of disorders with varying content. The mean age of onset is 40 years and although the majority of sufferers will be employed and married, there is a higher incidence among the lower social classes. Immigrants who are unable to speak the local language are at particular risk for developing a paranoid delusional system. There appears to be some familial clustering but the precise genetic basis for the condition remains unclear. Long-term follow-up reveals that the disorder remains stable over time and does not develop into a schizophreniform psychosis or mood disorder.

651. The answer is D (4). (Kaplan, 6/e, p 655.) The most common cause of formed visual hallucinations in the elderly is declining vision. This was first described in the eighteenth century by Charles Bonnet and the syndrome bears his name. Neuroleptics have not proved effective and patients usually respond to reassurance and correction, if possible, of visual deficits.

NEUROLOGY QUESTIONS FOR PSYCHIATRISTS

Directions: Each item below contains five suggested responses. Select the **one best** response to each item.

652. All the following would be considered part of normal aging in an 80-year-old man EXCEPT

(A) loss of vibration sense in the legs
(B) short, uncertain steps
(C) decreased stage 4 sleep
(D) decreased vocabulary
(E) loss of large cortical neurons

653. A 55-year-old man presents for evaluation of his behavioral change. His family describe his recently increasing belligerence, inappropriate social behavior, sexual promiscuity, and foul language. Examination reveals an intact memory and visuospatial functions, word-finding difficulties, and frontal lobe deficits. The most likely diagnosis is

(A) Alzheimer's disease
(B) neurosyphilis
(C) Pick's disease
(D) AIDS dementia complex (ADC)
(E) multi-infarct dementia

654. Following the resection of an anterior communicating artery aneurysm, a patient may exhibit each of the following EXCEPT

(A) amnesia
(B) personality change
(C) akinetic mutism
(D) expressive aphasia
(E) urinary incontinence

655. Each of the following is a true statement of AIDS dementia complex (ADC) EXCEPT

(A) the syndrome usually has a slow onset
(B) deficits in attention are usually significant
(C) behavioral changes are often prominent
(D) amnesia is usually the earliest clinical sign
(E) psychomotor slowing is usually pronounced

656. A young woman with a history of borderline personality disorder complains of a gradual loss of sensation extending from her shoulders to her hands. Examination reveals loss of pain sensation and position sense but intact touch perception in both hands. Reflexes are absent in both arms and the muscles of her hands are atrophied. The most likely diagnosis is

(A) tabes dorsalis
(B) vitamin B_{12} deficiency
(C) syringomyelia
(D) amyotrophic lateral sclerosis
(E) alcoholic neuropathy

657. Following a cerebrovascular accident, an elderly woman states that she recognizes the voices but not the faces of family members. The probable site of the lesion is

(A) bilateral occipitotemporal
(B) right hippocampal
(C) left hippocampal
(D) biparietal
(E) mediodorsal nucleus of the thalamus

658. If a patient displays complete paralysis of some muscles of an extremity with normal power in adjacent muscles of that extremity, it is most likely that the patient has a

(A) lower motor neuron lesion
(B) upper motor neuron lesion
(C) combined upper and lower motor neuron lesion
(D) motor cortex lesion
(E) myopathy

659. Persons with transient global amnesia

(A) are usually young and female
(B) know who they are
(C) usually have a psychiatric history
(D) are likely to have several episodes
(E) should have a sodium amytal interview

660. Each of the following is a true statement of narcolepsy EXCEPT

(A) clinical onset is usually during early adulthood
(B) the disorder is associated with HLA-DR2 antigen
(C) the disorder is characterized by an increased REM sleep latency
(D) tricyclic antidepressants have therapeutic benefits in narcolepsy
(E) the male:female incidence is equal

661. If an examiner shines a light in one eye of a normal person, which of the following pupillary responses occurs?

(A) Both pupils constrict equally
(B) The ipsilateral pupil constricts more than the contralateral one
(C) The contralateral pupil constricts more than the ipsilateral one
(D) Only the ipsilateral pupil constricts
(E) Only the contralateral pupil constricts

662. A 40-year-old man is able to stand upright with his feet close together. When asked to close his eyes, however, he begins to sway. Appropriate laboratory investigations include each of the following EXCEPT

(A) complete blood count
(B) VDRL test
(C) serum lead levels
(D) serum vitamin B_{12} level
(E) serum folate level

663. One month following a cerebrovascular accident, a 50-year-old man is asked to complete the letter cancellation test. His performance is shown below. The probable site of the cerebrovascular accident is the

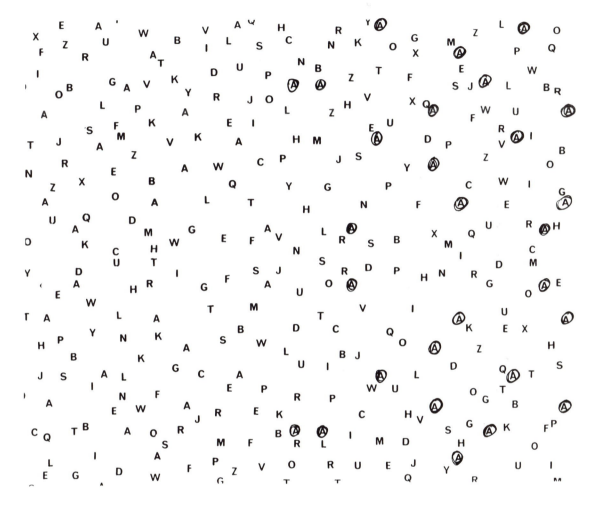

(A) frontal lobes
(B) left temporal lobe
(C) right parietal lobe
(D) right occipital lobe
(E) left occipitotemporal area

664. An elderly man was asked to reproduce the sample drawing. His performance suggests

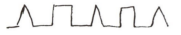

SAMPLE DRAWING

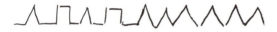

(A) Parkinson's disease
(B) a right parietal lobe lesion
(C) a right temporal lobe lesion
(D) occipital lobe lesions
(E) frontal lobe lesions

665. The combination of acalculia, right-left disorientation, finger agnosia, and agraphia without alexia suggests a lesion of the

(A) right posterior parasylvian region
(B) left medial temporal area
(C) left angular gyrus
(D) left calcarine cortex
(E) left prefrontal cortex

666. Complete interruption of the right optic tract produces

(A) bitemporal hemianopia
(B) right homonymous hemianopia
(C) left homonymous hemianopia
(D) right quadrantanopia
(E) left quadrantanopia

667. The most consistent and reliable sign of cerebellar dysfunction is

(A) unsteadiness of gait
(B) excessive swaying with the eyes closed
(C) nystagmus
(D) weakness
(E) tremor

668. Upon routine admission screening, a 70-year-old demented man is found to have a positive VDRL (Venereal Disease Research Laboratory) test. The most appropriate next step would be to

(A) treat the patient for neurosyphilis
(B) isolate the patient
(C) inform his wife that she, too, probably has syphilis and should be tested
(D) obtain CSF for another VDRL test
(E) obtain a fluorescent treponemal antibody absorption (FTA-ABS) test

669. A 35-year-old male executive presents with a complaint of irregular incapacitating headaches, which may last several weeks. He describes them as a steady pressure extending from his neck to the top of his head and says they are often associated with light-headedness. The pain, which is relieved by alcohol, is present in the morning and worsens as the day progresses. The most likely diagnosis is

(A) cluster headache
(B) tension headache
(C) classic migraine
(D) raised intracranial pressure
(E) temporal arteritis

670. A 17-year-old girl presents to the emergency room in an acute confusional state. She complains of double vision, difficulty swallowing, weakness of her legs, and abdominal pain. She had been treated with a sulfonamide for a urinary tract infection 3 days prior to admission but complained that her urine still appeared foul. On examination she was apyrexial with evidence for a motor peripheral neuropathy. CSF examination revealed only a mild elevation of protein. The most likely diagnosis is

(A) herpes encephalitis
(B) acute intermittent porphyria
(C) gonococcal meningitis
(D) multiple sclerosis
(E) mercury poisoning

671. A 70-year-old man is unable to follow simple multistep directions such as to fold a letter, place it in an envelope, and affix a postage stamp. He is, however, capable of performing each of these tasks individually. This is an example of

(A) motor apraxia
(B) an amnestic disorder
(C) ideational apraxia
(D) autopagnosia
(E) simultagnosia

672. True statements regarding diffuse Lewy body disease include that it

(A) usually presents clinically before age 40
(B) is inherited as an autosomal dominant trait
(C) frequently presents with thought disorder
(D) usually presents with prominent memory problems
(E) is associated with previous head trauma

673. A young man presents to your office complaining of rapidly increasing weakness, which began in his feet and is now affecting his legs and arms. He also complains of pain in the back, legs, and arms. Physical examination reveals diminished motor power and areflexia in the legs more than the arms, autonomic instability, and intact sensation. The most likely diagnosis is

(A) motor neuron disease
(B) polio
(C) conversion disorder
(D) Guillain-Barré syndrome
(E) multiple sclerosis

674. To elicit clonus, an examiner does which of the following?

(A) Quickly jerks a part of the body that is at rest
(B) Slowly pulls a part of the body that is at rest
(C) Quickly jerks a part of the body that is under voluntary tension
(D) Slowly pulls part of the body that is under voluntary tension
(E) Forces the body part back and forward

675. In a 20-year-old man with Gilles de la Tourette's syndrome (GTS), abnormal behavior

(A) is likely to improve with social stress
(B) may include echolalia
(C) is often reduced by caffeine
(D) seldom includes complex stereotypic motor behaviors
(E) frequently includes periods of catatonia

676. A patient with normal pressure hydrocephalus

(A) benefits from diuretic treatment
(B) exhibits gait apraxia early in the course of the illness
(C) should not have a lumbar puncture performed
(D) frequently develops papilledema
(E) exhibits significant cortical atrophy on MRI scanning

677. When asked to describe his problem after his stroke, a patient said, "I cannot sum gook sib fib trans anymore." The lesion is likely to be situated in

(A) the left temporoparietal area or arcuate fasciculus
(B) the left anterior temporal lobe
(C) the left prefrontal lobe
(D) the left parahippocampal gyrus
(E) the globus pallidus

678. The cognitive changes associated with Parkinson's disease

(A) primarily involve memory
(B) primarily involve cortical functions
(C) are late manifestations of the disease
(D) usually include deficits in visuospatial functioning
(E) are frequently associated with depression

679. A supranuclear palsy is characterized by each of the following EXCEPT

(A) clonus
(B) marked atrophy
(C) spasticity
(D) hyperreflexia
(E) normal electromyographic tracing

680. Occlusion of the posterior inferior cerebellar artery will cause

(A) ipsilateral paralysis and loss of pain and temperature sensation
(B) contralateral paralysis and ipsilateral cerebellar ataxia
(C) ipsilateral facial nerve palsy and cerebellar ataxia
(D) contralateral loss of pain and temperature sensation and ipsilateral ataxia
(E) pseudobulbar palsy

681. Causes of parkinsonism include each of the following EXCEPT

(A) carbon monoxide poisoning
(B) AIDS
(C) dementia pugilistica
(D) chronic alcoholism
(E) Wilson's disease

682. In persons with normal hearing, tests for efficiency of air and bone conduction of sound (Rinne test) demonstrate that

(A) air conduction is better than bone conduction for all frequencies
(B) bone conduction is better than air conduction for all frequencies
(C) bone and air conduction are equal for high-frequency sounds
(D) air conduction is superior for high-frequency sounds
(E) air conduction is better in children and bone conduction is better in adults

683. The single most important part of the motor examination is

(A) elicitation of the plantar reflexes
(B) inspection for fasciculations
(C) strength testing
(D) palpation
(E) observation of gait

684. A 40-year-old man is seen in the emergency room. He is unable to provide a clear history. On examination he is found to be in a confusional state with ataxia, nystagmus, and ophthalmoplegia. He is afebrile, his pupils are normal and reactive, funduscopy is normal, and he has a large hematoma on his forehead. As the treating physician your first order should be

(A) an immediate spinal tap and CSF evaluation for xanthochromia
(B) thiamine intravenously and intramuscularly
(C) intravenous line with a 10% dextrose infusion
(D) emergency head CT scan without contrast media
(E) emergency head CT scan with contrast media

685. A lesion of the cerebellum may be associated with each of the following EXCEPT

(A) ataxia
(B) dysmetria
(C) hypertonia
(D) titubation
(E) scanning speech

686. A 65-year-old woman, who has been referred for evaluation of dementia, walks into your office. You observe that her trunk is bent forward, her steps are short and shuffling, and her feet hardly clear the ground. Her legs are stiff and bent at the knees and she does not swing her arms. The probable diagnosis is

(A) peripheral neuropathy
(B) spastic diplegia
(C) parkinsonism
(D) astasia-abasia
(E) normal pressure hydrocephalus

687. A benign essential tremor

(A) is limited to the upper limbs
(B) occurs at rest
(C) may have an autosomal dominant inheritance
(D) is aggravated by alcohol
(E) has a frequency of 8 to 12 Hz

688. The most effective method of visualizing the demyelinating plaques of multiple sclerosis is

(A) contrast-enhanced MRI with a long T2 weighted image
(B) contrast-enhanced MRI with a short T1 weighted image
(C) contrast-enhanced MRI with a long T1 weighted image
(D) single proton emission computed tomography
(E) CT with contrast media

689. Lumbar puncture and cerebrospinal fluid examination reveal a normal opening pressure, mild turbidity, 50 lymphocytes per millimeter, protein of 100 mg/mL, and glucose of 50 mg/mL. The most likely diagnosis is

(A) fungal infection
(B) tuberculosis
(C) meningococcal meningitis
(D) viral meningitis
(E) Guillain-Barré syndrome

690. Huntington's disease is correctly described by which of the following statements?

(A) It frequently presents with personality change
(B) It is associated with degeneration of the red nucleus
(C) It is linked to a gene located on the short arm of chromosome 8
(D) It usually manifests in the second decade
(E) It produces cortical atrophy visible on MRI

691. To reinforce the stretch reflex of a hypoactive quadriceps femoris muscle, an examiner requests the patient to

(A) think about an emotionally stimulating event
(B) count slowly to 10
(C) close the eyes
(D) grasp one hand with the other and pull
(E) walk briskly around the room

Directions: Each item below contains four suggested responses of which **one or more** is correct. Select:

A	if	**1, 2, and 3**	are correct
B	if	**1 and 3**	are correct
C	if	**2 and 4**	are correct
D	if	**4**	is correct
E	if	**1, 2, 3, and 4**	are correct

692. Features of Broca's (expressive) aphasia include

(1) sparse, telegraphic speech
(2) absence of prepositions, articles, and conjunctions of speech
(3) dysprosody
(4) associated alexia and visual field defects

693. The Brown-Séquard syndrome is characterized by

(1) enduring loss of sphincter control
(2) contralateral loss of pain and temperature sensation
(3) ipsilateral cerebellar ataxia
(4) ipsilateral loss of position sense

694. Loss of position sense may be caused by lesions of the

(1) peripheral nerves
(2) dorsal roots or columns
(3) medial lemniscus
(4) parietal cortex

695. A tumor confined to the internal auditory canal would be very likely to cause

(1) facial palsy
(2) tinnitus
(3) vestibular dysfunction
(4) diplopia

696. Correct statements about the tremor of Parkinson's disease include which of the following?

(1) It does affect the tongue
(2) It is present during sleep
(3) It is present at rest
(4) It has a frequency of 6 to 8 Hz

697. Correct statements about the optic disc include which of the following?

(1) The palest sector is lateral
(2) The optic disc appears pink
(3) The pigment ring is more conspicuous laterally
(4) The large vessels pierce the disc peripheral to the optic cup

698. Which of the following may produce a leukoencephalopathy?

(1) Diffuse Lewy body disease
(2) Hypoxia
(3) Parkinson's disease
(4) HIV infection

699. The AIDS dementia complex (ADC)

(1) is secondary to opportunistic central nervous system infection
(2) is characterized by psychomotor slowing
(3) occurs in approximately 10 percent of patients with HIV infection
(4) usually has an insidious onset

SUMMARY OF DIRECTIONS

A	B	C	D	E
1,2,3	1,3	2,4	4	All are
only	only	only	only	correct

700. The Klüver-Bucy syndrome is characterized by

(1) hypometamorphosis
(2) amnesia
(3) compulsive rituals
(4) hypersexuality

701. A person with progressive supranuclear palsy

(1) usually has a flexed neck
(2) has difficulty reading
(3) often exhibits dyskinetic movements
(4) often appears anxious

702. A person with herpes simplex encephalitis

(1) usually has an abnormal electroencephalogram
(2) has often had symptoms for several months prior to initial presentation
(3) often exhibits personality change
(4) seldom survives with or without treatment

703. Seizures after head injury

(1) have an incidence of 50 percent after compound skull fractures
(2) usually occur in people with a family history of seizures
(3) are less likely to recur in patients who have their first seizure at the time of trauma rather than months later
(4) seldom generalize

704. A young woman is diagnosed as suffering from multiple sclerosis (MS). True statements about her illness include

(1) approximately one-third of patients with MS have no functional disability after 10 years
(2) cognition is almost always spared in MS
(3) the risk of recurrence is increased by stress
(4) optic neuritis almost always develops into disseminated MS

705. Central nervous system manifestations of Lyme disease include

(1) facial nerve palsy
(2) quadriparesis
(3) cerebellar ataxia
(4) behavioral change

706. Anoxic encephalopathy may result in

(1) an amnestic state
(2) a major depressive disorder
(3) a progressive dementing illness
(4) an acute psychotic episode

707. The neuropathologic changes of Alzheimer's disease

(1) are most commonly localized to the paralimbic areas
(2) do not usually include significant cortical neuronal cell loss
(3) are characterized by the presence of Lewy bodies
(4) usually involve the locus coeruleus

708. Which of the following would normally be found in a patient with a large meningioma of the olfactory groove?

(1) Amotivation
(2) Poor impulse control
(3) Unilateral optic atrophy
(4) Papilledema

709. Occlusion of the superior branch of the right middle cerebral artery may produce

(1) deviation of the eyes to the right
(2) left-sided motor weakness
(3) left-sided sensory deficit
(4) a left homonymous hemianopia

710. A left oculomotor nerve palsy produces

(1) diplopia on straight-ahead gaze
(2) a dilated unreactive left pupil
(3) lateral deviation of the left eye
(4) ptosis of the left eye

711. Features that are helpful in distinguishing multi-infarct dementia from Alzheimer's disease include

(1) age of onset
(2) abnormal reflexes
(3) CSF pleocytosis
(4) stepwise progression

712. Causes of tunnel vision include

(1) glaucoma
(2) migraine
(3) papilledema
(4) hysteria

713. Which of the following may cause absent knee and ankle jerks with an extensor plantar response?

(1) Transection of the cord at the level of T12
(2) Tabes dorsalis
(3) Lead intoxication
(4) Diabetes mellitus

714. Papilledema may be caused by

(1) lead poisoning
(2) hypertensive encephalopathy
(3) optic neuritis
(4) normal pressure hydrocephalus

715. The serum level of phenytoin is raised by the concomitant use of

(1) carbamazepine
(2) fluoxetine
(3) clonazepam
(4) sulfonamides

716. True statements regarding chronic subdural hematomas include

(1) they are normally associated with a normal electroencephalogram
(2) they very seldom cause focal neurologic signs
(3) they seldom cause significant symptoms
(4) they may resorb spontaneously

717. Infection of the nervous system with HIV may result in

(1) an acute onset paraplegia
(2) acute meningoencephalitis within a few days of exposure
(3) a peripheral neuropathy
(4) urinary incontinence

SUMMARY OF DIRECTIONS

A	B	C	D	E
1,2,3 only	1,3 only	2,4 only	4 only	All are correct

718. The cerebrospinal fluid of a patient with multiple sclerosis may demonstrate

(1) moderate mononuclear pleocytosis
(2) oligoclonal IgG bands
(3) an increased IgG index
(4) increased protein

719. Features of the Argyll Robertson pupil include

(1) small, equal pupils
(2) response to mydriatic drugs
(3) failure to constrict on accommodation
(4) failure to react to light

720. Typical features of cluster headaches include

(1) pain that wakes the patient at night
(2) focal neurologic deficits
(3) lacrimation and nasal congestion
(4) relief of the pain with alcohol

721. The afferent tracts and relays for transmitting pain sensation to the cortex include

(1) the posteromedial funiculus
(2) the lateral neospinothalamic tract
(3) the dorsomedial nucleus of the thalamus
(4) the spinoreticulothalamic tract

722. Which of the following would be expected to produce episodic "dyscontrol" or violence?

(1) Left prefrontal cerebrovascular accident
(2) Herpes encephalitis
(3) Raised intracranial pressure
(4) Meningioma of the olfactory groove

723. A 60-year-old man develops wasting of the small muscles of his hand. Before considering a diagnosis of amyotrophic lateral sclerosis, which of the following conditions should be considered as part of the differential diagnosis?

(1) Cervical spondylosis
(2) Multiple sclerosis
(3) Syphilis
(4) Myasthenia gravis

724. A person with vertebrobasilar migraine may present with

(1) temporary blindness
(2) staggering
(3) stupor
(4) quadriplegia

725. Causes of a mononeuritis multiplex include

(1) HIV infection
(2) chronic alcoholism
(3) diabetes mellitus
(4) lead poisoning

726. Nonmetastatic neurologic complications of bronchial carcinoma include

(1) personality change
(2) dementia
(3) psychosis
(4) parkinsonism

727. True statements regarding trigeminal neuralgia include which of the following?

(1) It usually has its onset in early adulthood

(2) It may be a manifestation of motor neuron disease

(3) It is associated with an area of sensory loss appropriate to the branch of the trigeminal nerve involved

(4) It is more common in females

728. A patient with the Dejerine-Roussy syndrome

(1) has a sensory loss

(2) has a thalamic lesion

(3) has unusual pain in the affected area

(4) usually recovers

729. Inappropriate and jocular affect is likely to be produced by a lesion in which of the following sites?

(1) Left prefrontal cortex

(2) Right posterior parietal cortex

(3) Left periventricular area

(4) Right prefrontal cortex

730. A patient has recently been diagnosed as suffering from tardive dyskinesia. Correct statements about the condition include

(1) approximately 40 percent of cases resolve over the first 12 months after discontinuing neuroleptics

(2) symptoms may be improved by increasing the dose of neuroleptic

(3) reserpine may reduce the intensity of symptoms

(4) symptoms will increase with sodium valproate

731. A 60-year-old man has just suffered a transient ischemic attack. He could accurately be told

(1) he has a 20 percent chance of eventually having a major cerebrovascular accident within 5 years

(2) he has a 20 percent chance of having a myocardial infarction within 5 years

(3) he will have no neurologic deficit from the episode

(4) he should have a carotid endarterectomy as soon as possible

732. Clinical features that suggest a subcortical rather than a cortical dementia include

(1) early onset of apraxia

(2) bradyphrenia

(3) language disturbance

(4) movement disorder

Directions: Each group of questions below consists of lettered options followed by a set of numbered items. For each numbered item select the **one** lettered option with which it is **most** closely associated. Each lettered option may be used **once, more than once, or not at all.**

Items 733–735

For each of the following clinical syndromes, select the artery that is occluded.

   (A) Anterior cerebral artery
   (B) Middle cerebral artery
   (C) Posterior cerebral artery
   (D) Carotid artery
   (E) Vertebrobasilar artery

733. Contralateral sensory loss, contralateral homonymous hemianopia, and alexia without agraphia

734. Urinary incontinence, paratonia, transcortical aphasia, and abulia

735. Contralateral hemiparesis, hemisensory loss, homonymous hemianopia, and aphasia syndromes

Items 736–740

For each of the neuropathologic findings listed below, choose the movement disorder with which it is most closely associated.

   (A) Hemiballismus
   (B) Chorea
   (C) Parkinson's disease
   (D) Wide-based gait
   (E) Akinetic mutism

736. Bilateral hemorrhage into the cingulate gyri

737. Lewy bodies

738. Degeneration of the caudate nuclei

739. Infarction of the subthalamic nucleus

740. Evidence of previous meningitis

Items 741–745

Match each clinical presentation of a seizure disorder with the likely cause.

(A) Hippocampal sclerosis
(B) Orbitofrontal lesion
(C) Left temporal glioma in Heschl's gyrus
(D) Occipital lobe infarct
(E) Lesion in the right supplementary motor area

741. A 40-year-old woman turns her eyes to the right. Initially the fingers of her left hand start to twitch, followed by her face, leg, and then her whole body. She then loses consciousness and is incontinent of urine

742. A 25-year-old man complains of a foul odor, epigastric discomfort, and dysphoria. He then exhibits a motionless stare for 1 min. He later denies any knowledge of this event

743. A 50-year-old man complains of brief periods of "flashing lights and strange colors"

744. A 17-year-old girl complains of episodes of flushing, excessive sweating, palpitations, and dry mouth

745. A 20-year-old man complains of brief periods during which he believes he is hearing Beethoven's Ninth Symphony

Items 746–750

Match the clinical syndrome with the site of pathology.

(A) Right temporoparietal area
(B) Left prefrontal lobe
(C) Orbitomedial frontal lobes
(D) Right anteromedial temporal lobe
(E) Right inferoparietal lobe
(F) Left peristriate area
(G) Hypothalamus

746. A 35-year-old man is referred by his internist. The family has recently noticed a change in his demeanor. They describe him as apathetic, slovenly, and lazy. He lies around the house all day and watches television or sleeps. However, he has also embarrassed his family by making sexual advances toward old family friends and upset the parish priest by telling dirty jokes outside church

747. A 25-year-old man is referred to the student counselor by his college professor. The professor states that he is "exhausted" by the young man's enthusiasm for his class. Each day, the student has voluntarily been handing in 30-page assignments on biblical texts and ruminates constantly over his subjective sense of personal destiny and his moral outrage over the decadence in the world. According to the professor, the student "never stops talking" and claims to have become celibate

748. A 16-year-old girl presents to the emergency department accompanied by the police. She apparently "ran amok" in the classroom and attacked several students without provocation. The episode lasted a few minutes and the girl denies any recollection of the incident

749. A 60-year-old man is found wandering the streets. He is confused and disoriented to time and place. There is no evidence for any substance or alcohol use. No abnormalities are found on metabolic screening

750. A 40-year-old computer expert is referred by his psychiatrist for a second opinion. Despite prolonged psychotherapy and appropriate psychotropic medication, the patient remains profoundly depressed

NEUROLOGY QUESTIONS FOR PSYCHIATRISTS

ANSWERS

652. The answer is D. (Adams RD, 5/e, pp 526–536.) Neurologic changes that are expected to occur with the process of aging include each of those mentioned plus presbycusis, decreased smell, decreased motor movement, small pupils, diminished pupillary reflexes, decreased upward gaze, impaired fine coordination and agility, and decreased muscle power. Although it was originally believed there is a linear decrease in cognitive abilities with age, this has not proved to be true. A decline in abstraction and the ability to process and store new material appear to be the changes associated with aging. Along with other pathologic changes, the population of large cortical neurons decreases with age.

653. The answer is C. (Adams RD, 5/e, pp 966–968.) Pick's disease is a rapidly progressive degenerative disorder primarily affecting the frontal and temporal lobes. Histopathology reveals marked loss of neurons in the first three cortical layers and argentophilic bodies (Pick bodies) within the remaining neurons. Clinical features essentially reflect the lobar distribution of these pathologic changes. Patients display apathy, amotivation, and shallowness alternating with periods of inappropriate stimulus-bound behavior. A gradual deterioration in language from an initial fluent aphasia into palilalia and finally mutism is typical. The cause of the disorder is unknown, but a genetic basis appears likely. The disease runs a rapid downhill course with death usually occurring in 2 to 5 years.

654. The answer is D. (Adams RD, 5/e, p 680.) The anterior cerebral artery supplies the medial, medial-orbital, and lateral surface of the frontal lobes. In addition the artery supplies most of the corpus callosum. Deep proximal branches also supply the head of the caudate, anterior limb of the internal capsule, and the anterior part of the globus pallidus. A bilateral lesion of this artery, such as the resection of an aneurysm, will produce profound deficits in the prefrontal lobe, such as personality change; urinary incontinence; gait apraxia; amnesia; paraplegia; sensory loss over foot, toes, and leg; and paratonia.

655. The answer is D. (Adams RD, 5/e, pp 661–665.) Approximately 60 percent of patients will exhibit clinical evidence of central nervous system involvement in AIDS. At postmortem almost 90 percent of patients will be found to have neuropathologic changes associated with the disease. The dementing illness associated with HIV infection essentially reflects the subcortical neuropathologic changes found in the illness. Patients usually display the gradual onset of a "dilapidated" cognition characterized by marked psychomotor slowing, impersistence, and confusion. It is important to remember that these patients may develop many of the other secondary complications of the illness (e.g., infection, lymphomas) and therefore present with virtually any possible constellation of signs and symptoms.

656. The answer is C. (Adams RD, 5/e, pp 1111–1113.) Syringomyelia is a progressive degenerative condition of the spinal cord caused by a congenital abnormality—a syrinx (tube), which occupies the central gray matter of the cervical spinal cord. Gradual enlargement of the syrinx causes compression of surrounding structures and a neurologic deficit. The syrinx initially extends into the anterior and posterior horns and later into the lateral and posterior funiculi. The onset of symptoms is usually insidious and characterized by a dissociative loss of pain and temperature sensation, but not touch, over a capelike distribution of the neck, shoulders, and arms. Other clinical signs include muscle weakness and atrophy, loss of reflexes, and ataxia. Eventually a spastic paraparesis may result from involvement of the corticospinal tracts. There are frequently other congenital abnormalities associated with syringomyelia, such as fused cervical vertebrae, platybasia, and the Arnold-Chiari malformation. The condition is easily identified by MRI.

657. The answer is A. (Adams RD, 5/e, p 406.) The inability to recognize a previously familiar face is known as prosopagnosia. This is an example of a visual agnosia, i.e., the inability to identify or categorize an object or stimulus despite an intact visual system. Other examples of visual agnosias include color agnosia, topographic agnosia (an inability to recognize geographic landmarks), and simultagnosia (an inability to synthesize all the components of a visual field).

658. The answer is A. (Adams RD, 5/e, pp 42–48.) Complete paralysis of a set of muscles with preservation of adjacent muscles is evidence of a lower motor neuron lesion. Upper motor neuron lesions, in principle, do not cause paralysis of individual muscles. Instead, following the dictum of Hughlings Jackson, upper motor neurons paralyze movements. This statement holds true whether the lesion affects the motor cortex, hemispheric white matter, internal capsule, brainstem, or spinal cord. Although the myopathies may have a predilection for certain muscle groups, they tend to involve all muscles to some degree.

659. The answer is B. (Adams RD, 5/e, pp 373–374.) Transient global amnesia usually occurs in middle-aged or elderly people. The period of amnesia lasts a few hours and does not involve personal identity. The person is capable of normal language and intellectual functioning. Attention is normal throughout the period of amnesia. The etiology of transient global amnesia is unknown but is postulated to be a transient ischemic attack in the posterior cerebral circulation. The disorder usually lasts a few hours and seldom recurs. No emergency treatment is indicated.

660. **The answer is C.** (Adams RD, 5/e, pp 304–305.) With an estimated prevalence of 50 per 100,000, narcolepsy occurs more frequently than has been previously appreciated. There is a genetic susceptibility to the disorder as disclosed by an almost universal association of narcolepsy with HLA-DR2 and HLA-DQw1 antigens. The disorder usually has a gradual onset between ages 15 and 35 with an equal distribution between males and females. The core clinical features of the disorder are sleep attacks, cataplexy, and sleep paralysis. In addition, patients with narcolepsy may experience periods of automatism and hynopompic and hypnogogic hallucinations. Diagnosis is confirmed by a decreased REM latency period. Treatment options include psychostimulants, tricyclic antidepressants, and multiple, brief naps.

661. **The answer is A.** (Adams RD, 5/e, pp 241–243.) In normal persons, both pupils constrict equally when light is flashed in one eye. The contralateral connections of the afferent retinal fibers disperse the pupillary reflex equally over both IIIrd cranial nerves. Any difference in the response of the two pupils is evidence of a lesion somewhere in the reflex arc, i.e., between the retinal receptor and pupilloconstrictor muscle of the iris. When the pupils react differently to light, the examiner must inspect the retina, the visual fields, the oculomotor nerve, and the sympathetic innervation of the iris and investigate for possible midbrain lesions.

662. **The answer is C.** (Adams RD, 5/e, pp 864–865.) The patient demonstrates a positive Romberg's sign. This is indicative of a loss of proprioception and therefore of dorsal column pathology. The most common cause of this syndrome is subacute combined degeneration of the cord (SACD) secondary to vitamin B_{12} deficiency. This produces a demyelination peripheral neuropathy and involvement of the lateral and dorsal columns of the spinal cord. Clinical signs are therefore a classic "glove and stocking" sensory loss, loss of position sense, muscle weakness, spastic gait, and absent ankle jerks. Late in the illness, optic atrophy may occur as well as other symptoms secondary to demyelination of the central nervous system. Chronic lead intoxication produces a peripheral neuropathy with no loss of proprioception. Tabes dorsalis can produce a clinical picture similar to SACD.

663. **The answer is C.** (Adams RD, 5/e, pp 398–399.) The letter cancellation test demonstrates a typical example of left hemineglect. This syndrome is typically caused by a lesion in the right parietal lobe and is characterized by an inattention to somatosensory experiences located in the person's left hemifield. The person with hemineglect will be oblivious to activity or stimuli in the left half of the visual field and will also be unaware of the left side of the body. Since lesions of the left superior parietal lobe do not cause neglect, it is postulated that the right hemisphere is dominant for directing attention.

664. The answer is E. (Adams RD, 5/e, pp 386–390.) The patient's drawing demonstrates perseveration and an inability to change set. This is suggestive of frontal lobe deficits. Other abnormalities that might be found in this patient are amotivation, apathy, poor impulse control, lack of insight, and emotional lability. Since the prefrontal lobes are primarily involved in the integration and execution of sophisticated motor and cognitive behavioral functions, it is difficult to evaluate their functioning within the confines of the structured neuropsychological laboratory. When considering the possibility of frontal lobe deficits, the examiner is well advised to observe the patient's behavior within the context of an ambiguous social environment.

665. The answer is C. (Adams RD, 5/e, p 398.) The tetrad of (1) agraphia without alexia, (2) finger agnosia, (3) loss of right-left discrimination, and (4) acalculia characterizes Gerstmann's syndrome. This results from a lesion in the left anterior parietal area (i.e., the left angular gyrus). The syndrome appears to represent a defect in cross-modal matching. For example, patient's with Gerstmann's syndrome can maintain appropriate conversation and can read but cannot understand a sentence if it contains complex statements about relationship (e.g., the man who came after the second woman). Similar processing difficulties explain the problems with calculation, finger agnosia, and left-right orientation.

666. The answer is C. (Adams RD, 5/e, pp 219–220.) Interruption of the right optic tract causes a left homonymous hemianopia. One optic tract contains the nondecussated axons from the lateral half of the ipsilateral retina and decussated axons from the medial half of the contralateral retina. Thus, the axons in one tract unite homonymous visual fields, and their interruption results in a contralateral homonymous field defect. A complete lesion of the visual pathway between the origin of one optic tract and the calcarine cortex will cause a complete contralateral homonymous hemianopia. Therefore, the localization of the lesion depends on the associated neurologic findings rather than on the visual field defect per se.

667. The answer is A. (Adams RD, 5/e, pp 78–81.) An unsteady gait is the most consistent sign of cerebellar dysfunction. The Romberg sign is a test of posterior column function. The interpretation of nystagmus is complex and often nonspecific. Lesions of the cerebellar vermis secondary to alcohol, in particular, will cause gait abnormality. Cerebellar lesions may also cause an intention tremor, an inability to perform rapid alternating movements (dysdiadochokinesia), past pointing (dysmetria), scanning speech, and truncal ataxia. Common causes of cerebellar dysfunction include chronic phenytoin (Dilantin) therapy and alcohol abuse.

668. The answer is E. (Adams RD, 5/e, p 15.) The VDRL test, which has a sensitivity of 85 percent, is currently the test used most frequently as a screen for neurosyphilis. False positives on the VDRL test may be found with old age, autoimmune disease, and addictive disorders. False negative results may occur many years after initial exposure or after previous treatment (even if inadequate). More specific, but more expensive, tests such as the fluorescent treponemal antibody absorption (FTA-ABS) or treponema micro-hemagglutination (MHA-TP) tests should be used if the VDRL test is positive or a false negative result is suspected. CSF testing should be performed when asymptomatic or symptomatic persons test positive on the FTA-ABS or MHA-TP or when a patient with HIV infection exhibits mental status change. CSF VDRL testing is highly specific and diagnostic for neurosyphilis but does have a high rate of false negatives.

669. **The answer is B.** (Adams RD, 5/e, p 16.) A thorough history and full physical examination are essential when evaluating the symptoms of headache. The pain of a tension headache is thought to be secondary to muscle contraction precipitated by fatigue, emotional stress, bright lights, or noise. The pain typically worsens as the day progresses and is often relieved by alcohol or exercise. The condition is more frequent in women and tends to run in families. Treatment is essentially empiric and includes simple analgesics, relaxation techniques, or low-dose tricyclic antidepressants.

670. **The answer is B.** (Adams RD, 5/e, p 1131.) Acute intermittent porphyria (Swedish-type porphyria) is an autosomal dominant metabolic disorder of hemoglobin synthesis resulting in excessive production and urinary excretion of porphobilinogen and Δ-aminolevulinic acid. Clinical symptoms include abdominal discomfort, dark urine, encephalopathy occasionally with seizures, polyneuropathy, cranial nerve palsies (e.g., dysphagia, facial palsy), and autonomic arousal. Attacks are precipitated by estrogens, sulfonamides, barbiturates, phenytoin, and succinimides. Treatment is supportive and intravenous glucose is administered to inhibit hemoglobin production. Pyridoxine supplements may also be beneficial.

671. **The answer is C.** (Adams RD, 5/e, pp 48–51.) Apraxia is the inability to carry out previously learned motor sequences despite intact motor ability. This group of disorders may be considered the motor equivalent of the aphasias. The apraxias are examples of disconnection syndromes in which different modalities are separated from one another (e.g., speech from motor functions). In *ideational apraxia* the subject cannot perform sequential motor tasks but can perform each component step; this is caused by dementia or other pathologic processes. In *ideomotor apraxia* the subject is unable to perform simple motor sequences (e.g., buttoning a shirt). This form is caused by dominant posterior frontal or anterior parietal lesions. And in *constructional apraxia* the subject is unable to put together the parts of the whole—a disorder caused by a right parietal lesion.

672. **The answer is C.** (Fogel, pp 816–817.) Diffuse Lewy body disease is characterized neuropathologically by the diffuse presence of Lewy bodies in cortical, subcortical, and brainstem regions. The disorder may occur in association with the characteristic neurofibrillary plaques and tangles of Alzheimer's disease. The etiology of the disorder is unknown. Patients typically present with a combination of cognitive and extrapyramidal signs and symptoms. Psychiatric symptoms, including mood and thought disorders, are common. The disorder runs an unpredictable, fluctuating course.

673. The answer is D. (Adams RD, 5/e, pp 1126–1130.) Guillain-Barré is an acute demyelinating polyradiculoneuropathy that manifests as a rapid ascending paralysis with autonomic neuropathy and minimal sensory loss. The onset is rapid and paralysis may ascend to involve the cranial nerves within days or weeks. Patients may require respiratory support secondary to phrenic nerve palsy. The condition is presumed to be an autoimmune response to host myelin, which has been linked to a number of infectious diseases, such as hepatitis, Lyme disease, and infectious mononucleosis. The disease has also been associated with lymphomas, insect bites, sarcoidosis, and connective tissue diseases. Plasmapheresis is currently the only therapeutic intervention but is of doubtful efficacy. Patients may require several months to regain their muscle power.

674. The answer is A. (Adams RD, 5/e, pp 47–48.) To elicit clonus the examiner quickly jerks a part of the body that is at rest. The quick jerk is necessary to stretch the muscle spindles to set off the repetitive series of stretch reflexes that constitute the clonus. The examiner should ensure that the part of the patient's body is at rest and placed in a position that allows control of the amount of tension and movement to be imparted.

675. The answer is B. (Fogel, pp 827–839.) GTS is found in all cultural and racial groups but is rare among African Americans. It is more common among males with a typical age of onset between 2 and 15 years (with an average of 7). Patients may exhibit both simple and complex motor and vocal tics. In addition to their tics, patients may also manifest echolalia and palilalia. Tics and vocalizations are typically aggravated by anxiety, stress, boredom, caffeine, and excitement, while sleep, alcohol, orgasm, relaxation, and concentration usually diminish the frequency and intensity of these abnormal behaviors. There appears to be an increased incidence of ADHD, depression, and obsessive-compulsive disorder in GTS patients.

676. The answer is B. (Adams RD, 5/e, pp 1012–1013.) Normal pressure hydrocephalus usually presents with the classic triad of gait apraxia, urinary incontinence, and dementia. The gait is typically "magnetic" (i.e., patients have difficulty shifting their weight forward) and wide-based and the patient often walks on tiptoes. Aberration in gait is typically the first sign of the disease and its severity is proportional to the stage of the disease. Urgency and frequency incontinence are typical, but patients may become completely incontinent. Although there is significant ventricular dilatation, the amount of cerebral atrophy is usually minimal. Lumbar puncture and CSF withdrawal may help the patient significantly. Surgical shunting is presently the only effective treatment.

677. The answer is A. (Adams RD, 5/e, pp 416–424.) The described patient exhibits the typical features of a fluent aphasia, that is, paraphasic errors, neologisms, clang associations, and circumlocution. The patient will be able to convey his emotional state by the use of nonverbal cues (i.e., prosodic behavior). Patients with fluent aphasias may be misdiagnosed as psychotic because of the similarities of their speech to schizophrenic speech. These patients may also experience paranoia. Fluent aphasia is caused by discrete lesions in the dominant temporoparietal area or arcuate fasciculus.

678. The answer is E. (Adams RD, 5/e, pp 369–370.) Parkinson's disease results in a subcortical dementia. The subcortical dementias are characterized by "dilapidated" cognition. Although neocortical systems are intact, the affected person appears to lack the motivation to engage in cognitive tasks. Patients will classically respond to questions with statements such as "I don't know. I just can't do it." Enthusiastic encouragement by the examiner will normally significantly improve the subject's performance. A significant percentage of patients with Parkinson's disease develop a major depressive disorder sometimes referred to as bradyphrenia. These clinical syndromes parallel the motor symptoms, which are normally the major focus of treatment.

679. The answer is B. (Adams RD, 5/e, pp 42–48.) An upper motor neuron or supranuclear palsy is characterized by (1) more than one muscle affected, (2) slight atrophy secondary to disuse, (3) spasticity with hyperreflexia, (4) normal nerve conduction studies, and (5) an extensor plantar response. Lower motor neuron palsy is characterized by (1) marked wasting, (2) fasciculations, (3) flaccidity and hyporeflexia, (4) the possibility of individual muscles' being affected, and (5) an abnormal EMG study.

680. The answer is D. (Adams RD, 5/e, pp 683–689.) Occlusion of the posterior inferior cerebellar artery produces damage in the lateral medulla and is therefore referred to as the *lateral medullary syndrome* (*Wallenberg's syndrome*). Damage is incurred by the cerebellar peduncle, trigeminal nerve nucleus, spinothalamic tract, nucleus ambiguus, and sympathetic fibers. Damage to these structures causes a complex clinical picture consisting of ipsilateral pain and numbness over the face; limb ataxia; vertigo, nausea, and vomiting; Horner's syndrome; dysphagia, hoarseness, vocal cord paralysis, and decreased gag reflex; hiccup; and numbness of arm, trunk, or leg. Contralateral signs are decreased pain and temperature sensation over half the body.

681. The answer is D. (Adams RD, 5/e, pp 975–982.) Apart from the idiopathic disease, the symptoms of parkinsonism have numerous possible etiologies. "Post encephalitic Parkinson's disease" was common following the encephalitis lethargica epidemic of 1914. There are many other causes of the syndrome, however, including carbon monoxide poisoning, anoxia, dementia pugilistica, Wilson's disease, AIDS, manganese poisoning, and dopamine blocking drugs. Recently, the "designer" street drug MPTP (methylphenyl pyridine) has caused several cases of fulminant parkinsonism and provided a possible research model for the disorder.

682. The answer is A. (Adams RD, 5/e, p 252.) Air conduction is better than bone conduction in normal persons of all ages. Thus, the usual channel for sound perception through the ear is better than the artificial channel of bone stimulation. If bone conduction is better than air conduction, there must be a problem in the external canal, eardrum, or ossicles. The Weber test consists of placing the tuning fork in the midline of the forehead. A normal person will hear the sound equally in both ears. In neural deafness the sound will be localized in the normal ear; in conductive deafness the sound is localized to the affected side.

683. The answer is E. (Adams RD, 5/e, pp 94–99.) The most important part of the motor examination is watching a patient walk. Unfortunately many examiners fail to do so. Since pathology of the central nervous system, peripheral nerves, muscles, or joints will manifest in the patient's gait, most motor system abnormalities can be diagnosed from simply observing the patient walk.

684. The answer is B. (Adams RD, 5/e, pp 851–888.) The patient presents with the classic symptoms of Wernicke's encephalopathy. This is a medical emergency and demands immediate parenteral thiamine supplementation. Since thiamine is a safe therapeutic agent, it can be prescribed before other possible differential diagnoses have been excluded. Despite the prompt use of thiamine, approximately one-fourth of patients with Wernicke's encephalopathy will develop an amnestic disorder. The use of intravenous glucose prior to thiamine may precipitate or aggravate a Wernicke's encephalopathy and should be avoided in confused or comatose patients until thiamine administration. A definitive diagnosis of thiamine deficiency is confirmed by a low erythrocyte transketolase level.

685. The answer is C. (Adams RD, 5/e, pp 78–81.) Cerebellar dysfunction may give rise to hypotonia, ataxia (incoordination affecting voluntary movement), and disorders of equilibrium and gait. Hypotonia is usually due to extensive lesions of the cerebellar hemispheres or peduncles and is more pronounced with acute lesions. For example, "pendular reflexes" are caused by decreased tone in the quadriceps and hamstrings. Examples of ataxia include dysmetria, dyssynergia, and dysdiadochokinesis. The cerebellar gait is typified by a wide base, lateral veering, irregular steps, and unsteadiness. Titubation describes the anteroposterior head nodding that these patients may exhibit. Disorders of equilibrium and gait are usually secondary to cerebellar vermis lesions.

686. The answer is C. (Adams RD, 5/e, pp 975–982.) The patient exhibits the festinating gait that is typical of parkinsonism. These patients also have difficulty initiating their gait and exhibit retro- and anteropulsion. The gait of normal pressure hydrocephalus is characterized by a short step and wide base. Patients with a sensory ataxia have to watch the floor to determine the position of their feet, which are raised high and often stamped down. The spastic diplegic has a classic "scissor gait" with no flexion at the hip, knee, or ankle and therefore limited movement and short steps.

687. The answer is C. (Adams RD, 5/e, pp 86–87.) An essential tremor may be familial and transmitted as an autosomal dominant trait, occur with old age (senile tremor), or occur on a sporadic basis in young people (essential tremor). It is an action tremor with a frequency of 4 to 8 Hz that usually affects the upper limbs but may also involve the axial and cervical musculature, causing a typical head nodding tremor. The tremor is relieved by alcohol. Beta blockers and primidone have both demonstrated efficacy in reducing the tremor, although the condition seldom requires treatment.

688. The answer is A. (Adams RD, 5/e, pp 20–21.) Tissue exposure to a powerful electromagnetic field causes its excitation. The energy of the electromagnetic pulse is absorbed by the tissue and subsequently released until the tissue once again relaxes completely. This period of relaxation (i.e., energy release) produces two relaxation constants that are tissue-specific—the T1 and T2 constants. The scan may be set to produce an image of either of these signals and also a balanced T1/T2 image. The long T1 weighted image demonstrates fluid with a low density and provides a better definition of brain tissue and anatomy. Since T2 weighted images ascribe a high density to fluid, they are useful in documenting tumors, inflammation, and infarction where edema is suspected. The paramagnetic contrast media such as gadolinium provide higher definition images and aid in the delineation of even small areas of inflammation.

689. The answer is D. (Adams RD, 5/e, pp 12–15, 550.) CSF examination provides reliable evidence for the type of intracranial infection. Viral meningitis causes a low-grade pleocytosis, moderately elevated protein, and possibly a mild decrease in glucose. The appearance of the CSF is normal or mildly turbid and Gram stain is negative. Bacterial infections cause a marked polymorphonuclear leukocytosis, decreased glucose, and elevated protein; Gram stain frequently demonstrates the pathogen. TB and fungal infections produce a greater lymphocytosis and protein elevation than does a viral infection; special stains and antigen studies (e.g., cryptococcal) may be diagnostic. Guillain-Barré syndrome may produce mild elevation in serum protein with a very low pleocytosis.

690. The answer is A. (Adams RD, 5/e, pp 969–973.) Although the motor components are the most visible clinical aspect of the disorder, it is important to consider all the aspects of Huntington's disease (HD). Degeneration of the caudate nucleus produces deficits in cognition, behavior, and movement. The personality changes are usually the first to appear and are characterized by shallowness, lability, poor planning, and poor impulse control. Patients with HD may develop mood disorders and thought disorders. Because of the extensive reciprocal connections between the head of the caudate and the prefrontal lobes, the dementia is primarily subcortical with features suggestive of prefrontal deficits. HD is an autosomal dominant disorder with occasional sporadic cases. The responsible gene has been identified on the short arm of chromosome 4.

691. The answer is D. (Adams RD, 5/e, pp 5–8.) To reinforce a quadriceps femoris muscle stretch, the examiner may try the maneuver of Jendrassik in which the patient grasps his or her own hands and pulls hard, while the examiner attempts to elicit the stretch reflex. The voluntary innervation of the part not being tested "overflows" to augment the innervation of the lower motor neurons of the quadriceps. Some persons normally have such a high threshold for the muscle stretch reflex that reinforcement is necessary to demonstrate that the reflex arc is intact and that no pathology exists.

692. The answer is A (1, 2, 3). (Adams RD, 5/e, pp 416–432.) Features of a Broca's aphasia are sparse, telegraphic speech; absence of prepositions and conjunctions in speech; and dysprosody. Alexia and visual field defects are associated with lesions in the parieto-occipito-temporal region (posterior parasylvian region) and therefore are more likely to occur in association with a Wernicke's aphasia. Patients with a nonfluent aphasia are aware of their inability to communicate and this may aggravate or precipitate a major depressive disorder. Most patients also exhibit dysgraphia with letters misspelled or poorly formed.

693. The answer is C (2, 4). (Adams RD, 5/e, p 143.) The Brown-Séquard syndrome describes a hemisection of the spinal cord. This results in ipsilateral loss of dorsal column function with loss of position sense and in contralateral loss of pain and temperature. Interruption of the ipsilateral corticospinal tract causes hemiplegia and therefore precludes testing cerebellar function. Tactile sensation is not affected since the fibers from one side of the body are distributed via the posterior columns and anterior spinothalamic tract to both sides of the body.

694. The answer is E (all). (Adams RD, 5/e, pp 138–139.) Loss of position sense may occur following lesions to the peripheral nerves, dorsal roots or columns, medial lemniscus, thalamus, internal capsule, and parietal cortex. The clinician should therefore consider this pathway when determining the etiology in a particular case. Abnormalities of position sense are determined in a number of ways: with arms outstretched and eyes closed the affected arm will stray from its position; outspread fingers will change posture ("piano playing" movements); and a positive Romberg's sign will be present.

695. The answer is A (1, 2, 3). (Adams RD, 5/e, pp 580–583.) A tumor confined to the internal auditory canal would affect only the VIIth and VIIIth cranial nerves, producing a facial palsy and disturbances of both the vestibular and auditory components of the VIIIth nerve. An acoustic neuroma would cause diplopia only if extended out of the canal into the adjacent cerebellopontine angle, thereby compressing the VIth nerve and eventually the Vth, IXth, Xth nerves; brainstem; and cerebellum. The earliest symptom is usually hearing loss, but by the time of the first neurologic examination, the clinical picture is quite complex.

696. The answer is B (1, 3). (Adams RD, 5/e, pp 975–982.) The tremor of Parkinson's disease is a resting tremor that is aggravated by emotional stress. It is absent during sleep. Tremors occurring with action (i.e., intention tremors) are usually secondary to a lesion in the cerebellum or its pathways. The parkinsonian tremor is coarse with a frequency of 3 to 5 Hz and is often referred to as a "pill rolling tremor" because of the characteristic movements of the thumb and fingers. The tongue, eyelids, and jaw are all subject to the tremor, which has a constant frequency.

697. The answer is B (1, 3). (Adams RD, 5/e, p 209.) The normal optic disc is palest laterally and has the most conspicuous pigment deposition along the lateral boundary. The large vessels of the retina pierce the disc within the optic cup. The cup itself appears white. The clinician must be familiar with these normal anatomic features of the disc in order to identify lesions or congenital abnormalities of that area. Other significant features of the disc that should be noted during the ophthalmoscopic examination include the size of the disc, the color of the nerve fiber layer and its degree of capillarity, the size of the vessels, and the distinctness of the disc margins.

698. The answer is C (2, 4). (Fogel, p 916.) The introduction of magnetic resonance imaging (MRI) has greatly enhanced the clinician's ability to identify patients suffering from white matter disorders. Although multiple sclerosis is a common etiology for leuko-encephalopathy, many other disorders should be considered as part of the differential diagnosis. These include demyelinative disorders (multiple sclerosis), vasculopathy (subcortical encephalopathy), toxins (toluene, alcohol, irradiation, chemotherapy), metabolic (vitamin B_{12} deficiency, hypoxia, central pontine myelinosis), infections (HIV, progressive multifocal leukoencephalopathy, Lyme disease), trauma, and gliomatosis cerebri. The leukoen-cephalopathies may result in cognitive deficits as well as mood and thought disorders.

699. The answer is C (2, 4). (Adams RD, 5/e, pp 661–665.) Approximately 50 percent of patients with HIV infection will eventually develop clinical evidence of an HIV encephalitis. This is currently referred to as the AIDS dementia complex (ADC) and is not considered to be a manifestation of an opportunistic infection. The disease normally has an insidious onset and has the features suggestive of a subcortical dementing process. It is therefore characterized by apathy, psychomotor slowing, and impersistence as well as motor abnormalities and ataxia. Neuropathologic features are a diffuse multifocal rarefaction of the cerebral white matter with perivascular infiltrates of lymphocytes and multinucleated cells.

700. The answer is C (2, 4). (Kaufman, 3/e, p 331.) The Klüver-Bucy syndrome describes the behavioral changes following bilateral anterior temporal damage. The most common causes of the syndrome are herpes encephalitis, trauma, bilateral lobectomies, infarction, and end-stage Alzheimer's disease and Pick's disease. Clinical features include indiscriminate hypersexuality for both animate and inanimate objects, aggression, amnesia, hyperorality, and hypermetamorphosis (excessive exploration of the environment).

701. The answer is C (2, 4). (Adams RD, 5/e, pp 982–984.) Progressive supranuclear palsy usually occurs in people over age 60. Pathologic changes are the loss of neurons and gliosis in the periaqueductal gray matter, superior colliculus, subthalamic nucleus, red nucleus, pallidum, dentate, pretectal and vestibular nuclei, and oculomotor nucleus. Clinical features include difficulty in downward gaze and later in horizontal gaze; axial dystonia; dysarthria and dysphagia; gait ataxia; and extension of the neck. The patient often exhibits personality changes characterized by anxiety, dependency, and dysphoria. The ocular changes and cervical extension give the patient an "apprehensive" appearance.

702. **The answer is B (1, 3).** (Adams RD, 5/e, pp 652–654.) Herpes simplex encephalitis may occur at any age. Although the disease is probably due to the dissemination of a reactivated cold sore virus, the presence of these sores is not helpful in making a diagnosis. Patients may present with a wide range of nonspecific symptoms and signs including fever, personality change, delirium, seizures, ataxia, cranial nerve palsies, and hemiparesis. About one-third demonstrate the amnesia classically associated with the condition. The disease is usually rapidly progressive over 1 to 2 weeks. A brain biopsy is required to confirm or dispute the diagnosis, which may have been incorrect in as many as half the clinically suspected cases. Acyclovir has reduced the mortality of the disease from 70 to approximately 20 percent. As many as 45 percent of patients have made a successful recovery by 6 months.

703. **The answer is A (1, 2, 3).** (Adams RD, 5/e, pp 288–292.) The incidences of seizures after closed and open head injuries are approximately 5 and 50 percent, respectively. Patients who experience their first seizure at the time of injury are less likely to experience recurrence than those who have a delayed onset of seizures. The frequency of seizures tends to decrease with time and as many as 30 percent will remit completely.

704. **The answer is B (1, 3).** (Adams RD, 5/e, pp 777–790) Approximately 20 to 40 percent of patients with solitary optic neuritis will eventually go on to develop the clinical features of multiple sclerosis. The initial manifestations of the disease range from mild to severe. About 10 percent of patients will develop a steadily progressive downhill course; however, approximately one-third of patients will not be functionally disabled after 10 years. The majority of patients with progressive disease will develop cognitive deficits. The chance of relapse is markedly increased by emotional or physical stress.

705. **The answer is E (all).** (Adams RD, 5/e, pp 627–628.) Lyme disease is caused by the spirochete *Borrelia burgdorferi,* whose usual vector is the deer tick. The peak incidence of the disease is between June and September. Patients usually present with the insidious onset of malaise, low-grade fever, and arthralgias. The classic skin rash associated with the illness is erythema chronicum migrans, which consists of a central red spot surrounded by a ring of erythema. Like another spirochete, *Treponema pallidum, Borrelia burgdorferi* is a great imitator and may present with diverse multisystem pathology. Neurologic involvement may produce peripheral and cranial nerve palsies, meningoencephalitis, seizures, and headache. The peripheral neuropathy may resemble a Guillain-Barré syndrome and rapidly progress to a quadriparesis. The lethargy, malaise, and dysphoria may sometimes be misinterpreted as a major depressive disorder. Dementia and psychosis have both been attributed to Lyme disease.

706. **The answer is B (1, 3).** (Adams RD, 5/e, pp 878–881.) Anoxia results in the catabolism of neurons and the accumulation of catabolic products that cause further cellular destruction. The areas of initial and major destruction are the watershed zones. The permanent neurologic sequelae of anoxic encephalopathy are persistent coma, dementia, amnesia, extrapyramidal and choreoathetoid syndromes, myoclonus, and cerebellar ataxia. A progressive postanoxic encephalopathy may produce delayed and progressive neurologic deficits. Although patients may develop a chronic confusional state, they will not exhibit psychosis.

707. **The answer is D (4).** (Adams RD, 5/e, pp 959–966.) The pathology of Alzheimer's disease is characterized by the following: cortical atrophy and neuronal loss usually involving the frontal, temporal, and parietal lobes; neuritic plaques; neurofibrillary tangles; and granulovacuolar degeneration of neurons. These cellular changes are normally most pronounced in the temporoparietal association areas and in the hippocampus and subicular and presubicular regions. Lewy bodies are normally found in Parkinson's disease. Despite the apparent clarity and specificity of the above pathologic changes, individual variations are not unusual.

708. **The answer is E (all).** (Adams RD, 5/e, pp 567–569.) Mengiomas of the olfactory groove often reach massive proportions before coming to the attention of the physician. They initially grow into the inferior orbitofrontal lobes, where they produce the personality changes of amotivation, jocularity, poor impulse control, and low insight. Compression of the ipsilateral optic nerve will produce optic atrophy, while the raised intracranial pressure will produce contralateral papilledema (the Kennedy syndrome). Patients may therefore develop unilateral or total blindness. Despite their size, these tumors can usually be successfully excised.

709. **The answer is A (1, 2, 3).** (Adams RD, 5/e, pp 676–682.) Most occlusions of the middle cerebral artery are embolic and usually involve one of the branches of the artery, i.e., the superior or inferior divisions and their branches. The superior branch supplies the rolandic and prerolandic areas, while the inferior branch supplies the inferior parietal and lateral temporal areas. Occlusion of the superior division causes a dense contralateral sensorimotor deficit and deviation of the head and eyes to the side of the occlusion. Left-sided lesions produce a motor aphasia with deficits in the comprehension of written and spoken words. Occlusion of the inferior branch produces a Wernicke's aphasia and a homonymous hemianopia.

710. **The answer is E (all).** (Adams RD, 5/e, pp 226–231.) Disruption of the oculomotor nerve produces ipsilateral ptosis; a dilated, unreactive pupil; and diplopia. The ipsilateral eye is deviated downward and outward because of paresis of the medial rectus, inferior oblique, inferior rectus, and superior rectus. Diplopia is aggravated by attempting to adduct the affected eye. The third nerve nucleus is situated in the midbrain and passes through the red nucleus and corticospinal tract.

711. **The answer is C (2, 4).** (Adams RD, 5/e, pp 370–371.) It is difficult to distinguish completely between an Alzheimer's dementia and multi-infarct dementia. Many patients have evidence for both pathologies. Features that may help to distinguish the two conditions include a history of hypertension or transient ischemic attacks; stepwise progression of the illness; the presence of neurologic signs such as abnormal reflexes or motor and sensory abnormalities; and pseudobulbar signs. The amnesia of the multi-infarct dementia is seldom as dominant a part of the clinical picture as that of Alzheimer's disease. The presence of multiple white matter lesions on MRI will support a diagnosis of multi-infarct dementia.

712. The answer is E (all). (Adams RD, 5/e, pp 219–220.) Tunnel vision describes a concentric diminishment of the visual field. Apart from hysteria, there are several causes of tunnel vision. These include glaucoma, retinal disease (retinitis pigmentosa and choroidoretinitis), papilledema, bilateral lesions of the anterior calcarine cortex, acute ischemia (e.g., migraine), and chronic syphilitic optic neuritis. A useful clue to distinguishing hysterical from true tunnel vision is to remember that, even with tunnel vision, the area of the visual field will increase with distance from the object.

713. The answer is C (2, 4). (Adams RD, 5/e, pp 39–42.) The combination of absent ankle and knee jerks and an extensor plantar response suggests a mixed upper and lower motor neuron pathology. Conditions that may produce this clinical picture are subacute combined degeneration of the cord, syphilitic taboparesis, Friedreich's ataxia, motor neuron disease, diabetes mellitus, or a lesion at the level of the conus medullaris.

714. The answer is B (1, 3). (Adams RD, 5/e, pp 216–217.) The pathogenesis of papilledema is not fully understood but is currently thought to involve swelling of the optic nerve fibers due to stasis of anterograde axoplasmic flow. The later vascular changes (i.e., hyperemia of the disc, capillary dilatation, and hemorrhages) are secondary to edema of the disc. Anything that induces axoplasmic stasis of the optic nerve can therefore cause papilledema. Recognized causes include raised intracranial pressure, arterial hypertension, optic neuritis, obstructed retinal venous drainage (e.g., from a tumor or cavernous sinus thrombosis), hypercapnia, hypoparathyroidism, vitamin A poisoning, lead poisoning, and exophthalmos.

715. The answer is C (2, 4). (Adams RD, 5/e, p 268.) Phenytoin is metabolized by the liver. The plasma half-life is about 17 h. Anything that inhibits the microsomal metabolism of phenytoin will effectively raise its blood level and increase the risk of side effects. Among those agents demonstrated to increase levels are disulfiram, chloramphenicol, and fluoxetine.

716. The answer is D (4). (Adams RD, 5/e, pp 762–764.) The incidence of chronic subdural hematoma is highest in the elderly and often follows an apparently trivial head injury. In the weeks that follow, headache, dizziness, confusion, and occasionally seizures are the principal symptoms. Patients may develop a gradual onset of hemiparesis and aphasia. As the condition progresses, the patient will display a fluctuating level of consciousness. EEG may demonstrate slow high-voltage waves. Lumbar puncture will demonstrate an elevated pressure with normal protein and xanthochromia. CT will normally demonstrate the fluid collection, but this may sometimes be isodense and therefore not discernible. MRI provides a clear but more expensive alternative.

717. The answer is E (all). (Adams RD, 5/e, pp 661–665.) HIV has become "the great impersonator" and may produce virtually any constellation of acute or chronic neurologic signs and symptoms. These may result from the virus itself or the presence of an opportunistic infection or other complication of infection with the HIV. Currently documented syndromes include an acute meningoencephalitis shortly after exposure to the virus, a dementia (ADC), peripheral neuropathy, mononeuritis multiplex, myelopathy, polymyositis, and aseptic meningitis.

718. The answer is E (all). (Adams, RD, 5/e, p 786.) Approximately one-third of patients with MS (particularly during the acute phase) will have a mild/moderate CSF pleocytosis. Pleocytosis is the only CSF marker of disease activity. Other CSF changes include an increase in the ratio of CSF IgG to total CSF protein (the IgG index). An IgG index above 1.7 indicates a high probability for MS. Discrete IgG proteins (oligoclonal bands) are also frequently detectable. The combination of increased IgG index and oligoclonal bands has a 90 percent sensitivity for MS. The total CSF protein is raised in 40 percent of patients and is usually less than 100 mg/dL.

719. The answer is D (4). (Adams RD, 5/e, p 243.) The Argyll Robertson pupil is characterized by small, unequal pupils; failure to react to light or mydriatic drugs; constriction on accommodation; and occasional atrophy of the iris. Similar signs are occasionally seen with diabetes, Lyme disease, multiple sclerosis, and pinealomas.

720. The answer is B (1, 3). (Adams RD, 5/e, p 160.) Cluster headaches usually occur in men aged 20 to 40. They consist of episodes of pain involving, and localized to, the eye on one side and are often associated with lacrimation and nasal congestion. Occasionally the patient exhibits a partial Horner's syndrome. The pain characteristically lasts 20 to 30 min and awakens the patient several hours into sleep. The pain is usually aggravated by alcohol. Each "cluster period" lasts about 6 weeks and tends to recur at the same time each year. Possible treatments are steroids, propranolol, methysergide, or lithium.

721. The answer is C (2, 4). (Adams RD, 5/e, pp 114–116.) Axons from the secondary nociceptive neurons decussate in the anterior spinal commissure and ascend in the anterolateral funiculus. There are two major ascending spinal pathways: the lateral spinothalamic tract, which acts as a fast relay system, and a slower spinoreticulothalamic pathway. The fast system, the (neo)spinothalamic system, projects to discrete areas of the sensory cortex and is responsible for discriminative functions. The slower (paleo)reticulothalamic tract projects via the laminar and intralaminar nuclei to diffuse limbic and frontal projections and is involved in determining the affective or motivational relevance of a nociceptive stimulus.

722. The answer is C (2, 4). (Strub, pp 456–459.) No clear definition of *episodic dyscontrol* exists. In simple terms one may state that the more primitive or the more inappropriate the violence is, the more likely it is that a neuropathologic substrate for the behavioral change will be found. Nonpurposeful rage attacks are often associated with lesions in the area of the hypothalamus. Orbitofrontal deficits will result in lack of impulse control and a "short fuse" and violence that is typically triggered by a perceived threat or insult. These patients are often remorseful after they have calmed down. Patients with chronic confusional states are often involved in aggressive behavior that is nonpurposeful and short-lived. The relationship between epilepsy and violence remains controversial. Patients may be violent as a consequence of their ictal/periictal confusion. It is most unlikely that a seizure can manifest as a nonstereotypic violent act. Interictal personality change may result in a hypermoral personality that feels justified in pursuing violence as a means to an end.

723. The answer is B (1, 3). (Adams RD, 5/e, pp 993–994.) It is important to rule out treatable causes of muscle wasting before accepting a diagnosis of amyotrophic lateral sclerosis. The most common cause is cervical spondylosis, and myelography or MRI is indicated to evaluate this possibility. Other conditions that should be excluded are cervical cord tumor or compression, syringomyelia, meningovascular syphilis, Klumpke's paralysis, cervical ribs, and ulnar or median nerve palsies. Disuse secondary to local injury or arthritis will also produce wasting.

724. The answer is E (all). (Adams RD, 5/e, pp 152–157.) Vertebrobasilar migraine most commonly occurs in young women. Symptoms include transient blindness, vertigo, ataxia and perioral tingling. Occasionally, patients may develop an atypical psychosis, alteration in consciousness, or even quadriplegia. These symptoms usually precede the headache and last about 30 min.

725. The answer is B (1, 3). (Adams RD, 5/e, pp 1156–1165.) Mononeuritis multiplex describes a lesion in two or more nerves. Conditions that may produce this pattern are diabetes, HIV infection, leprosy, sarcoidosis, rheumatoid arthritis, polyarteritis nodosa, and carcinoma.

726. The answer is A (1, 2, 3). (Adams RD, 5/e, pp 592–595.) Apart from intracranial seeding of metastases, bronchial carcinoma may produce a number of varied nonmetastatic syndromes (paraneoplastic disorders). These include limbic encephalitis, which may produce changes in mood, comportment, thought processes, and cognition; peripheral neuropathy; cerebellar degeneration; myopathy; and myasthenia gravis.

727. The answer is D (4). (Adams RD, 5/e, pp 1171–1172.) Trigeminal neuralgia usually has its onset in middle or late adult life and is three times more common in females. Patients experience 10- to 30-s paroxysms of stabbing or burning pain in an area supplied by a branch of the trigeminal nerve. These paroxysms may persist for several weeks and there may be a chronic low-grade hypersensitivity or dull ache in the area between attacks. There is no associated motor or sensory loss.

728. The answer is A (1, 2, 3). (Adams RD, 5/e, p 685.) The Djerine-Roussy syndrome is caused by a lesion in the posterolateral thalamus. The immediate consequence is a contralateral sensory loss. After a delay of several weeks or months, with or without the return of sensory function, the patient experiences unusual pain in the area of original sensory loss. This dysesthesia is aggravated by factors such as change of temperature or touch. There is no simple or effective treatment and the condition is usually chronic.

729. The answer is D (4). (Adams RD, 5/e, pp 383–390.) Inappropriate and jocular affect (so-called pseudohypomania) is found in patients with right-side lesions. In particular, patients with right frontal lesions may exhibit an inappropriate response to their illness and appear almost impervious to the consequences of any resultant disability. This is referred to as *anosognosia* and may be mistaken for a mild hypomania. Right subcortical and periventricular lesions have also been found in association with hypomanic states. Patients with a left prefrontal lesion usually develop dysphoria that may meet criteria for a major depressive disorder.

730. The answer is A (1, 2, 3). (Adams RD, 5/e, pp 934–935) Tardive dyskinesia usually occurs after at least 1 year of neuroleptic treatment. The symptoms remit in 40 percent of patients after discontinuing the neuroleptic. Numerous drugs have been used to treat the condition; reserpine is usually considered the most effective. Other agents used include clonazepam; acetylcholine precursors such as deanol, lecithin, and choline; sodium valproate; baclofen; and diltiazem.

731. The answer is A (1, 2, 3). (Adams RD, 5/e, pp 703–710.) Transient ischemic attacks (TIAs) are almost always associated with atherosclerotic thrombosis. By definition, they produce no neurologic deficit beyond 24 h. TIAs indicate significant atherosclerotic disease and therefore predict a higher incidence of myocardial infarction and cerebrovascular accidents. The patient may experience only a single TIA or many hundred and a major occlusive event may occur at any time. The use of surgical resection remains controversial and should probably be limited to those patients who have severe extracranial stenosis or ulcerating plaques.

732. The answer is C (2, 4). (Strub, p 228.) In simple terms, patients with cortical dementia have lost the cortical "hardware" to perform complex cognitive tasks while patients with subcortical dementia have lost the "drive" necessary to perform. Patients with a subcortical dementia will therefore present with a "dilapidated" cognition characterized by apathy and dysphoria, and their performance will be influenced by the emotional valence of the situation (or the enthusiasm of the examiner). Cortical dementias will present early with deficits in cortical function: apraxia, agnosia, language deficits, and memory deficits. Subcortical dementias will be accompanied by other evidence of the primary disease process, e.g., movement disorder.

733–735. The answers are 733-C, 734-A, 735-B. (Adams RD, 5/e, pp 676–696.) Because each of the major cerebral arteries supplies a specific territory, it is possible to delineate the site of a cerebrovascular accident. The anterior cerebral artery supplies the frontal pole, anterolateral frontal lobe, anterior limb of the internal capsule, the head of the caudate nucleus, and the putamen. Obstruction of this system produces contralateral motor and sensory loss and behavioral changes associated with frontal lobe lesions.

The middle cerebral artery splits into superior and inferior divisions and supplies the insula; posterior limb of the internal capsule; external capsule; caudate, frontal, and temporal lobes; and part of the parietal and occipital lobes.

The posterior cerebral artery supplies the midbrain, thalamus, and inferomedial portions of the temporal and occipital lobes.

The vertebral arteries supply the spinal cord and give rise to the basilar artery, which in turn supplies the pons, midbrain, and cerebellum.

736–740. The answers are 736-E, 737-C, 738-B, 739-A, 740-D. (Adams RD, 5/e, pp 66, 67, 303, 545, 978.) Lewy bodies are eosinophilic cytoplasmic inclusions found in the cell bodies of the substantia nigra in patients with Parkinson's disease. Close scrutiny will often detect similar bodies in cortical neurons and the sympathetic ganglia.

Obliteration of the subarachnoid space by previous or low-grade meningitis may result in normal pressure hydrocephalus (NPH). The classic triad of NPH is a wide-based gait, urinary incontinence, and dementia. Other etiologies of NPH include previous subarachnoid hemorrhage, achondroplasia, and Paget's disease.

Chorea describes an involuntary, jerky, arrhythmic movement. Grimacing and peculiar respiratory sounds may also be associated with the condition. Muscle tone tends to be reduced in all limbs and the reflexes are pendular. Chorea is caused by damage to the caudate nuclei. Possible etiologies include Huntington's disease, pregnancy, Sydenham's chorea, and use of neuroleptics.

Hemiballismus is characterized by wild flinging movements of the arm or leg. It is caused by a lesion of the subthalamic nucleus.

Akinetic mutism describes a state in which the patient is awake and vigilant but makes no attempt to communicate or interact with the outside world. The state has also been called a "coma vigil." This clinical picture may be caused by lesions of the basis pontis or bilateral cingulate cortex.

741–745. The answers are 741-E, 742-A, 743-D, 744-B, 745-C. (Adams RD, 5/e, pp 273–295.) A thorough history will often provide reliable information about the site of a seizure focus. Describing what he witnessed in his own wife, Hughlings Jackson described the features of a seizure spreading from its origin in the prefrontal motor area. The so-called Jacksonian march manifests as a tonic-clonic seizure starting in the extremity and spreading to involve all muscle groups. The patient will deviate the eyes to the side opposite to the focus if area 8 of the prefrontal cortex is involved. Generalized spread will produce a loss of consciousness.

Hippocampal sclerosis results in damage, and therefore a seizure focus, in the mediotemporal areas. This produces a number of complex abnormal subjective experiences and bizarre motor behavior. An ictus confined to the mediotemporal area will produce context-inappropriate affective experience often associated with a rising epigastric discomfort and olfactory or gustatory hallucinations. The patient will often stare motionlessly and may also exhibit lip smacking or other bizarre orofacial movements.

Spread from the mediobasal temporal area to involve temporal neocortical areas may produce auditory hallucinations (Heschl's gyrus), visual hallucinations, or aphasia.

An ictal focus in a primary sensory cortex will produce unformed sensory experiences. Since the orbitofrontal lobe is a paralimbic association area, a seizure arising from this region will have autonomic manifestations.

746–750. The answers are 746-C, 747-D, 748-G, 749-E, 750-B. (Strub, pp 253–301.) Lesions in the orbitomedial frontal lobes are characterized by stimulus-bound behavior and an inability to suppress limbic drives. Patients will therefore exhibit a lack of motivation and drive (abulia) if left to their own devices. However, in social situations they will fail to modulate their behavior and will act outside accepted social norms. They will be angered easily and may be involved in violent outbursts. They typically display a shallow facetiousness (witzelsucht) and disregard for the consequences of their actions.

Lesions in the inferoparietal lobule may produce a chronic confusional state. Since this area is considered to be a heteromodal association cortex, any small lesion of the area will have a profound influence on higher cognition and therefore behavior.

Temporolimbic epilepsy produces a classic constellation of symptoms including hyperreligiosity, hypergraphia, hyperviscosity (an inability to change the subject), a sense of personal importance, hyposexuality, and persistent dysphoria.

Discharging diencephalic lesions produce "rage attacks" consisting of brief, non-purposeful, violent outbursts, which often include biting. These are often precipitated by hunger. Patients often exhibit other neuroendocrine abnormalities.

Left prefrontal lesions, particularly in the opercular area, usually produce a depressive disorder that usually responds to psychotropics. Right prefrontal lesions typically produce a "pseudohypomania" that is essentially an anosognosia (a blatant disregard for the gravity of a situation).

BIBLIOGRAPHY

NEUROLOGY

NEUROLOGY

Adams RD, Victor M: *Principles of Neurology,* 5/e. New York, McGraw-Hill, 1993.

American Psychiatric Association (APA): *Diagnostic and Statistical Manual of Mental Disorders,* 4/e (*DSM IV*). Washington, DC, American Psychiatric Press, 1995.

Bird TD, Bennett RL: Why do DNA testing? Practical and ethical implications of new neurogenetic tests. *Ann Neurol* 38:141–146, 1995.

Bodner RA, Lynch T, Lewis L, Kahn D: Serotonin syndrome. *Neurology* 45: 219–223, 1995.

Browne DL, Gancher ST, Nutt JG, et al: Episodic ataxias with myokymic syndrome is associated with point mutations in the human potassium gene. *Nature-Genetics* 8:136–140, 1994.

Brust JCMB: *Neurological Aspects of Substance Abuse.* Stoneham, MA, Butterworth-Heinemann, 1993.

Carpenter MB: *Core Text of Neuroanatomy,* 4/e. Baltimore, Williams & Wilkins, 1991.

Cogan DG: Visual hallucinations as release phenomena. *Graefes Arch Klin Exp Ophthalmol* 188: 139–150, 1973.

Cooper JR, Bloom FE, Roth RH: *The Biochemical Basis of Neuropharmacology,* 7/e. New York, Oxford University Press, 1996.

Daly BD, Pedley TA: *Current Practice of Clinical Electroencephalography*, 2/e. New York, Raven, 1990.

DeAngelis LM: Primary central nervous system lymphomas. *Neurology* 41:619–621, 1991.

Elble RJ, Koller WC: *Tremor.* Baltimore, Johns Hopkins, 1990.

Erenberg G, Fahn S: Tourette syndrome. *Arch Neurol* 53:588, 1996.

European Atrial Fibrillation Trial Study Group: Optimal oral anticoagulation therapy in patients with nonrheumatic atrial fibrillation and recent cerebral ischemia. *N Engl J Med* 333:5–10, 1995.

Fischer HW, Ketonen L: *Radiographic Neuroanatomy: A Working Atlas.* New York, McGraw-Hill, 1991.

Glaser JS: *Neuroophthalmology,* 2/e. Philadelphia, Lippincott, 1990.

Goetz CG, Tanner CM, Klawans HL: Pharmacology of hallucinations induced by long-term drug therapy. *Am J Psychiatry* 139:494–497, 1982.

Haerer AF: *DeJong's The Neurologic Examination*, 5/e. Philadelphia, Lippincott, 1992.

Hardman JG, et al (eds): *Goodman and Gilman's The Pharmacological Basis of Therapeutics,* 9/e. New York, McGraw-Hill, 1995.

Jankovic J, Brin M: Therapeutic uses of botulinum toxin. *N Engl J Med* 324:1186–1194, 1991.

Johns DR: Mitochondrial DNA and disease. *N Engl J Med* 333: 638–644, 1995.

Jones HR, Siehert RG: Neurological manifestations of infective endocarditis. *Brain* 112: 1295–1315, 1989.

Kandel ER, Schwartz JH: *Principles of Neural Science,* 2/e. New York, Elsevier, 1985.

Kaplan HI, Sadock BJ: *Comprehensive Textbook of Psychiatry,* 6/e. Baltimore, Williams & Wilkins, 1995.

Kaplan HI, Sadock BJ: *Kaplan and Sadock's Synopsis of Psychiatry,* 7/e. Baltimore, Williams & Wilkins, 1994.

Kelly JJ, Adelman LS, Beckman E, Bhan I: Polyneuropathies associated with IgM monoclonal gammopathies. *Arch Neurol* 45:1355–1359, 1988.

Langston JW, Irwin I: MPTP: Current concepts and controversies. *Adv Neurol* 9:485–507, 1986.

Logigian EL, Kaplan RF, Steere AC: Chronic neurologic manifestations of Lyme disease. *N Engl J Med* 323:1438–1443, 1990.

Lucas MJ, Leveno KJ, Cunningham F: A comparison of magnesium sulfate with phenytoin for the prevention of eclampsia. *N Engl J Med* 333:201–205, 1995.

McLean MJ: Clinical pharmacokinetics of gabapentin. *Neurology* 44 (suppl. 5):S17–S22, 1994.

Mesulam MM, Waxman SG, Geschwind N, Sabin T: Acute confusional states with right middle cerebral artery infarctions. *J Neurol Neurosurg Psychiatry* 39:84–89, 1986.

Meyers MG, Norris JW, Hackinski VC, et al: Cardiac sequelae of acute stroke. *Stroke* 13: 838–842, 1982.

Miller GM, Stears JC, Gugenheim MA, Wilkening GN: Schizencephaly: A clinical and CT study. *Neurology* 34:997–1001, 1984.

Musher DM, Hamill R, Baughn RE: Effect of human immunodeficiency virus (HIV) infection on the course of syphilis and on the response to treatment. *Ann Intern Med* 113:872–881, 1990.

Newell FW: *Ophthalmology: Principles and Practice.* St. Louis, Mosby, 1992.

Okazaki H: *Fundamentals of Neuropathology: Morphologic Basis of Neurologic Disorders,* 2/e. New York, Igaku-Shoin, 1989.

Osborn AG: Diagnostic Neuroradiology. St. Louis, Mosby, 1994.

Parkinson Study Group: Effects of deprenyl on the progression of disability in early Parkinson's disease. *N Engl J Med* 321:1364–1371, 1989.

Plum F, Posner JB: *The Diagnosis of Stupor and Coma,* 3/e. Philadelphia, Davis, 1980.

Poirier J, Gray F, Escourolle RE: *Manual of Basic Neuropathology,* 3/e. Philadelphia, Saunders, 1990.

Pruitt A, Rubin RH, Kerchmer AW, Duncan GW: Neurologic complications of bacterial endocarditis. *Medicine* 57:329–343, 1978.

Quality Standard Subcommittee of the American Academy of Neurology: Practice parameters for determining brain death in adults (summary statement). *Neurology* 45:1012–1014, 1995.

Rosenberg RN: Triplet repeats and neurologic disease. *N Engl J Med* 335:1222–1224, 1996.

Rowland LP: *Merritt's Textbook of Neurology,* 9/e. Baltimore, Williams & Wilkens, 1995.

Samuels MA, Feske S (eds): *Office Practice of Neurology.* New York, Churchill Livingstone, 1996.

Siegel G, Agranoff B, Albers RW, Molinoff P: *Basic Neurochemistry,* 4/e. New York, Raven, 1989.

Simpson DM, Tagliati M: Neurologic manifestations of HIV infection. *Ann Intern Med* 121: 769–785, 1994.

Victor M, Adams RD, Collins GH: *The Wernicke-Korsakoff Syndrome and Other Disorders due to Alcoholism and Malnutrition,* 2/e. Philadelphia, Davis, 1989.

Weiger WA, Bear DM: An approach to the neurology of aggression. *J Psychiatr Res* 22:85–98, 1988.

Wijdicks EFM: Determining brain death in adults. *Neurology* 45:1003–1011, 1995.

Winker MA: Tacrine for Alzheimer's disease. Which patient, what dose? *JAMA* 271:1023–1024, 1994.

PSYCHIATRY

Adams RD, Victor M: *Principles of Neurology,* 5/e. New York, McGraw-Hill, 1993.

American Psychiatric Association (APA): *Diagnostic and Statistical Manual of Mental Disorders,* 4/e (*DSM IV*). Washington, DC, American Psychiatric Press, 1995.

American Psychiatric Association (APA)—Task Force Report: *Benzodiazepine: Dependence, Toxicity, Abuse.* Washington, DC, American Psychiatric Press, 1990.

American Psychiatric Association (APA): *Treatments of Psychiatric Disorders,* vols 1–3. Washington, DC, American Psychiatric Press, 1989.

Cooper JR, Bloom FE, Roth RH: *The Biochemical Basis of Neuropharmacology,* 7/e. New York, Oxford University Press, 1996.

Davis K, Klar H, Coyle JT: *Foundations of Psychiatry.* Philadelphia, Saunders, 1991.

Fischer HW, Ketonen L: *Radiographic Neuroanatomy: A Working Atlas.* New York, McGraw-Hill, 1991.

Fogel BS, Shiffer R, Rao S: *Textbook of Neuropsychiatry,* Baltimore, Williams & Wilkins, 1996.

Jenike MA: *Geriatric Psychiatry and Psychopharmacology.* Chicago, Year Book Medical, 1989.

Kaplan HI, Sadock BJ: *Comprehensive Textbook of Psychiatry,* 6/e. Baltimore, Williams & Wilkins, 1995.

Kaufman DM: *Clinical Neurology for Psychiatrists,* 3/e. Philadelphia, Saunders, 1990.

Physicians' Desk Reference (PDR). Oradell, NJ, Medical Economics, 1996.

Schatzberg A: *The American Psychiatric Press Textbook of Psychopharmacology.* Washington, DC, American Psychiatric Press, 1995.

Simon RI: *Clinical Psychiatry and the Law.* Washington, DC, American Psychiatric Press, 1987.

Strub RL, Black FW: *Neurobehavioral Disorders—A Clinical Approach.* Philadelphia, Davis, 1988.

ISBN 0-07-052535-8